1989

NURSING HOME ADMINISTRATION

James E. Allen, M.S.P.H., Ph.D., N.H.A., is Associate Professor of Health Policy and Administration at the University of North Carolina at Chapel Hill. He has 16 years' experience teaching and conducting research in the field of health care administration. He is a licensed State of North Carolina nursing home administrator.

Nursing Home Administration

James E. Allen, M.S.P.H., Ph.D., N.H.A.

Springer Publishing Company
New York

Springer Publishing Company, Inc.
536 Broadway
New York, NY 10012

    89   90   91 / 5   4   3   2

Library of Congress Cataloging-in-Publication Data
Allen, James E. (James Elmore), 1935–
  Nursing home administration.

  Includes bibliographies and index.
  1. Nursing homes — Administration. I. Title.
[DNLM: 1. Nursing Homes — administration & dosage.
WX 150 A427n]
RA999.A35A45 1987   362.1'6'068   87-9629
ISBN 0-8261-5390-9

Printed in the United States of America

Contents

PART ONE   General Administration

PART TWO   Personnel

PART THREE   Budgeting and Finance

PART FOUR   Laws and Regulatory Codes

PART FIVE   Patient Care

PART SIX   Marketing the Long-Term Care Facility

Special Contributors

Special contributions were made to this text by the following persons:

Philip S. Brown, Th.M., M.A., N.H.A.
Administrator, Episcopal Home for the Aging
Southern Pines, North Carolina

Philip Brown contributed uniquely to this text, playing major roles in the process that led to its completion. In the summer of 1983 he served as the author's preceptor during the administrator-in-training period required of the author for licensure as a nursing home administrator in the state of North Carolina. During this period Mr. Brown shaped the author's thinking about the practice of nursing home administration. His insights particularly influenced the final section of Part Five: "Personal and Social Aspects of Institutional Living." He contributed heavily to conceiving the final sequencing of materials in this book: a combining of the test areas of the national nursing home examination with the core areas of knowledge required of nursing home administrators. Mr. Brown helpfully critiqued each section of the text as it emerged, especially Part 1: General Administration.

Philip S. Brown brings more than two decades of experience as a licensed administrator in not-for-profit and life-care community administration, as well as extensive national involvement in training nursing home administrators. He has held national office in the National Association of Boards of Examiners for Nursing Home Administrators and is a former chairman of the North Carolina State Board of Examiners for Nursing Home Administrators. He has held numerous offices in the North Carolina Health Care Facilities Association, including its vice-presidency for four years. He owns his own long-term care consulting firm and has lectured nationally on long-term care topics.

Catherine Chase, A.B., M.S.P.H.
Houston, Texas

While working as a research assistant for the author, Catherine Chase contributed the first full draft of Part 3: Budgeting and Finance. Although Part 3 went through five subsequent editings by the author, it appears substantially as originally written. Ms. Chase offers a background in financial management in both theoretical analysis and practical applications.

Kathleen Connors, B.S., M.S.P.H., R.N.
Health Care Financing Administration
Baltimore, Maryland

Working as a research assistant for the author, Kathleen Connors wrote the first draft of Section 5.3, "The Aging Process As It Relates to Diseases Common to the Nursing Home Population." Although this section also was subjected to numerous later editings by Ms. Connors and others mentioned below, the final text appears substantially as originally written by Ms. Connors.

Ms. Connors has professional nursing experience in both for-profit and not-for-profit sectors of the health care industry. She is currently a long-term care project specialist for the federal Health Care Financing Administration.

James F. Leach, A.B., N.H.A.
Administrator, Hawthorne Nursing Center
Charlotte, North Carolina

James F. Leach served as an invaluable sounding board during the writing of this book. In addition, he contributed early drafts of Section 1.11, "Organization of the Nursing Facility," and Section 1.12, "Legal Aspects and Business Forms." Mr. Leach reviewed, commented on, and helped edit all parts of the book.

For more than ten years Mr. Leach has been a licensed nursing home administrator of skilled and intermediate-care facilities that are part of nursing home chains, as well as individually owned. He has lectured extensively on topics discussed in this book.

Gene B. Tarr, B.A., J.D., N.H.A.
Attorney at Law
Winston-Salem, North Carolina

Gene B. Tarr edited the final version of Section 1.12, and twice edited the legal definitions for accuracy. He also suggested the addition of a number of terms.

Dr. Tarr offers a unique combination of professional and educational experiences. He is a legal specialist in the nursing home field and has a full-time legal practice as a partner in a major North Carolina law firm. He has professional experience as the administrator of skilled nursing facilities and is a licensed North Carolina nursing home administrator. Dr. Tarr has delivered numerous lectures to professional groups on the legal aspects of skilled-nursing-facility operation.

Foreword

It is unusual to comment on a text that so many students have already used. Dr. James Allen teaches the course "Basic Nursing Home Administration" at the University of North Carolina at Chapel Hill (UNC-CH). The information in this book was developed for the course, and has been continuously refined with each presentation.

Dr. Allen's association with the North Carolina State Board of Examiners for Nursing Home Administrators began in late 1982. In March of the following year he applied for licensure as a nursing home administrator in this state. He was motivated by several factors: a desire to experience the licensing process in order to better assist his students who wished to become licensed nursing home administrators; the conviction that it would enhance his teaching in the area of long-term care; and the recognition that the administrator-in-training (AIT) program of the licensing process provided an opportunity to interact with nursing home administrators and thereby gain greater insight into his field of work.

Dr. Allen completed all of the requirements for licensure, which then included an AIT program and both the national (NAB) and state examinations. His dedication to his AIT program was abundantly clear from his reports to the Board of Examiners. Not only did he work more than the required number of hours a week in the facility, but he was also very ingenious in devising ways to experience the roles of the staff in each discipline working in the nursing home, and in viewing its operations from the patient's point of view.

After receiving his license Dr. Allen invited the State Director and members of the Board of Examiners to assist him in informing his students at the UNC-CH School of Public Health about requirements for licensure, functions of the Board, and the profession in general.

These exercises proved of value to both students and licensing agency representatives. At that time the Board was exploring possible changes in the course of study required for the AITs to complete licensure requirements. Dr. Allen proposed that a program be developed for presentation at UNC-CH that would serve to involve the AITs with each other and to establish for them a course of study at the college level. The Board was very receptive to the idea, and the first group of AITs began the course in January 1985. Dr. Allen introduced an academic program to enable administrators to cope with the responsibilities of their positions and to prepare them to provide the highest quality of patient care possible.

Fully informed of each revision of the book by the author, the Board of Examiners has monitored and reviewed the sections at regular intervals. Encouraged by the students and AITs enrolled in his classes, as well as by members and staff of the Board of Examiners, Dr. Allen ultimately decided to seek publication of the material. This finished product is a testimonial to his purpose of adding other dimensions to the knowledge base of applicants for licensure, nursing home administrators, and others interested in this burgeoning field.

During the period when he was devoting considerable time and energy to this project, Dr. Allen was, of course, carrying this full teaching assignments at the School of Public Health. He also assisted the Board with the presentation of seminars for nursing home administrators seeking preceptor certification and in continuing education of other administrators in North Carolina.

We feel that this text will be helpful not only in this state, but across the country as well. Because of its substantial contribution to their knowledge, individuals entering the field who rely on this book will find themselves better prepared to accept the challenges of this dynamic and demanding profession. Both the UNC-CH School of Public Health and the North Carolina Board of Examiners for Nursing Home Administrators have and will continue to benefit from Dr. Allen's work and commitment.

Mrs. Sue B. Payne, Chairman, 1982–1985

Mr. William Moon, Director

North Carolina State Board of Examiners for
Nursing Home Administrators

Preface

The study of nursing home administration is a relatively new field. Prior to the 1960s there were few nursing facilities, and their administrators tended to be untrained owners of small-size freestanding facilities. Administrators of these homes were not required to be licensed.

In February 1970 the federal government mandated that, beginning in that year, nursing home administrators (in this text we use the terms "nursing home" and "nursing facility" interchangeably) not only be licensed by the states but also be trained in nine core knowledge areas. The federal core knowledge areas are (1) environmental health and safety, (2) local health and safety regulations, (3) general administration, (4) psychology of patient care, (5) principles of medical care, (6) personal and social care, (7) therapeutic care, (8) departmental organization, and (9) community interrelationships.

The nursing home industry has expanded rapidly since the 1960s. Today there are more than 23,000 nursing homes in this country, more than three times the number of hospitals. Long-term care facilities are expected to continue to increase in response to the ever larger proportion of the American population who are 65 years of age and older. To meet these growing demands, an active, identifiable professional group of nursing home administrators has come into existence.

For licensure, 50 states currently require that the candidate have a certain minimum academic training and pass a state examination. In all states except Texas an additional requirement is a passing grade on the examination offered by the National Board of Examiners for Nursing Home Administrators.

In November 1986 the Board of Governors of the National Association of Boards of Examiners for Nursing Home Administrators, Inc. (NAB) specified six content areas (which it calls "domains of practice") for the national licensure examination. These content areas are expected by the NAB to be effective through 1991 when they will be reevaluated for timeliness (Mid-Year Meeting, November 11–12, 1986, p. 59).

The areas of management in which the NAB expects to examine are as follows,

Personnel (22% of exam, 33 questions), includes such topics as recruitment, interviewing, employee selection, training, personnel policies, health and safety (covered in Part Two of this text).

Finance (18% of exam, 27 questions), includes topics such as accounting, budgeting, financial planning and asset management (covered in Part Three of this text).

Marketing and Public Relations (6% of exam, 9 questions), topics such as public relations activities and building a marketing program (covered in Part Four of this text).

Physical Resource Management (10% of exam, 15 questions), such topics as safety procedures, fire and disaster plans, maintenance of the building and its environment (covered in Parts One and Four of this text).

Laws, Regulatory Codes, and Governing Boards (18% of exam, 27 questions), covering such topics as the federal Conditions for Participation (also covered in Part Four of this text).

Patient Care (26% of exam, 39 questions), covering services such as nursing, food, social and recreational services, pharmacy, rehabilitation, physician services and medical records (covered in Part Five of this text).

This text addresses both the nine federally recommended core of knowledge and the six domains of practice.

This work is more than a mere delineation of the federally mandated core of knowledge and the NAB domains of practice. Not only the fundamentals for acquiring licensure as a nursing home administrator are given, but also an introduction to practice in that challenging field.

The unique contribution of this text, then, is the presentation under one cover of the material needed for a basic understanding of nursing home administration, together with an interpretative explanation of the materials for use in the classroom or the facility setting.

To provide the reader with the essential knowledge of the laws themselves, federal regulations and legislation that govern the industry are presented in their original wording. All terms are defined when first used.

Long-term care is a complex service industry. We have attempted to furnish sufficient information for comprehension of its development, current status, and trends.

Managing a health care facility requires at least the following skills: planning, organizing, staffing, directing, controlling, innovating, and representing. Each of these is discussed in Part One, together with a brief review of the development of management philosophy and practice.

Four additional areas are covered in Part One. First, the organizational pattern of a hypothetical 100-bed skilled nursing facility is presented, with explanations of each of the 17 possible departments. This is followed by perspectives useful in approaching the long-term care field: (1) the historical evolution of the industry over a 400-year period; (2) implications of the most recent major legislation, including an overview of the continuum of long-term care; and (3) the current profile of the industry.

Part Two outlines the basic personnel functions, which include the recruitment, hiring, training, and retention of employees. Additional personnel topics discussed are forecasting employment needs; writing job descriptions; evaluating, paying, and disciplining employees; and controlling employee benefits.

Financial management of the facility is a major responsibility of the nursing home administrator. Part Three provides a full introduction to the fundamentals of financial management. Basic principles of maintenance of financial records are discussed, followed by explanations of approaches to accounting, the accounting process in general, concepts and procedures available to help maintain control over finances, depreciation, "costing," and budgeting.

Long-term care is a heavily regulated industry. Numerous government regulations apply to health care facilities. These are presented, together with explanations of the origins of and rationale for the regulations themselves, in Part Four. Topics include the laws establishing the nursing home industry, fire safety regulations, regulations assuring access by the handicapped, and the federal Conditions of Participation for Skilled Nursing Facilities.

Several additional types of legislative regulation are dealt with; among these are labor legislation, occupational health regulations, health planning requirements, and voluntary standards appropriate to the nursing facility. Additional topics covered in Part Four are marketing, public relations, and physical resource management.

Nursing home administrators are legally responsible for the quality of care given to patients in the facility. The administrator must be able to evaluate this care and direct the staff in its provision. To accomplish this goal, basic understanding of the patient care process is crucial.

A number of patient care topics are covered in Part Five: the basic theories of aging; an introductory level explanation of the body systems and how they are thought to be affected by the aging process; health care terminology commonly used in the long-term care facility, including medical specialties, abbreviations, prefixes, and suffixes.

In the final section of Part Five the personal and social aspects of living in an institution are explored. Approaches to administrative planning for patient care to achieve a satisfactorily high quality of life for each resident are suggested.

The skilled-nursing-facility administrator is rapidly becoming an identifiable new health professional. The emergence of chains now offers middle- and upper-level management opportunities that did not exist 20 years ago.

Administration of a long-term care facility differs from that of an acute-care facility (hospital) in the necessity for dealing creatively with the effects of extended institutionalization on its residents.

The acute-care administrator focuses on the need for the short-term and manages technologically intense care. The long-term-care administrator is responsible for a less technologically intense but equally compelling problem: meeting the social as well as the health-related needs of the patients, whose stays are measured in months and, for many, the remainder of their lives.

Long-term care administration is a uniquely challenging management opportunity. Although the skilled nursing facility is a complex organization, it is small enough for the administrator to influence each dimension of its activities. The goal of long-term care administration is high quality of patient life. This would embrace more than excellence of physician and nursing care. Quality of patient life includes the full range of social aspects of the resident's day-to-day existence in the facility.

For these reasons, the author has addressed the problems of person-centered management. In his view the whole patient is the appropriate focus of the nursing home administrator. This requires interpersonal and social management skills, as well as technical competence.

OPTIONS FOR USERS OF THIS TEXT

The basic design of the text is a sequential presentation of material to provide the reader with a logical progression in learning the fundamentals of nursing home administration. However, each of the six parts of this text can be approached independently. The individual interested in learning about patient care, for example, can profitably study Part Five without having read the earlier sections.

A potential disadvantage of using these six topical areas is delaying presentation of the majority of laws and regulations until Part Four. To overcome this possibility, at various points in the earlier sections the author asks the reader to turn to Part Four and read the relevant passages on law or regulations influencing the topic under discussion.

Portions of Part Four, then, serve as a resource document for the rest of the text. This has an important advantage. Presenting verbatim the current legislation governing the industry gives the reader the opportunity to study the original material, thus approaching the legislation as written and not as interpreted by others.

Acknowledgments

The author also wishes to acknowledge particularly valuable contributions to this effort by other persons who have made the final product a reality.

Ms. Irene Rosenfeld devoted hundreds of hours to the careful editing of this book. Her interest in the project and willingness to assist in blending the efforts of several persons has resulted in a text that benefits from the insights of persons representing several disciplines and professional experience, without the discontinuities that can occur in such a joint effort.

Members of the North Carolina Board of Examiners for Nursing Home Administrators read and offered helpful suggestions on the many versions of the manuscript over a period extending beyond 2 years. Without the particular encouragement of the Board Chairman, Ms. Sue B. Payne, and the Board Director, Mr. William Moon, the project might never have been achieved.

At the invitation of the State Board of Examiners, several nurses offered helpful critiques of the patient care section. Thanks are due to Ms. Elizabeth Gilbert, R.N., Ms. Christine Coley, R.N., Ms. Winnie Jo Brock, R.N., Ms. Ann Hall, R.N., Ms. Gwen Butler, R.N., and Ms. Connie Hopkins, R.N.

Appreciation is acknowledged also to the students (more than 100) who took this course in its early versions and helpfully critiqued the materials. Ms. Mei Ling Tsing devoted many hours to Section 5.2, "Medical and Related Terms."

Thanks are also due to Dr. Sagar C. Jain, my department chairman, who allowed me the time required to accomplish this project.

Finally, appreciation is due to my wife, Janet, in whose study the IBM PC-XT computer on which I typed and continuously revised all of this material was located. Many hours of her privacy were preempted by the noisy sounds of the printer grinding out yet one more version of one of the sections.

One personal note: When I went through the administrator-in-training experience, I experienced a high level of frustration as I attempted to find materials to assist me in my effort to become a knowledgeable skilled-nursing-facility administrator. This book was born out of that frustration. It is hoped that these materials will be of assistance to persons seeking to master the skills and knowledge expected of those who seek excellence in skilled-nursing-facility administration.

List of Figures

List of Tables

PART ONE

General Administration

1.1 Administrative Functions

The skilled administrator of a long-term care facility is a person capable of organizing the resources and finances available to the nursing home facility to best meet the needs of the patients. In successfully accomplishing this, the administrator makes innumerable decisions.

Management is decision making (Dale, p. 5; Barnard, p. 232). What the administrator does for the nursing home is make decisions about what ought to happen in the facility (Falek, 8). Although there is by now an extensive literature describing the field of management theory, authors have returned again and again to a basic set of activities as the best explanation of what managers do (Drucker, p. 352; Dale, pp. 5–6). Luther Gulick, an early 20th-century author, defined the manager's tasks as planning, organizing, staffing, directing, coordinating, reporting, and budgeting (Gulick, & Lyndall, p. 13).

Several decades later Earnest Dale, in his textbook *Management: Theory and Practice,* differed only slightly in his description. He agreed on the importance of the first four tasks, but consolidated the last three under three rubrics: controlling, innovating, and representing (Dale, pp. 5–7). We will discuss these concepts in much greater detail, but very briefly this is what an administrator does:

Plans—finds out what needs to be done and makes a set of plans to accomplish it.

Organizes—once a plan has been made, decides how to structure a suitable organization to implement the plan, put it into action. This will include the money available for the enterprise, the number of people needed for the staff, and the materials with which to build or work.

Staffs—attempts to find the right person for each well-defined job.

Directs—provides direction (preliminary training and ongoing supervision) to each employee, who thereby learns what is expected of him/her.

Controls—evaluates the employee's performance of the job as instructed; if this is unsatisfactory, takes steps to assure that the job is done as planned.

Innovates—is responsible for developing new ideas for the facility to enhance its attractiveness in the community served.

Represents—is responsible for communicating the work and accomplishments of the nursing home to the outside world (public relations).

Note: The two terms "manager" and "administrator" are used interchangeably to mean exactly the same function or set of behaviors. (See Levey & Loomba, p. 491, for an opposite view.) Sometimes managers are thought of as upper-level policymakers and administrators as lower or middle-level policymakers, and sometimes vice versa (Rogers, p. 7). There is also a tendency to use "administrator" to mean the chief person of a public agency and "manager" to mean the chief officer in a private business. But directors of hospitals, whether public or private, are called administrators.

Another explanation of the manager's function is that "management is getting things done through other people" (Levey & Loomba, p. 494). A staff member who becomes a manager may or may not continue to give direct care, but does assume new duties that are entirely managerial in character (Dale, p. 4). The new manager is no longer directly responsible for doing specific work, such as patient care, but ensures that such care is accomplished. For example, when a charge nurse who has been giving direct care to patients becomes the director of nurses, this new job entails supervision of other employees to provide the nursing care needed by the patients/residents.

The manager's job is to ensure that the appropriate employees do the tasks of the organization at an acceptable quality level (Dale, p. 4). Many volumes have been written about managing because it is one of the more complex tasks in modern society. Three professors at the Harvard Graduate School of Business Administration (Roland Christensen, Norman Berg, and Malcolm Salter), in the eighth edition of their text *Policy Formulation and Administration* (p. 12), state that what managers do is ask three questions: Where are we now?, Where do we want to go?, and How do we get there?

A DETAILED LOOK AT WHAT MANAGERS DO

We have described in very general terms what administrators do. What is actually involved is planning, organizing, staffing, directing, controlling, innovating and representing. We consider the following the basic functions of the manager:

Planning (deciding what is to be done)

The manager decides what is to be accomplished, sets short- and long-term objectives, then identifies the means for achieving them. This requires forecasting the economic, social, and political environment expected for the organization and the resources that will be available to it.

Organizing (deciding the scheme of the organization and the staffing it will require)

The manager decides on the structure the organization will take, the skills that will be needed, and the staff positions and their particular duties and responsibilities. This includes coordinating the work assignments, i.e., the interrelationships between workers.

Staffing (the personnel function)

The manager attempts to find the right person for each defined job.

Directing (providing daily supervision)

The manager provides day-to-day supervision of subordinates, makes sure that subordinates know what results are expected, and helps the staff to improve their skills. In short, the administrator explains what is to be done and the employees do it to the best of their abilities.

Controlling (evaluating)

The manager, first of all, determines how well the jobs have been done and what progress is being made to achieve the organization's goals; second, takes necessary corrective actions; and third, uses the management information system to assess the need for changes.

Innovating (the effective manager is always an innovator)

The manager develops new ideas him/herself, combines old ideas to form new ones, searches for useful ideas from other fields and adapts them, or acts as a catalyst to stimulate others to be as creative.

Representing (to the public)

The manager speaks on behalf of the organization in dealings with outside groups.

According to Christensen, Berg, and Salter (p. xvi), the general manager (such as a nursing home administrator) performs five functions:

- planning for future operations
- designing and administering decision making structures [organizing]
- developing human resources and capabilities [staffing, directing]
- supervising current operations [controlling]
- representing and holding an organization responsible to its various constituencies (p. xvi)

These are the basic functions of managers/administrators. The reader may wish to use other words and concepts to describe these functions, or even improve on the model. Certainly managers do much more than has been described (Pressman & Wildavsky, p. xiii). However, if planning, organizing, staffing, directing, controlling, innovating, and representing are not successfully accomplished, the minimum responsibilities of a nursing home administrator have not been fulfilled.

The skilled long-term care administrator is capable of accomplishing each of these tasks in a manner that meets both financial and patient-care needs.

1.1.1 Levels of Management

Two additional concepts are worth noting at this point: the concept of upper–middle–lower levels of management and the concept of line–staff relationships. The administrator of a large nursing home might assign some of these responsibilities to others.

In a large home of perhaps 300 to 400 patients the administrator might assign coordination of the hiring, evaluating, and firing of employees to a personnel director. The administrator need not personally perform each of the management tasks, but rather must assure that these tasks are successfully carried out. To accomplish this, management is often divided into three layers: upper management, middle management, and lower management (Katz & Kahn, pp. 318–323).

UPPER-LEVEL MANAGEMENT

The upper-level manager is responsible for the overall functioning of the facility, normally interacting directly with the board of directors and/or owners. This person is responsible for formulating policies that will be applied to the entire facility. The nursing home administrator is an excellent example of upper-level management (Mintzberg, pp. 25–26).

MIDDLE-LEVEL MANAGEMENT

Middle-level managers report to upper-level managers and at the same time interact significantly with lower-level managers. A good example in nursing homes is the director of nursing, who reports to the facility administrator and in turn has managers—e.g., nurse supervisors and charge nurses—reporting to him/her (Mintzberg, pp. 26–29).

As the name implies, this staff member interfaces between upper-level and lower-level managers. The middle-level manager normally does not make policies affecting the entire facility, as does the facility administrator. However, the middle-level manager does make decisions of policy for managers responsible to him/her. The middle-level manager must have good communication skills to deal successfully with both the administrator of the facility and the lower level workers.

The emergence of nursing home chains has implications for the type of management role local nursing home administrators are being assigned. Some chains allow local facility administrators wide latitude in decision making, in which case the local administrator functions primarily as an upper-level manager. In other chains, decision making is centralized in the corporate offices, in which case the local administrator's role more nearly resembles that of the middle-level manager.

LOWER-LEVEL MANAGEMENT

As a rule, lower-level managers have direct supervisory responsibilities for the staff who do the actual work, e.g., the nurses who physically take care of the patients in their rooms. The nurse supervisor or charge nurse is a good example of lower-level management in a nursing home facility (Mintzberg, pp. 31–32). At this level managers deal directly with those at the middle level but not with administrators at the upper level. That is, they are expected to conduct their business through the channel of their middle-level managers.

If the charge nurse wants a change in a policy, he/she will discuss the matter with the supervisor, who in turn will bring it to the attention of upper-level managers, should this be desirable. The middle-level manager might also make a policy decision without consulting upper-level management, e.g., to change the bathing schedule to accommodate an additional workload due to increased occupancy.

Management decisions in nursing home facilities are more complicated than the simple establishment of lower, middle, and upper levels of management. The presence of several professions, e.g., physicians, nurses, physical therapists, dietitians, and others, causes decision making in nursing home facilities to be a complex and often delicate task. This is explored later in this section.

1.1.2 Line–Staff Relationships

Line–staff relationships constitute a second important concept in understanding management functions (Dale, p. 196). A person who is empowered by the administrator to make decisions for the organization is said to have line authority. A person is said to have a staff role if he/she is advisory to the manager and does not have authority to make decisions for the organization (Robey, p. 51).

A LINE POSITION

The administrator must assign to other employees some of the decision-making authority to accomplish the work of the organization. Such employees are line managers. They are empowered to make decisions on behalf of the administrator. The director of nurses is a line position. Therefore, decisions by the director of nursing have the same force as if the administrator made them. The administrator still remains responsible for all decisions made on his/her behalf by persons to whom decision-making authority has been delegated.

A STAFF POSITION

A staff position, on the other hand, is an advisory role. None of the administrator's authority to make decisions on behalf of the facility is delegated to persons in a staff position. An accountant in the business office is an example of a staff position. Persons who are paid consultants, such as a local pharmacist or a nutritionist, hold staff positions. These persons are expected to advise the administrator or others in the facility on what to do, but they have been given no authority by the administrator to make decisions on behalf of the facility.

Smaller nursing home facilities typically do not employ as their food services director a person eligible for registration by the American Dietetic Association. Consequently, to meet federal regulations, they hire such a person as a consultant on a periodic basis. Although the consulting dietitian may be the better trained person, if the nursing home administrator allows this consultant to give direct orders to the food service director, lines of authority in the facility may become confused, and staff morale will suffer.

Or, again, in a very large facility the administrator might hire a specially trained geriatric nurse to advise the administrator on nursing functions in the facility. This nurse would have no authority to ask or order anyone to do anything in the facility.

It is the director of nursing to whom power and authority to make nursing decisions has been delegated and who therefore makes decisions on behalf of the administrator in the nursing area. The director of nurses can hire and fire, assign work, and give whatever orders are needed to make the facility nursing activities function because line authority to do so has been delegated to that employee.

In practice, line and staff authority and functions are often blurred. Many administrators do not sufficiently appreciate the importance of keeping line and staff authority relationships clear.

If, for example, the administrator permitted the geriatric nurse, to whom a staff role had been assigned, to tell the director of nurses what to do or to give orders to nurses on the halls, the authority of the director of nurses would be undermined. The director of nurses and the nursing staff would be understandably confused about the role of the director of nurses: Does the director of nurses represent the authority of the administrator or is the staff advisory nurse actually the manager of the director of nurses?

We turn now to a more detailed discussion of some of the activities and skills involved in the management functions. We will begin to explore some of the complexities of these functions.

1.2 Planning

The administrator's planning for the nursing facility's future is not necessarily different from the planning individuals do for their own careers. Most persons devise some kind of plan to arrive at a career goal. Take, for example, making a career decision to become a nursing home administrator. This is a conscious act of planning—deciding what one wants to achieve. Long-term and short-term goals are probably set up in the process. The long-term goal could be "becoming an effective and successful nursing home administrator." To achieve this long-term goal one needs to achieve a short-term goal: to be trained and licensed.

It is also likely that other key steps in successful planning are taken, e.g., forecasting the economic, social, and political environment. Individuals considering a career in long-term care administration will try to find out about the economic future. "Will good jobs be available?"

Will society continue to need more nursing home administrators? Are politicians likely to support provision for financial assistance to the increasingly larger proportion of Americans who are 65 and older? In short, persons engage consciously and unconsciously in a planning process when making career decisions.

VARYING STYLES

Much of this deliberation about entering a profession such as the long-term-care field may have been based on hunches, intuition, or knowledge of the work obtained from a family member or acquaintances engaged in that field. For some, the planning process may have been very orderly and methodical, for others more haphazard or based on chance.

Organizations, just like individuals, have planning needs to come into existence and remain in operation. A well-managed organization does not improvise as it goes along, meeting each situation as it arises or dealing with crises instead of forestalling them with thoughtful planning. All of this is the responsibility of the administrator.

Although a person may have the option to be casual and even haphazard in making personal career plans, this degree of informality is not appropriate for the functioning administrator. Planning for the long-term care facility must be conscious, carefully designed, and then successfully communicated to the employees.

1.2.1 Why Plan?

AN INTEGRATED DECISION SYSTEM

The purpose of planning is to provide an integrated decision system that establishes the framework for all facility activities (Rogers, pp. 37–38; Levey & Loomba, pp. 269–274; Dale, p. 5). Organizations must have plans in order to function. Plans provide the limits within which members of the nursing home staff make decisions. Plans, in essence, are statements of the organizational goals of the facility.

A MEANS OF COPING WITH UNCERTAINTY

Plans are a means of coping with the uncertainty of the future (Levey & Loomba, p. 271; Katz & Kahn, p. 271). All organizations must deal with the outside world in order to survive. Inevitably, events beyond the control of the nursing home will shape the range of options available to the facility and set the context within which it will be obliged to function.

A plan is a prediction of what the facility's decision makers believe they must do to cope with the future. A carefully developed plan makes it possible to compare what happens to what was expected to happen. Then the plan may be altered to achieve the set goals when external conditions change. We will discuss this aspect of planning more thoroughly in the section dealing with systems.

1.2.2 Steps in Planning

PHASE ONE: DECIDE WHAT OUGHT TO BE DONE

Not many people have the opportunity to plan for an organization from the very outset. Typically, in the nursing home field, an individual accepts the job of administrator of an ongoing facility. For the purposes of illustration, however, let us follow the planning process that might occur in the creation of a new nursing home.

Suppose that one is assigned by the management of a group of nursing homes the task of evaluating a medium-size community for the purpose of recommending or advising against the building of a nursing facility there. Assume that sufficient funds are available if a decision is made to build a facility. The assumption is further made that, if a home is built, the person doing the assessment would serve as its initial administrator.

This individual must appraise the present competitive, economic, and political environment in that community. We will not attempt to provide a complete checklist for arriving at an assessment of a community. Among the major planning considerations would be the following factors.

Governmental Permission

If Certificate of Need legislation exists, the likelihood of obtaining a certificate to build a facility must be an early consideration.

Competition

What is the level of unmet need for long-term care beds in the community? How many competitors are there? What are their present and projected bed capacities? Is there enough unmet bed need to expect that a new nursing home would fill up sufficiently quickly and maintain the desired level of occupancy over an extended period of at least 5, preferably 10, years?

Economic Considerations

Are the expected patients/residents likely to have the present and future income to keep the occupancy level high and with the desired mix of private and public paying patients? Is the community itself likely to maintain or improve its economic condition over the next several years?

Other Political Considerations

Will approval of all required federal, state, and local governmental permits be forthcoming (Miller, 1982, pp. 5046–5047; Boling et al., p. 198)? What is the political climate in the town? Is the proposed nursing facility likely to be welcomed, or if not, would any needed permits probably be delayed, disapproved, or interpreted so strictly that costs rise unacceptably?

Next, the person assigned this task must visualize the desired role of the proposed nursing home in this environment. The considerations mentioned amount to conducting a *needs assessment* for the proposed nursing home. The perceived unmet needs will influence the role planned for the proposed nursing facility.

Let us say that the need for a nursing facility of about 150 beds with both skilled and intermediate levels of care in that community has been formally recognized. The role this facility can be expected to play may then be planned. If the requirements for long-term care services are correctly estimated, it becomes possible to begin developing short- and long-range objectives for the proposed nursing facility.

PHASE TWO: SET SHORT- AND LONG-RANGE OBJECTIVES

A next step is to develop broad goals, objectives, and plans that will direct the efforts of the proposed nursing facility. A broad goal might be to build it in keeping with the architecture of the community, in a location near the local hospital and physicians' offices, in a residential section of the town.

From this broad goal statement, more specific objectives and plans can be developed. A short-range objective (Kotter, pp. 13–14) might be set to have a 150-bed facility in operation within 18 months and, as a long-range objective, a second facility of an additional 100 beds in operation within 5 years.

PHASE THREE: DECIDE ON THE MEANS TO ACHIEVE THE OBJECTIVE

The next logical step is to translate broad planning goals into functional efforts on a more detailed basis. It is at this level that a building site is chosen, allowable cost levels determined, and detailed plans for the building drawn.

The planning process has moved from the general to the specific: from broad goals to detailed architectural plans that are specific enough to direct every person connected with the project. In this way, broad goals are translated into specific and detailed behaviors for everyone who takes part in realizing those goals.

THE ULTIMATE PLANNING DOCUMENT

The ultimate planning document, one that everyone seems to understand, is the budget (Wildavsky, pp. 2–3; Dale, p. 334). In the end, all plans have to be translated into dollars allocated in the budget. It is the budget that offers the skillful administrator the most powerful planning and control tool. Budgeting is discussed more fully below in the section dealing with "Control," and in detail in Part 3: Budgeting and Finance.

HIERARCHY OF PLANNING

Planning in Phase 1 is done by the upper-level policymakers. They are the owners, the board of directors, or the chief administrator to whom they have delegated decision-making authority (Miller & Barry, pp. 4–5). They set broad policy, e.g., the decision to build a nursing facility of 150 beds with both skilled and intermediate levels of care.

Christensen, Berg, and Salter have described upper-level policymaking as follows (p. 11):

$$\left.\begin{array}{l}\text{Facility Environment} \\ \text{Facility Resources} \\ \text{Management's Values} \\ \text{Facility Responsibilities}\end{array}\right\} \leftrightarrow \text{Facility Strategy}$$

Broad goals, e.g., to build a facility within such and such a time frame, are translated into more specific goals by the next level of managers, who decide on the location of the proposed building and the general style of architecture. Finally, at the third level of planning, highly detailed plans are drawn up by which the actual work is directed and controlled on a day-to-day basis.

PLANNING FOR NEXT YEAR

We have used planning for a new facility as the example because this demonstrates the entire planning process. Most planning is short-range (done for the next year). As a practical matter, this planning is usually accomplished when the budget for the next fiscal year (next 12 months) must be developed. An extensive example of the steps of planning for the next fiscal year through the budgeting process is given in Part 3: Budgeting and Finance.

Once plans have been made, the next step is to take the necessary actions to put them into effect, to make them operational. This is the process of giving plans an organizational form. The form depends on the administrator's perception of that organization in particular and the nature and behavior of organizations in general.

1.3 Organizing

Organizing is a method of ensuring that the work necessary to achieve a goal is broken down into segments, each of which can be handled by one person (Dale, p. 178). There must be no duplication of work. Efforts are then directed toward accomplishing the goal by, first, dividing the work up so that each job can be done by one person, and second, providing a means for coordinating the jobs done by different people—the task of the managers.

Descriptions are written for each job. A job list for each position usually includes the following:

- the objectives (result to be accomplished)
- the duties and authorities of the position
- its relationship to other positions in the organization

As a rule, an organizational manual containing all job descriptions and several charts is prepared.

It is argued in William Glueck's text that job analysis consists of answering the following questions (p. 103):

- What does the worker do? (worker functions)
- How does the worker do it? (methods and techniques)
- What aids are necessary? (machines, tools, equipment)
- What is accomplished? (products, services produced)
- What knowledge, skills, abilities are involved? (qualifications)

Organizing is the first step in implementation of a plan. It is the process of translating plans into combinations of money, materials, and people.

All administrators organize their facilities according to some theory of organization. Their understanding of organization is reflected in their day-to-day and year-to-year direction. For some administrators this is a very thoughtful process; for others it is quite superficial. Nevertheless, all of them apply their concept of organization through their behavior in daily decision making.

DIAGNOSING ORGANIZATIONAL PATHOLOGIES

In caring for their patients, physicians base their treatment judgments on their medical diagnoses, which they interpret from the patient's symptoms. In the same way administrators are organizational diagnosticians who manage the nursing home facility by using judgment based on their interpretation of organizational symptoms. Physicians diagnose and treat patient illnesses; administrators diagnose and treat organizational illnesses. In the literature, organizational illnesses are often referred to as organizational pathologies. Organizational pathology is the study and diagnosis of what is believed to be a problem adversely affecting the nursing facility.

In the following pages we provide an introduction to organizational theory, which should be useful in assisting nursing home administrators to make effective and successful decisions.

SYSTEMS

Organizations are systems of interactions among the three available inputs: people, materials, and money (Robey, pp. 28–30).

A great deal has been written in recent decades about *systems theory*. This literature appeared after World War II and has paralleled the development of computer applications to management tasks (Levey & Loomba, p. 106; Katz & Kahn, p. 30; Boling et al., p. 47). The systems concept is primarily a way of thinking about the task of managing any organization. It offers the manager a framework for visualizing the internal and external environment of the organization (Katz & Kahn, p. 17).

A system has been defined as an organized or complex whole, an assembling or combining of things or parts forming a complex or single whole. Stated more simply, *the idea of systems helps us to figure out how things are put together.* How, for example, do all of the departments in the nursing home relate to each other, to the community, and to the rest of the world that affects them?

Systems theory is a tool for making sense out of our world by helping to make clearer the interrelationships within and outside of the organization. The administrator uses systems theory to figure out what is going on inside the facility and between the facility and the larger outside community.

1.3.1 Description of the Organization as a System

Systems descriptions vary from completely nonmathematical to highly sophisticated mathematical models demanding specially trained personnel and computers (Mintzberg, pp. 37–44; George, pp. 165–166). The model we present does not require quantification, although numerical weights could be given each of its elements (Zmud, p. 87; DeGroot, p. 3).

OVERVIEW

In Figure 1-1 we illustrate a systems model that may be useful to the nursing home administrator in daily management of the facility. This model consists of the following elements: inputs, processor, outputs, control, plans of action, feedback, and environment. (For an equally simplified model, see Miller 1982, pp. 4015, 4018; see also Robey, pp. 134–135).

Organizations such as nursing homes use *inputs* to get work done, which results in *outputs*. The outputs are evaluated by the public, which then reacts, and the facility receives this feedback. The outputs are also evaluated by the administrators and compared to what was sought. If the results, or outputs, do not conform to organizational policy and action

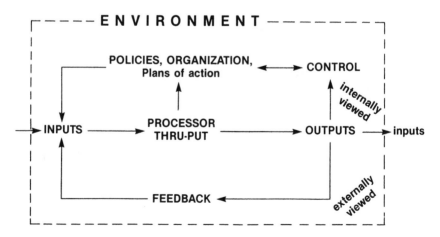

FIGURE 1-1. Simplified systems model.

plans, the administrators take control actions to bring the outputs in line with those plans. All of these activities occur within the constraints placed on the organization from the external environment.

This is a superficial view of the parts of a functioning system. We now take a closer look at the parts of a functioning nursing home organization.

INPUTS

The inputs in any organization can be described as three elements: money, people, and materials. Two of the elements at the disposal of a nursing facility are known and predictable: (a) a stipulated amount of money to work with (the budget) and (b) the amount of materials (buildings, supplies, etc.) with which to work. The number of patients with whom a facility will be working may be less predictable, depending on whether facilities in that area have lists of people waiting to be admitted, or are competing for patients. Inputs are things the facility administrators can change and use to advantage.

How Can Inputs Be Increased?

A primary concern of the system's administrator is, how can inputs be increased? To accomplish this, organizations take in resources (Katz & Kahn, p. 20). Just as the human body must have oxygen from the air and food from the environment, the nursing facility must constantly draw renewed supplies of energy from other institutions, people, or the material environment.

As patients are rehabilitated and return home, or die, more patients must come into the facility if it is to continue to function. As food is consumed in the dining rooms, more food supplies must be brought in, so that the work of the facility (caring for patients/residents) may continue. As employees leave for other jobs, new staff must be recruited. As the month's cash income is spent paying the facility bills, more revenue from patients must be brought in.

PROCESSOR

The processor is the work the organization accomplishes. Organizations transform the energy (inputs) available to them, just as the human body converts starch and sugar into heat and action. The nursing facility cares for patients/residents. Work gets done. Inputs are reorganized. This is sometimes called the *throughput*. It is the actual work that the organization performs (Katz & Kahn, p. 20).

The nursing facility takes its inputs (staff, money, and materials) and reorganizes them into active caring for patients/residents. In essence, what nursing facilities do is take money resources from patients/residents and other sources and use that money to hire staff and provide materials needed (buildings, beds, food, syringes, tissues) to give patient care.

OUTPUT

The results of the work (caring for patients) that nursing facilities do is the *output, the product of the work accomplished by the organization.* They export some product to the environment.

Nursing homes produce cared-for patients/residents. This care may take many forms, as we have noted elsewhere, such as day care as the output for an adult day program, improved mobility as the output of a physical therapy program, meals served to senior citizens in the community, and so forth. Nursing homes can and do provide a variety of outputs to the community.

The benefits of thinking about the administrative tasks within a systems framework will become evident as we describe the complex ramifications of the work of nursing homes (patient care) that is produced for the community. Later in this section we will examine a number of additional insights provided by viewing organizations as systems.

CONTROL

Control will be discussed at greater length below. For the purposes of exploring the systems diagram in Figure 1-1, it will be described only briefly here. Control is the single most important tool available to administrators in the process of keeping the organization on course. *Control is the evaluation by the organizational decision makers of the results of the organization's work, its output.*

In the nursing home the administrator exercises control by comparing the actual care given patients with the care called for in the organization policies and plans of action. This, in our view, is at the very heart of what administrators do. Just as important, every nursing home administrator has the responsibility of comparing the ultimate financial results with the expected financial results. We deal with this in depth in Part 3: Budgeting and Finance.

Administrators compare the results of the care given patients with the care called for in the policies of the facility. Put simply, control is the process of asking if the work accomplished by the facility is up to expected standards and, if not, taking corrective actions to remedy the problem (Dale, p. 6). Here we are discussing the actual standards the organization has established for itself through its policies and plans of action.

There are several "standards of care" that exist for nursing homes. Among them are the federal standards for care in homes licensed as skilled nursing facilities and the standards imposed by each state for a license to operate (Robey, p. 367).

POLICIES AND PLANS OF ACTION

Policies and plans are discussed in greater depth elsewhere in this text. For the purpose of illustrating the system configuration we use, let us simply refer to policies and plans of action as *the guidelines the administrator uses to compare the output* (e.g., actual patient care or financial results achieved) *with the expected* (i.e., the policies and plans of action developed and put into operation by the facility). As the arrows in Figure 1-1 indicate, the administrator uses the organization's policies (broad statements of goals and procedures) and plans of action, which are the more specific procedures designed to govern the implementation of the policies.

There are numerous organizations geared to set policies and impose plans of action for nursing homes in the United States (Rogers, p. 55; Miller & Barry, pp. 21–24; Boling et al., pp. 191–221). This has been a response, in part, to the financing of nursing home care by the Social Security Administration.

Congress imposed detailed operating requirements, called Conditions of Participation (see Part 4), on facilities prepared to accept Medicare patients (Miller, 1979, p. 23). Individual states, at the request of Congress, have also issued very specific sets of policies and detailed requirements for facilities that wish to serve Medicaid patients (Rogers, p. 59). A number of states leave little room for the exercise of discretion, while others have dealt with a more permissive hand (Boling et al., pp. 214–215).

Nevertheless, there are many areas in which nursing facilities must develop and implement their own policies and plans for action. One such area is food services. Every facility develops policies by which it hopes to control the quality of food served its patients/residents.

To summarize: administrators compare the results obtained with the results expected and then take steps to reorganize the inputs and/or reorganize the processor (the work itself) to conform to the expected standards.

FEEDBACK

Feedback is a form of control, but feedback is used here to refer to *the external responses to the output* (patient care provided, etc.) by the nursing facility.

Nursing facility outputs have many dimensions, such as roles played in long-term care in the community and in providing short-term care to patients who have been hospitalized, before they return home. For the purpose of simplicity we refer to care given patients/residents as the primary output of nursing facilities.

Congressional Feedback

Inevitably, members of the community and other individuals, such as state inspectors, evaluate the results of nursing home efforts to provide quality care to patients/residents. Two decades ago Congressional feedback to the nursing home industry resulted in considerable reshaping of the inputs in the industry when these lawmakers established the Conditions of Participation.

Through the laws passed by Congress and the subsequent regulations prescribing how nursing homes must configure inputs (e.g., the minimum number of staff hours per patient day, square feet of floor space per patient), the potential freedom to determine operating policies is reduced. We devote Part 4 to these concerns.

External Feedback

Typically, external feedback to an industry is not manifested in powerful and influential terms. This feedback is normally expressed through feelings in the community about quality of work (outputs) being produced. This appears in

- word of mouth evaluations
- newspaper articles and radio and TV comments
- the reputation enjoyed by the facility's staff that leads potential employees to consider the nursing home as a desirable or undesirable place to work
- the number of potential residents applying for admission to the facility

The reader can doubtless add to the list. All of these elements constitute what is referred to in Figure 1-1 as the environment.

ENVIRONMENT

The environment consists of all relevant external forces that affect the nursing home facility, but over which the facility has no effective control.

Defining the Environment

Defining the *relevant environment* of one's organization is perhaps the most complex and least obvious aspect of viewing organizations as systems. One way to conceptualize this is to ask two questions:

1. Does it relate significantly to my objectives?
2. Can I do anything about it?

If the answer to the first question is yes and the second is no, it is in the relevant environment. From the systems perspective the entire world is interconnected in one large network. The challenge is to identify the aspects of the external world that now affect or may eventually affect the facility in its attempt to achieve objectives, such as serving patients and making a profit.

Sometimes the environment is viewed as a set of constraints within which the organization must function. It is also a set of opportunities that the organization may seize (Pfeffer & Salanick, pp. 14–15).

Another difficult distinction is that between environment and inputs. If a thing can be changed and used by an organization to its own advantage, it can be thought of as an input and no longer in the organization's environment.

Some easily recognizable components of a nursing facility's environment are

- federal, state, and local regulations
- the number of other facilities operating in the area
- the availability of qualified applicants for positions to be filled in the home
- the availability of foods at affordable prices
- state Medicaid practices and reimbursement policies
- availability of funds
- inflation or deflation rates

1.3.2 Identifying Systems

The outputs of one system normally become inputs for the next system (Levey & Loomba, pp. 58–65), for example, the set of relationships that normally exists among hospitals, nursing homes, and home health agencies.

Hospital patients who need facility-based skilled nursing care (the outputs of the hospital) become the inputs of the skilled nursing facility—new patient admissions. The rehabilitated nursing home patient who no longer needs facility-based skilled nursing care but requires follow-up home care (the nursing home output) becomes the input of the home health agency.

We have been using the nursing home as an entity to illustrate the systems concept. We could have selected another level of function within the facility, for instance, the department of nursing.

WHO DEFINES THE SYSTEM?

The selection of what is to be viewed as the system is left entirely to the discretion of the person who describes or analyzes it. This may be one of the more subtle concepts in systems theory. The fact is that the user decides what to designate as a system for his/her own purposes. For example, the chief executive officer of a large nursing home chain is accustomed to thinking of the several hundred homes as the system. The individual nursing home administrator may conceive of the departments operating in the facility as the system. The maintenance chief may consider his/her department as the system for working within the organization.

One of the virtues of the systems concept is that it is almost infinitely adaptable to the needs of the individual user. Anybody can define any set of interrelationships as the system for purposes of description or analysis. All of us use systems analysis in our everyday thinking about the inter-relationships of things around us. The systems theory and model described here is an analytical tool that the administrator can use to think through organizational problems as they arise.

1.3.3 Other Characteristics of Systems

Social science researchers have identified several characteristics of systems that the reader may find useful as an analytical tool.

The output of each system furnishes the stimulus for repeating the cycle (Katz & Kahn, p. 20). In the case of nursing care facilities, the successfully cared for patient (the output of the nursing home's efforts) furnishes the source of more inputs: other persons apply for admission to the facility to replace the patient who has left. The new resident brings renewed energy in the form of a renewed source of continuing income to the facility and thereby furnishes a renewal of the capacity of the facility to continue to pay employees and provide services.

The administrator can view the nursing facility as a dynamic system whose essence is the cycle of activities (providing care to patients, making a profit) for which he/she is responsible.

ORGANIZATIONAL CHARTS

Organizations are pictured through organizational charts, which show the structure of authority. These charts resemble a snapshot of an organization at any given moment, but they cannot capture the constant motion of the organization. For this reason, organizational charts, while very useful managerial tools, are only one of many clues to the actual functioning of the nursing home organization (Dale, p. 180).

It is very difficult to put an organization in all its complexity on a piece of paper. Organizational charts are and will remain important to administrators attempting to understand, manage, and interpret the organization to others, but they must respect the limitations inherent in these charts.

ORGANIZATIONAL GROWTH

A nursing home and similar social organizations can grow without any time limit.

Scientists speak of the entropic process, a universal law of nature that all organisms move toward death (Katz & Kahn, p. 21). All of us, for example, realize that one day we will die because one or more of our vital systems comes to a halt.

In sharp contrast, a nursing facility or chain not only does not have to die, but it can keep on growing, with no time constraints, as long as it receives more energy from the environment than it consumes. In this way organizations can be said to acquire negative entropy (Robey, pp. 174–177).

Organizations tend to try to grow; not in every case, of course, but in general. Organizational theorists have called this the tendency of organizations to maximize the ratio of imported to expended energy. This concept helps to explain the current tendency for nursing home chains to attempt to grow larger and larger and to compete with one another for the purchase of individual homes as they come up for sale.

One social scientist (Miller, pp. 513–531) has observed that the rate of growth of an organization, within certain ranges, is dramatic if it exists in a medium that makes available unrestricted amounts of additional inputs. The small family-owned nursing home is an example. We may be nearing the end of the period when small "mom and pop" freestanding nursing homes are available precisely because the chains, in their desire to constantly expand, have systematically bought them up whenever they come on the market.

This may further help to explain why nursing home chains are not only buying individual homes but also other chains. This is a phenomenon occurring in the hospital field as well. The significance for administrators is that organizations, unlike people, are not subject to disintegration as long as they can keep adding to their resources, and that organizations, like people, tend to try to grow. This growth may be qualitative (better care) or quantitative (a larger patient census or more and more facilities being added to the chain).

MAXIMIZING BASIC CHARACTER

Another important factor is that organizations, as they grow, want to shape the world around them to look just like themselves (Katz & Kahn, p. 24). For example, in planning for an ambulatory care system, the nursing home associations place the nursing home at the heart of the system. The American Hospital Association, on the other hand, envisions the American health care system with the hospitals at its core. The insurance companies are similarly convinced of their own strategic importance at the very center of such a system.

MAINTENANCE FUNCTIONS

Once in place, organizations become creatures of habit and develop a tendency to resist change. There can be a strong effort to keep the current pattern of relationships with others from changing at all. Sometimes this is called organizational hardening of the arteries. Organizations that have become set in their ways will try to maintain the status quo through several devices:

1. Any internal or external situation that threatens to force a change in the organization is countered by employees seeking to keep their old patterns and ways of doing things. For example, the nursing home faced with a "disruptive employee" agitating for changes will dismiss the disruptive employee, will resist change (Bradley, pp. 56–65).

2. Administrators, when confronted with external changes that might

force changes in the organization, will try to ignore them. For example, if the patient census declines while that of other nearby homes increases, the tendency will be to find excuses rather than asking what is causing this reduction or seeking to discover if the other homes are offering better services.

3. In trying to resist change, many organizations will attempt to cope with external forces that might force them to change by acquiring control over them. For example, if a nursing home chain is losing patients to competing freestanding facilities, the chain might attempt to acquire those other facilities, rather than remedy its own situation (Katz & Kahn, p. 24).

Finally, two other characteristics of organizations should be briefly mentioned.

ORGANIZATIONS GROW INCREASINGLY COMPLEX

New organizations tend to be simple at their start, then become more and more complex as they grow. The human personality is similar. As infants we have few perceptions. As we grow, we begin to build ever more complex and complicated perceptions of the world around us. The personality we develop is a system with no physical boundaries. A social organization such as the nursing home is also a system with no physical boundaries (Katz & Kahn, p. 24; Allport, 1962, pp. 3–30).

Just as the human personality becomes progressively more sophisticated, social organizations move toward the multiplication and elaboration of roles with greater specialization of functions. For example, the mom-and-pop nursing homes of two decades ago are giving way to increasingly larger and more sophisticated chains.

The federal government is another good example of this process. In the early part of this century there were only a handful of federal bureaus. Today, to administer the thousands of bills Congress has passed, there are literally hundreds of federal bureaus imposing ever more complicated sets of rules on businesses.

The organization of American medicine provides another illustration. In 1870, 80% of all American physicians were general practitioners. Only a few were specialists. Today, with the explosion of medical technology, the reverse is true: 80% of American physicians are specialists, and only 20% are general practitioners.

The process of nursing homes grouping into increasingly larger and competing chains (i.e., multiplication and elaboration of roles) has led to multiplying the number of possible management jobs available to persons interested in a career in nursing home management. Middle- and upper-level positions are now available in corporate nursing home management offices.

ORGANIZATIONS ARE DIFFICULT TO PREDICT

There need not be a single strategy for an organization to achieve an objective. We have argued that organizations are dynamic systems of social interactions. Because the situation is so volatile, there is low predictability (Bertalanffy, p. 521 ff.).

An organization can reach its goals from differing starting points and by a variety of routes. If, for example, a small, financially weak nursing home chain management staff wanted to take over a financially stronger and larger chain, there are many possible alternatives. They could try to compete more successfully, thus weakening the larger chain, making it more susceptible to takeover. They could attempt to raise enough venture capital to buy out the larger group. They could arrange to be taken over by an unrelated corporation with large assets, thereby enabling them to buy out the currently stronger and larger chain.

The listing of the ten largest nursing home chains has changed rapidly over the past several years, constantly producing surprise moves in which smaller chains have taken over larger ones. Predictability is equally low in a number of fields; e.g., the hospital field and the computer industry are experiencing unexpected takeovers and ownership changes.

SUMMARY

In the process of looking at the function called organizing we have suggested that thinking of organizations as systems is a useful approach to the task of understanding how a nursing facility functions. We have argued that the systems model is a useful way to visualize the inputs (money, materials, and people) that are available to administrators. We have shown that the way in which administrators configure and use money, materials, and people will depend on their beliefs about how organizations function.

1.4 Staffing

Staffing is hiring the right persons for the jobs in the organization. It is one of the most difficult tasks the administrator faces because it is seldom possible to predict from an interview and recommendations how a person will work out on the job. The number of variables is almost infinite, and many of them are difficult to recognize beforehand.

Staffing patterns of nursing homes are more prescribed than they are for most other health care institutions. This is the result of the federal Conditions for Participation and state regulations, which carefully delineate qualifications for each type of staff position and require minimum staffing in nearly every area of the facility.

One thing is quite clear: the success of the nursing home depends directly on adequate staffing. Nursing care is looking after people. The interactions between patient and staff determine the quality of life in the nursing home. Physical facilities are important, but once they are in place at a minimally adequate level, the patient's satisfaction with the facility varies directly with his/her satisfaction with the staff performance.

As mentioned earlier, the administrator may choose to delegate co-ordination of the hiring process to a personnel director or assign it to the individual department heads with the advice and consent of the administrator. In every case, the staffing function is critical to the successful operation of the nursing facility. The National Board of Examiners for Nursing Home Administrators has recognized this and has devoted an entire section of the national examination to the staffing responsibilities carried by nursing home administrators. For this reason, we mention the staffing function at this point. The reader is referred to Part 2 for a detailed discussion of staffing tasks.

1.5 Directing

Directing is the process of communicating to employees what is to be done by each of them and helping them to accomplish it. An earlier step, organizing, included breaking down the work necessary to achieve the organizational goals into work assignments that can be handled by one person. Directing is a portion of the organizational activity in which the actual work is done.

Several important management concepts should be included under this heading:

- policymaking
- decision making
- leadership
- power and authority
- communication skills
- organizational norms and values
- additional related concepts

Directing involves reference to each of these key concepts to arrive at the goal of a successful program.

1.5.1 Policymaking

The ultimate goal of each administrator is to have a program in which every member of the organization makes the same decisions given the same set of circumstances. That is, the administrator's goal is to persuade the entire staff to carry out their responsibilities exactly as the administrator would like them to.

PURPOSE AND FUNCTION

It is impossible for the administrator to be everywhere at once, 24 hours a day throughout the facility. It is possible, however, for the administrator to make policies that direct the activities of the employees everywhere in the facility 24 hours a day. The purpose and function of these policies is to communicate to each employee as exactly as possible what the management expects in any situation on the job.

It is, of course, neither possible nor desirable to establish policies for every conceivable situation. However, a person can provide guidelines or policies that become the framework within which the employee decides what to do in each situation requiring action on behalf of the nursing home facility. G. R. Terry, in his book *Principles of Management*, has defined policy as a verbal, written, or implied overall guide that sets up boundaries supplying the general limits and direction in which managerial action will take place.

Policies are used to help keep decisions within the areas intended by the planners, since they provide for some consistency in what employees decide in particular situations usually under repetitive conditions. Policies reveal the facility administrator's intentions with respect to the behavior of employees, patients/residents, and the public for future time periods. Policies are decided before the need for employee knowledge arises. A simple illustration might be useful.

It is not possible for management to know when, where or even whether a fire will break out in the facility. By developing a complete set of procedures for personnel to follow in case of fire, the administrator is able to communicate before the occasion arises precisely what each employee in the facility must do if a fire should occur.

DEFINING POLICIES AND PROCEDURES

The reader may have noticed the use of the word *procedures* above, rather than *policies*. Writers in the field of management use *policies, procedures,* and *plans of action* as terms to indicate movement from generalized statements of intention (policies) to specific spelling out of the method, step by step (procedures), for carrying out those policies or plans of action.

It may be useful to think of the following set of concepts, which moves from the general to the specific setting forth of behaviors the manager wishes the employees to exercise.

EXAMPLE OF POLICIES AND PROCEDURES

General goals or objectives may be stated for the facility. In the area of fire preparedness a goal statement might be: "Our goal is to have our facility employees completely prepared to take appropriate action in case of fire." The administrator might then write a general *policy statement* indicating that the head of the housekeeping department would develop a step-by-step plan of action for every department to follow in case of fire. This step-by-step plan of action developed by the head of housekeeping is a *set of procedures*, a highly detailed plan of specific actions that each employee would be expected to follow in case of fire.

Notice that at each level the degrees of freedom within which decisions could be made were reduced. The head of housekeeping could develop a variety of configurations for employee responsibilities, but by the time the individual employee became involved, the degrees of freedom had nearly vanished. The responsibility in case of fire had moved from the general goal or policy of fire preparedness to a detailed set of instructions or procedures to be followed to the letter (e.g., "the moment you hear the fire alarm, proceed immediately to station J on Wing B and report to the nurse in charge" is an example of a procedure).

The board of directors might set a policy goal of offering an outstanding selection of first-quality food to the residents of the facility. It becomes the responsibility of each of the progressively lower levels of management to actually implement this policy. The food service director must take this communicated policy or goal and develop a series of policies for decision making by the kitchen staff that result in the actual service of an outstanding selection of first-quality food to the residents.

General policies are developed at each level of management. Normally, the amount of specificity increases at each lower level. The food service manager may, for example, announce a policy to the food service supervisor responsible for salads that there be a sufficient variety with a specified proportion of crisp fresh lettuce every evening. The supervisor may then write out a step-by-step set of procedures for the kitchen worker who prepares salads. The set of steps the salad worker is to follow at 4:00 P.M. each afternoon, beginning, perhaps, with removing the lettuce from the refrigerator, is an example of a set of procedures. The broad policy of excellence in food service set by the administrator has now been translated into a set of procedures or individual steps for the salad worker in the kitchen to follow at 4:00 P.M. each afternoon to assure the crispness of the lettuce to be served each evening.

SUMMARY

Policies serve as general statements or understandings that guide or channel subordinates' thinking as they make decisions. Policies limit the area within which a decision is to be made and assure that it will be consistent with the overall objectives. Policies tend to decide issues ahead of time by establishing the framework and scope of the actions.

The decisions made at each level of management establish the framework for decision making at each successively lower level of management, generally with progressively less and less discretion to do so. However, each level of management does participate in the policymaking process, and policies *are* made at every level of management. Policy is made by persons at upper, middle, and lower levels of management within the nursing home facility. Defining policymaking is complicated by this fact.

When do policies become procedures? Sometimes this is a fine line and hard to distinguish. Generally, a policy is a statement that contains some degree of freedom, some further need for interpretation by the person implementing the action. A procedure, in contrast, has few if any degrees of freedom and little if any latitude for interpretation. Procedures are step-by-step instructions on how a specific task is to be carried out.

1.5.2 Making a Decision

Although decision making can be synonymous with managing, it is difficult to define. G.L.S. Shackle (p. 105) defines "deciding" as the focal creative psychic event in which knowledge, thought, feeling, and imagination are fused into action (see also Dale, chapter 23). Both Dale and Shackle point out the impossibility of a useful formula for decision making. Inevitably, we are left with an imprecise definition of the process. Even so, administrators do make numerous decisions every day.

To make the "right" decision in a given situation is often difficult. It is the nursing facility administrator's job to assure that all employees make the right decisions for the organization as often as possible (Kotter, p. 9).

We define a successful manager as a person who is able, on balance, to make enough right decisions for the organization and *no* disastrously wrong ones. Similarly, the organization's goal is to have employees make as many correct decisions as possible and *no* disastrously wrong ones. The manager's task is to provide enough direction to assure that employees make decisions that conform to the organization's goals.

1.5.3 Leadership

Decision making is an act of leadership for the organization. When the manager decides something, he/she is providing leadership to the facility (Pfeffer & Salancik, p. 17).

DEMOCRATIC LEADERSHIP

Over the past few decades a body of management literature in the United States has been accumulated, supporting the concept of democratic leadership in preference to other styles of management (Likert, 1961, pp. 97–104). This might have been predictable, given the commitment to a democratic way of life in this country.

The democratic leader is a person who encourages maximum feasible participation by others in organizational decisions, assuring that decisions are made at the lowest level of competence to arrive at the judgment. Aside from its democratic overtones, this approach was believed to be the most functional. Those with the greatest technical expertise would participate appropriately in the decision process. Clearly, there is a lot to be said for this approach.

How Functional Is It?

The democratic leader is always faced with the problem of how to be democratic in relationships with subordinates and yet maintain necessary authority and control.

When is it best for the facility administrator to decide? When the subordinates are encouraged to make many decisions, is the manager behaving democratically? This would depend, to some extent, on the nature of the decisions the administrator allows the lower-level managers to make.

Beyond this there is the serious question of whether the facility administrator can ever relinquish total responsibility for the facility by delegating. The issue of delegation will be discussed in greater detail in the section on Power and Authority.

In our view there is no simple answer to these questions. Several of the organizational characteristics we have discussed earlier must be taken into account. The problem for the organization's administrator is how to achieve employees' compliance with management's goals. Once the planning process has been achieved, and the board of directors or the owners have set forth the goals and objectives of the nursing care facility, the administrator's work begins. The search for personnel who will implement the plans that have been made by the organization's chief decision makers is undertaken.

THE ORGANIZATION'S LEADERSHIP DILEMMA

The dilemma faced by the administrator is to deal with staff who will exercise leadership for the benefit of the organization while being guided by the policies that have been set forth. This is a situation in which both strict conformity to the organizational goals and policies and encouragement of creativity among its employees are desirable behavior patterns.

We hold that the debate about how democratic an administrator "ought" to be is not very useful in the search for an appropriate leadership style for oneself as the administrator of a nursing care facility. The question that must be addressed is, how can the administrator best assure that the goals and objectives of the facility are achieved by the employees? In some situations the best method might be to take a highly authoritarian approach, while in others a more lenient one might lead toward a more effective realization of the facility's goals. In short, the style of leadership needed within the organization will probably vary from situation to situation and over time.

An administrator might be more effective by practicing a highly participative and democratic style with one group of employees, yet be much more directive with employees in another department in the same facility. For us, it is a question of whatever is practical.

There is no value in committing oneself to any particular style of leadership for its own sake (Katz & Kahn, pp. 330–331). The question must always be, what leadership behaviors are needed to assist this organization, given its present circumstances, to achieve its goals?

CHOOSING A LEADERSHIP STYLE

In *Leadership and Organization,* Tannenbaum et al. (p. 311) discuss a continuum of leadership styles. This allows us to characterize seven possible positions along the continuum, from manager-centered to employee-centered leadership. Several dimensions are portrayed in Figure 1-2. Under manager-centered leadership, the manager retains a high degree of control and uses authority extensively.

Manager centered leadership					Employee centered leadership	
Use of authority by manager					Areas of freedom for employees	
manager decides and announces decision	manager sells, persuades acceptance	manager presents ideas & invites questions	manager presents tentative decision	manager presents problem, takes suggestions, makes decision	manager defines the limits, tells group to make decision	manager permits employees to function within policies set by manager
1	2	3	4	5	6	7
Manager retains a high degree of control					Manager shares decision making	

FIGURE 1-2. Range of decision-making strategies open to the manager.

Manager-Centered Leadership

Position 1. The manager simply makes the decision, then announces it (autocratic style).

Position 2. The manager attempts to convince the employees of the value of the decision made.

Position 3. The manager presents ideas and invites questions, in effect engaging the employees actively in the decision-making process for the first time.

Employee-Centered Leadership

Position 4. The manager presents a tentative decision, subject to change; the employees are further involved in the decision-making process itself.

Position 5. The manager presents the problem requiring solution, invites suggestions, then makes the decision.

Position 6. The manager defines the problem, sets the limits within which the decision must be made, then asks the group to make the decision.

Position 7. The manager permits subordinates to make the decision and function within the limits defined by the manager (laissez-faire leadership style).

DECIDING HOW TO LEAD

Three levels should be taken into account by the administrator who is selecting the leadership style for a particular situation.

First level Forces in the manager:

- his/her own values
- confidence in subordinates
- own feeling of security

Second level Forces in the subordinates: permit greater freedom of subordinates:

- have great need for independence
- are ready to assume responsibility for decision making
- have relatively high tolerance for uncertainty
- are interested in the problem and feel it is important
- understand and agree with the goals of the organization
- have the necessary knowledge and experience
- are conditioned and expect to make decisions

Third level Forces in the organization:

- expectations of the organization's management
- ability of the subordinates to function as a group
- the problem itself
- time constraints

THREE LEVELS OF LEADERSHIP SKILL REQUIREMENTS

We have already discussed the three levels of management: upper level, middle level, and lower level, each with its own particular skill requirements. Figure 1-3, adapted from Katz and Kahn, shows these three different levels of leadership skills.

The Upper-level Manager (the nursing facility's upper level administrator) is primarily responsible for creating and changing the organization's structure.

The Middle-level Manager (the director of nurses, for instance) is responsible for development of more specific policies that interpret administration policy implications for the nursing department.

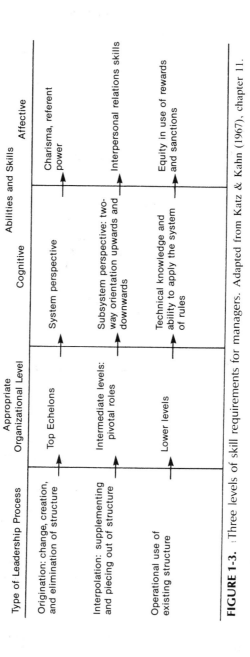

FIGURE 1-3. Three levels of skill requirements for managers. Adapted from Katz & Kahn (1967), chapter 11.

Type of Leadership Process	Appropriate Organizational Level	Abilities and Skills	
		Cognitive	Affective
Origination: change, creation, and elimination of structure	Top Echelons	System perspective	Charisma, referent power
Interpolation: supplementing and piecing out of structure	Intermediate levels: pivotal roles	Subsystem perspective: two-way orientation upwards and downwards	Interpersonal relations skills
Operational use of existing structure	Lower levels	Technical knowledge and ability to apply the system of rules	Equity in use of rewards and sanctions

The Lower-level Manager (e.g., the charge nurse who supervises a specific group of nurses) has the responsibility of applying the policies provided by the director of nursing to the actual care given to the patients.

As Figure 1-3 suggests, different skills are needed at the three different levels of management.

Upper Level Management's Job. The chief administrator must understand not only how the organization accommodates to the external environment but also the functions of all the subsystems within the nursing facility itself.

Middle Management's Job. The middle-level manager is responsible for implementing the policies of the administration by devising ways to put them into action within the facility. This level of management translates the broader institutional policies by developing more specific ones to control employee behavior. This requires the middle-level manager to understand how the subsystems of the organization fit together to achieve the overall goals. He/she has the difficult task of respresenting to upper-level management the needs of those supervised. To function effectively, middle-level managers must realize that they are the conduit through which action travels in both directions.

Lower Management's Job. Lower-level managers guide employees according to the established policies of the nursing facility. To accomplish this, the rules must be thoroughly understood and applied evenhandedly to all employees under their direction. One particularly important key to effective leadership at the lower level is the sense the employees have of their manager's advocacy. It is not enough to be their advocate, however; the manager must be their *effective* spokesperson.

Procedures can be written by any level of management, but typically, procedures are written at times by middle-level managers and most often by lower-level managers.

CHARACTERISTICS OF THE EFFECTIVE LEADER

Katz and Kahn (pp. 325–327) have characterized an effective leader as a person who

- mediates and tempers the organizational requirements to the needs of persons in a manner that is organizationally enhancing (the organization and the persons both profit from the relationship)
- promotes group loyalty and personal ties (working for the facility becomes a personally satisfying experience)
- demonstrates care for individuals

- relies on referent power (respect from employees and patients/ residents) rather than the power of legitimacy and sanctions alone (discussed below)
- encourages employees to develop a positive identity with the facility
- creates a high degree of personal commitment to the facility among the peers and subordinates

Tannenbaum (chapter 5) concludes that a successful leader is a person who is keenly aware of relevant forces in the situation, understands him/herself and the individuals with whom he/she is dealing, but also is able to behave appropriately vis-à-vis the situation, making decisions where needed and sharing the decision-making where appropriate.

Tannenbaum considers the successful leader as being neither strong nor permissive but rather as endowed with a strong instinct for determining appropriate personal behavior and capable of acting accordingly.

Day-to-Day Leadership Requirements

In the daily administration of the typical long-term care facility the administrator will face a variety of situations with differing leadership needs. Recognition of appropriate leadership behavior for any specific situation is a valuable insight; the capacity to behave in differing leadership styles is an accomplishment of a high order indeed. Much of the flexibility the administrator can exercise in distinctive leadership styles depends on how comfortable he/she is in wielding power and authority in the management of the facility.

Charismatic Leadership

Although charismatic leadership cannot be consciously chosen by the administrator, it is worth mentioning here. Charismatic leadership has been described by Max Weber as a magical aura with which people sometimes endow their leaders. It appears when a group has an emotional need for a person who, they feel, will make the right decision for them. The acts of charismatic leaders are typically unexamined. Their followers do not scrutinize their acts as they would those of their immediate supervisors. Charisma is not an objective assessment by the followers and normally requires a psychological distance between the followers and the leader. When charisma is assigned to a leader, the power and authority of the organization is enhanced.

1.5.4 Power and Authority

Power is the ability to control others. A person has power when he/she is able to make other people do what he/she wants them to. The administrator of a nursing facility has the power to order employees to act to implement the goals of the facility as expressed in the policies and plans.

Webster's *New World Dictionary* gives 14 definitions for the word *power*. An additional half-dozen synonyms indicate that power denotes the inherent ability or the admitted right to rule, govern, determine, control, regulate, restrain, and curb. Power is a complex concept in our culture.

The administrator has the power (from the board or the owners) to tell employees what to do and to expect them to do it. It is well known that although an organization theoretically provides equal legitimating power to all administrators at the same level, the administrators do not in fact remain equal.

If, for example, board of directors controlled five nursing facilities, the board, in theory, delegates equal authority to the administrators to act on its behalf in the five facilities. Some of these five administrators might have firm control over employee behavior, while others might be having difficulty convincing employees to do what they request. Why?

RECIPROCITY

Power is a reciprocal relationship. The board of directors or the owners can confer power on the administrator, but the employees and patients/residents must accept that power as permissible if it is to be meaningful. This does not imply disrespect or chaos. The concept of authority or power is more complicated than the mere announcement that power has been given to the administrator by the board or the owners.

French and Raven (pp. 607–623) and Robey (p. 147) have suggested that there are at least five types of power: legitimate, reward, punishment, referent, and expert.

Legitimate Power. This describes power given to a particular person or position, recognized as such, accepted as appropriate not only by the wielder of power, but by those over whom it is wielded and by the other members of the system. Organizations expect each person (employee, resident/patient) to yield to the appropriate authority of others in the organization.

Reward Power. The fact that reward is a second type of power is testimony to the idea that employees do not always do what the administrator asks of them. Administrators are given reward power to induce or persuade employees or patients/residents to do what the administrator wishes. If not, certain desired rewards will be withheld (Robey, pp. 382–383). For example, if the administrator has the authority to give a 15% year-end cash bonus to the three supervisors who have best achieved the facility's goals (translate: those who most often responded correctly to the administrator's instructions), then he/she has reward power.

Punishment Power. Administrators are also given punishment power to help bring employees or patients/residents in line with organizational policy. The ultimate punishment power is firing the employee or requiring the patient to leave the facility, but there are many intermediate, less drastic means. The employees who do not observe the administrator's rules for functioning in the facility may receive a written warning, a copy of which is placed in the personnel file. Additionally, the administrator may threaten to withhold any positive job recommendation as long as the warning remains in the file.

Other types of punishment available to the administrator are verbal reprimands, failure to give a raise, and the like.

Referent Power. Power to influence is often based on liking or identifying with another person. When the employees like the administrator and identify with him/her, they are far more apt to do what the administrator wishes. This is both simple and powerful. Employees who do not admire an administrator or do not identify with him/her are more difficult to control, i.e., to make them do their work as the organization wishes.

Expert Power. Power can derive from recognition by the employees and residents/patients that the administrator is very skillful, has had considerable training, and is quite knowledgeable in the field of nursing home administration. For the nurse, this acknowledgment comes from the RN (registered nurse) license; for the physician, the license to practice medicine.

POWER FROM OUTSIDE THE ORGANIZATION

It is important to note that expert and referent power, to the extent they are present in the facility, are additions to the power of organizationally given rewards and punishments because *expert and referent power cannot be conferred by the organization* (Katz & Kahn, pp. 302–303). There is literally an increase in the amount of power or control that can be exerted over the personnel and patients/residents, and it is a persistent factor in increased organizational performance.

Expert and referent power can be *substituted* for power based on punishment. This can mean fewer negative or undesired or unintended organizational consequences. It is desirable to promote referent power in addition to, or instead of, power based on rewards and punishment or organizational dictates. Remember, the goal of the administrator is to motivate the members of the organization to achieve the organization's goals.

Expert and referent power are available to all members of the staff. Referent power, in particular, depends on personal and group characteristics and is available to peers (persons at the same level) in the organization. Peer influence is often more readily accepted than influence from superiors. If, for example, one of the nurses is particularly skillful in providing patient care, his/her leadership through referent power gives the nursing facility greater control over the quality of nursing achieved.

THE ADMINISTRATOR'S POWER IS REAL

Administrators do have power over other people's lives. Christensen, Berg, and Salter have characterized the power of the chief administrator as potentially "irresponsible" (p. 49), not necessarily because of the use of power in any particular decision or even because of the motives of the administrators, but because those affected by the decisions (the employees, patients/residents, and even the board or owners) very often have little or no real voice in the making of those decisions. This can be especially true when most of the power is centralized in the office of the administrator. There are limitations, however.

THE ADMINISTRATOR'S POWER IS CONSTRAINED

As we discuss elsewhere, nursing facilities have quite complex lines of authority because of the presence of several professional groups within the facility: physicians, nurses, dietitians, physical therapists, and others. All of these groups have professional organizations and loyalties that influence their behavior in the nursing facility. They have "authority" within their professional spheres.

The facility administrator's authority is constantly constrained or limited by the influence of the medical, nursing, and other professions, respectively, over the behavior of its physicians, nurses, nutritionists, and other professionals within the facility. Membership in these professional groups means that, in the last analysis, the doctors' behavior may be governed more by professional standards enforced by the medical profession than by policies or goals of the nursing facility (Williams & Torrens, pp. 277–279). Similarly, nurses are governed by professional nursing standards rather than by policies or goals of the nursing facility. The same, of course, is true of the other professionals. This does not mean that the administrator has little or insufficient control but rather that the authority or power to act is always circumscribed or constrained by the presence of the controls over behavior exerted by the professional groups (Gorden, pp. 136–137). The task of achieving control over the behavior of the professional employees is a complicated one, requiring tact and ingenuity on the part of the administrator.

1.5.5 Communication Skills

Directing is also the process of communicating the organizational objectives to the staff and residents/patients. *Communication is the exchange of information and the transmission of meaning.*

Communication is essential for the survival of any social system. The skill of the administrator in communicating what is to be accomplished and the manner in which it is to be carried out have much to do with the success of the administration in achieving the plans for the facility. Unless the plans of action are successfully communicated to the staff, the plans will, at worst, not be implemented at all, or at best, only partially carried out.

Steps in the communication process are as follows: (a) someone initiates it; (b) it is transmitted from its source to its destination; and (c) it has an impact on the recipient. Unless and/or until a communication has made its intended impact on the recipient, it has, for all intents and purposes, not taken place.

COMMUNICATION = INFORMATION = POWER

Communication is the transmission of information, and information is power because it provides sounder bases for judgments. The informed person is on sturdier ground and therefore more powerful. The withholding of information is also a form of power, inasmuch as the person with the information is in a superior position to make decisions.

SYSTEMS OF COMMUNICATION

Typically, organizations are described as having at least two systems of communication existing side by side: the formal and the informal communication process.

The *formal communication* process closely resembles the formal organizational structure of the nursing facility (Dale, p. 286). The administrator may send memoranda to the department heads, or the department heads may send memos to their staff.

The *informal communication* process exists in nearly every organization. The social groups within the facility define the informal communication process (Mintzberg, p. 49; Dale, p. 285). Nurses chatting in their lounge communicate informally and exchange much important information in the course of their casual conversation.

Communication is the flow of information in the organization, which social scientists describe as flowing upward, downward, and horizontally. As the words themselves suggest, upward communication flows from subordinates upward to the next level(s) of administration. Downward communication flows from upper-level management to lower-level members of the staff. Horizontal communication is information flowing between peers or persons of equal rank or status.

The closer a person gets to the organizational center of control, the more pronounced the emphasis on the exchange of information. Administrators process information and use it in their decision making. Communicating is at the heart of the management process.

Communicating is an art that managers must master. Most communications between administrators and personnel are full of subtleties and shades of meaning. Most acts of communication also have numerous levels of meaning and function and are essential to building a relationship. Any act of communication may answer a question at the moment, but it has different meanings to the persons involved. Managers need to be aware that there are many barriers to full, clear communication. Seldom does any single communication have only one level of meaning (Kotter, p. 126).

BARRIERS TO COMMUNICATION

Agenda Carrying.   Each person carries his or her own agenda into every communication situation, preoccupied with his/her own concerns and life experiences. Each individual filters what is communicated by means of his/her own perceptions.

Selective Hearing.   Persons hear selectively; that is, they tend to hear what they want to hear, thereby filtering out the unpleasant. A nursing supervisor may wish to communicate to an aide dissatisfaction with one aspect of the aide's performance. To soften the effect, the supervisor may first praise the employee for some other work. The employee may hear the praise and effectively screen out the criticism.

Phases in Knowledgeability.   If a test of the role of the nurse's aide were given to all the aides in the facility, the novices might answer in one way, those who were somewhat familiar with expected practice in another, and the fully trained, who were familiar with policies, quite differently—that is, degrees of sophistication vary among listeners, and their answers will similarly vary.

The Filter Effect.   The manager is told what the employees believe he/she wants to hear. It is not easy to give a superior bad news when one already knows such news is not welcome. Ancient Greek literature recounts how frequently the messenger bringing bad news to the king was killed. The implications of this reaction have not been lost on most organizational members.

It seems that no matter how much middle- and upper- level administrators insist they want to hear bad as well as good news, the employees filter the information toward the known bias of the next level(s) of management. When there are several layers of management through which unwelcome news must filter, the upper management may receive relatively little accurate information.

Sub Group Allegiance.   Each one of the sub groups in the organization (nurses, housekeepers, patients) demands allegiance from its members. Tangible and intangible rewards are given in each group, so when a communication arrives, it is interpreted in light of the goals and needs of each subgroup and usually *not* from the viewpoint of the organization as a whole.

Jay Jackson, in *The Organization and Its Communication Problems* (pp. 443–456), concluded that

- people communicate far more with members of their own subgroup than with any other persons (e.g., the nurses have difficulty in learning what the nurses' aides are thinking and feeling)

- people prefer to communicate with someone of higher status than themselves (the aides prefer to talk to the nurses)

- people try to avoid having communication with those lower in status than themselves (the nurses prefer to talk to the doctors, not to the aides except when giving instructions to them)

- people will communicate with those who will help them achieve their goals—higher status persons have power to create either gratifying or depriving experiences

- people communicate with those who can make them feel more secure and avoid those who make them anxious

Status Distance. It is difficult for lower-level employees to communicate upward.

Language Barrier. Doctors and nurses speak "medicalese." The pharmacists speak yet another language. In short, given the large variety of professional specialists who must by regulation be employed or retained as consultants, the nursing home administrator and the staff who deal with these many jargons have an especially difficult task.

Self-Protection. Persons fail to communicate anything that might reflect badly on them, their friends, or the organization (translated: the administrator should assure her/himself that the accident report portrays what actually occurred).

Information Overload. The overabundance of information flowing in most nursing facilities (as many as 50 to 100 forms) produces an information overload that may result in the staff's inability to distinguish among communications requiring their attention.

Others. The administrator must bear in mind that all communication is multidimensional, needing appropriate interpretation to be of use.

In sending out a memorandum to employees or in engaging in any communication, the administrator must take into account that its effect depends on the following:

- feelings and attitudes the parties have toward each other
- expectations
- how well the subordinate's needs are being met by the organization—if the nursing facility is supportive, the employee receiving administrative communications will be less defensive and more problem-oriented, that is, readier to absorb the communication and comply with the organization's request

1.5.6 Organizational Norms and Values

DEVELOPING LOYALTY TO FACILITY GOALS

Administering an organization such as a nursing home facility is a complicated process. We have discussed some of the problems encountered by administrators as they attempt to lead employees to do the tasks required. One of the impediments to accomplishing this is that the organization can never count on the individual employee's undivided attention. This is known as the concept of partial inclusion, or the segmental involvement of people in the job role.

Limitations on Employee Participation

The nursing home defines behaviors that require only a portion of a person's attention. The facility asks only that during each shift employees perform the tasks or roles prescribed for them and that they have agreed to do (Pfeffer & Salancik, pp. 29–32). Unavoidably, however, the whole person must be brought into the work situation (Katz & Kahn, p. 50). To deal with this, the employee is asked to set aside the non-job aspects of life while at work. This is literally a depersonalizing demand, which most employees find difficult to accomplish, so informal "organizations within the organization" develop in defense of personal identity.

The result is that people behave less as members of the nursing facility and more in terms of some compromise of their many commitments. For example, when asked about the sources of satisfaction from their jobs, employees typically rate their interpersonal relationships with their fellow employees as the most important aspect of their work. Association with the patients follows, with the goals and values of the nursing home facility itself tending to be somewhat low on the list of employee motivation. Administrators and supervisors engage in a constant struggle to gain loyalty from employees to the goals of the facility.

There is yet another important limitation to employees' full participation. People tend to interpret the facility as a whole from the viewpoint of their particular section of the organization. This is another reason why upper-level administrators who collect information only from their immediate subordinates may never know what is really going on.

People tend to exaggerate their importance to the organization as a whole. Loyalties develop to the work area rather than to the whole facility. This is a major source of conflict between departments. The nursing department views the organization from its unique perspective, as do the maintenance, food service, and other sections.

To enable staff to accomplish necessary work, organizations develop and specify *roles* (job descriptions) that are carefully prescribed forms of behavior associated with the tasks the organization wants performed. Roles are standardized patterns of required behavior (Katz & Kahn, p. 49). The nurse's aide is told very clearly what his/her role is during the 8 hours on the job.

Connecting Roles to Norms

To build loyalty, organizations try to identify roles and the persons filling them with the *norms* or values of the organization, general expectations for all employees.

Professional standards for nurses and nurse's aides are examples of such norms. They are behavior patterns to which all members of the group are expected to adhere. Respecting the personal privacy of patients would be an example of such a norm.

Norms are justified by *values*, which are more generalized statements about the behavior expected from staff members. Values furnish the rationale for the normative requirements. Treating all patients with complete respect for their rights as persons is an example of a broad value statement, justifying the more specific norm that nursing personnel ought to respect each patient's personal privacy.

System norms and values are attempts to connect employees with the system so that they remain within it while carrying out their role assignments. It could be said that norms and values furnish "cognitive road maps" (ways to think about the organization and its goals). Norms help personnel to adjust to the system.

Moral and Social Justification of the Facility

Another major contribution of organizational norms and values is the moral or social justification for the activities of the nursing facility. This is useful for both the staff and members of the community and has been particularly important to long-term-care employees over the past two decades.

When nursing homes have been attacked in the newspapers and subjected to public criticism, their staff members have a special need of administrators who are able to reinforce their positive feelings about their workplace. This can be accomplished by helping employees understand and internalize the values—e.g., excellent quality of patient care—held by the facility.

WHY ORGANIZATIONS NEED ADMINISTRATIVE LEADERSHIP

Once all the plans have been developed and staff hired and trained, why doesn't the organization just run by itself? Although there are a number of dimensions to any answer to this question, we will discuss only a few that seem especially relevant.

All organizational designs are imperfect (Demski, p. 58). Differences between the organizational chart, the written policies, and the organization's actual functioning are easily seen. It is commonly recognized that the new worker, who has been instructed by the supervisor, turns to the group members to learn what the job requirements really are.

Actual behavior, the actual functioning of the organization, is infinitely more complex, inconclusive, and variable than the plan. An illustration of this is organizational sabotage. Any worker who wants to sabotage the facility can do so by merely following organizational law to the letter —doing what is formally stipulated, no more and no less.

Nursing facilities, like all organizations, need administrative leadership to cope with the constantly changing external environment that requires internal adjustments. When, for example, three new nursing facilities open in an area and one's own occupancy rate drops from 92% to 72%, organizational leadership is in order.

Organizations also need leadership to accommodate to the changes constantly occurring within them. Employees retire or find work elsewhere, staff and residents' needs change, conflicts develop, physical systems break down, and decisions to repair or replace are called for.

1.5.7 Additional and Related Concepts

We turn now to several additional concepts worth reviewing in any consideration of attempts by administrators to direct the efforts of the organization.

DELEGATION

The concept of delegation is to permit decisions to be made at the lowest possible level. Decision-making authority is given to middle-level and lower-level managers, allowing them to make decisions for the organization, as appropriate. The essential issue is the determination of the nature of the decisions to be made at whatever level (Meal, pp. 102–111; Mintzberg, pp. 212–213).

Delegating can be both beneficial and disadvantageous. At optimum operation, delegation channels decision making to staff members who are best informed and most skilled to make a particular decision or set of decisions. The negative aspect of this practice is that since the managers have only a partial view of the organization, they consciously or unconsciously may make decisions in a manner that maximizes their area of the organization, to the possible detriment of the facility as a whole.

Ultimate responsibility cannot be delegated. The chief administrator is held accountable for the acts of all persons working under facility auspices.

UNITY OF COMMAND

The concept of unity of command emphasizes the importance of each person being accountable to only one supervisor (Simon, 1960, pp. 23–26). Since it is functionally difficult for any employee to answer to two managers, the facility must be organized to assure this relationship (Robey, p. 51).

SPAN OF CONTROL

How many immediate subordinates with interrelated work should a manager supervise? This has been a point of argument for decades. The British World War I general, Sir Ian Hamilton, insisted that six was the maximum span of control. Others have proposed different numbers. In the last analysis, the administrator must be certain that each employee is effectively supervised (Robey, p. 311).

SHORT CHAIN OF COMMAND

This principle asserts that there should be as few levels of management as possible between the chief administrator and the rank and file (Dale, p. 190). Certainly, for the communication purposes of upper-level management, this seems a good principle to follow. It minimizes the number of interpreters through whom information for upper-level managers must be sifted.

BALANCE

Advocates of the principle of balance (Dale, pp. 190–191) assert that there is a need for continual surveillance to maintain balance among the following:

- size of the various departments
- standardization of procedures and flexibility
- centralization and decentralization
- span of control and short chain of command

MANAGEMENT BY OBJECTIVES

In theory, objectives are set by the chief administrator in consultation with middle- and lower-level managers. The efforts of the entire organization are then focused on achieving them. Control measures are set in place, monitoring progress toward ultimate success.

Management by objectives (MBO) was first put into practice on a large scale by Lyndon Johnson. As President of the United States, he wished to gain meaningful control of the largest bureaucracy under his management: the Department of Health, Education and Welfare (HEW; later renamed the Department of Health and Human Services).

James E. Swiss, a North Carolina State University political scientist, analyzed President Johnson's managers at the Department. He observed that the real effect of using MBO was to shift power from middle and lower managers to the office of the upper-level manager (the Office of the Secretary of HEW) (Swiss, p. 238). He found the influence of outside interest groups to be generally reduced at Health and Human Services through the use of MBO.

We agree with his conclusion that MBO is used by managers who value internal power highly. The effect of MBO is to place more final decision making into the hands of the chief administrator.

In short, the announced purpose of MBO is to enable employees to efficiently and effectively focus all of the organizational energies on achieving the announced objectives, giving maximum direction to the organizational decision making. But the ultimate effect of using MBO, in our opinion, is to concentrate more decisions in the hands of the upper-level manager(s).

MANAGEMENT INFORMATION SYSTEMS

The phrase *management information system* (MIS) originally came into the literature as a description of computer-based information processing for managers in making their decisions (Dearden & McFarlan, p. 18). Withington (p. 3) defined MIS as the study of how the organization communicates and processes information to maximize the effectiveness of management and to further the objectives of the organization.

The point recognized in MIS is that the manager needs a constant rationalized and organized flow of information in order to make appropriate decisions. In Levey and Loomba's view (pp. 386–387), developing an MIS is as simple as

- determining one's need for information
- identifying the sources of information
- deciding on the amount, form, and frequency of information needed for communication
- choosing the means of information processing
- implementing the system

Under the headings of the individual departments of the nursing facility discussed below, we will offer our own ideas on appropriate management information systems for the departments individually and the nursing facility as a whole.

EVALUATION

There has been an unfortunate tendency in health management literature to separate evaluation and control. To evaluate is to make a judgment of worth. It is the process of comparing one thing with another and then making a decision based on the comparison. This, in our view, is the control function in managing.

Separate discussion of evaluation is due to the emergence of what has been called program evaluation (Levey & Loomba, p. 422). As program after program was authorized by the federal and state governments, a cry arose for someone to "evaluate" them: to tell the funders and the public whether the programs were worthwhile and/or achieving their stated goals.

According to Levey and Loomba (p. 422), the purpose of evaluation is to examine the effectiveness of organizational plans. We have described this as the control process.

QUALITY ASSURANCE

The nursing home industry has become increasingly concerned with controlling the quality of care patients/residents receive in a facility. A number of homes and chains are inviting nongovernmental agencies to judge quality of care through the accreditation process of the Joint Commission on Accreditation of Hospitals and through similar mechanisms that are discussed elsewhere in this work. Management is addressing more attention to quality assurance programs. This, in a sense, is the nursing home industry's own effort toward program evaluation.

SUMMARY

In this section, we have examined a number of concepts: policymaking, decision-making, leadership styles, power, authority, need for communication skills, norms, and values. We have touched lightly on a number of concepts guiding the administrator in attempts to direct the efforts of the nursing facility and have indicated that the administrator, in providing day-to-day guidance for the staff, assures that they know what is expected of them.

Having done this, administrators may be tempted to rest on their oars. This could be a fatal error in judgment. We have demonstrated that organizations are volatile systems that may or may not respond to the administrator's direction. The only way an administrator can be certain that the nursing facility is in fact making appropriate progress toward implementing its policies and plans of action is by comparing the outputs (results of organizational work) with the intended results. This is the process of controlling.

1.6 Controlling

Perhaps the most difficult, yet absolutely essential, function managers perform is controlling. Controlling, *in theory*, is not too difficult; controlling is comparing the actual results of the facility's efforts with the outcomes proposed in the plans.

The problem in controlling is that it obliges the manager to take unpleasant corrective actions to keep the facility on target. This may involve advising the staff that the work result is not suitable, or informing managers that the actual outputs are unsatisfactory. This is invariably an awkward business and avoided by managers who hope the situation will correct itself or that the problem will simply disappear. But matters usually get worse and require attention for solution.

1.6.1 Requirements for Effective Control

In our view, there are several ways in which the administrator can achieve effective control:

1. Goals must be translated into policies and plans of action that are *clearly stated, known, and measurable.*

2. The appropriate measurements must be identified. If the wrong measurements to compare actual to expected outputs are used, no management information system, however sophisticated, can truly inform and control.

3. Limits to deviations from the goal/policy/plan of action have to be set.

The manager must have predetermined and known outside limits for each output being controlled.

4. Information in useful form must go to the controllers at the appropriate levels. The information should be timely, easily understood, and unambiguous, so that the employee cannot use lack of clarity as a pretext for nonconformity.

Policies of actions to be taken when limits are exceeded must be known to the managers responsible for controlling outputs. Clear statements of policies are crucial for influencing staff members to take corrective actions when needed.

5. Corrective actions must be taken. To maximize the probability that managers will take corrective actions, an effective system of rewards and punishments is needed to encourage them to do so. When middle- and lower-level managers sense any softening in the administrator's determination to enforce the control policies, there will be a simultaneous softening of the control system.

6. A system must be set up for constant renewal of control measures to account for any changing organizational goals (as expressed in different or modified plans of action) that are responses to changes in the external or internal environments of the organization.

Middle- and lower-level managers may interpret portions of the control system being discarded as evidence that *all* of the control system is no longer in force. Eternal vigilance is the price of a control system that remains effective over an extended period of time.

7. The control mechanisms themselves must be functional and valued at each level of management to remain effective. If the staff responsible for enforcing controls does not feel the measures are acceptable and productive, excuses will be found not to rely on them.

8. Limitations of the scope and capabilities of the control system itself must be kept constantly in mind. They are never perfect. It is not possible to devise an organizational control system that does not need the good judgment of concerned employees to arrive at an interpretation of what the organization "really wants" in any situation (Zmud, pp. 87–90).

1.6.2 Management by Exception

One of the most useful control devices available to managers is to focus attention on the exceptions that occur. Every day the manager receives numerous verbal and written reports, which typically contain routine information about the functioning of the facility.

Managers can effectively use their time by giving their attention to exceptions to the plan. If the patient census, the number of meals served, or their costs are within plan, there may be no need for action. There are multitudes of detailed tasks being accomplished in acceptable fashion by the staff every day. What merits the administrator's atttention are the exceptions to the policies and plans of action originally established for the organization.

The budget is one of the most useful control mechanisms available to those adhering to the management by exception principle (Gordon & Stryker, pp. 100–113). Getting information about the amount of money that has been spent in the last time period is a reasonably exact control measurement. As long as any department is spending within the agreed-on budget there *may* be no need for the administrator's attention. Whenever a departmental budget falls short or exceeds the amounts allocated to it, the administrator should give attention to the exception and take whatever steps may be necessary to bring expenditures back within the budgeted limits. For example, if the administrator is concerned that the quality of food be kept up to a certain level, too little expenditure by the food service might be as much as cause for alarm as too great.

Management by exception does not mean that the routine and within-specifications behaviors of the facility remain unexamined. It is the routine behaviors of the organization that are being examined for deviations from the norm.

1.6.3 Concepts of Efficiency and Effectiveness

Efficiency is the ability to produce the desired effect with a minimum of effort, expense, or waste (Webster's New World Dictionary). Efficiency can be measured by the ratio of effective work to the energy expended in producing it. In systems terms this simply means getting the maximum outputs with the minimum inputs (Pfeffer & Salancik, pp. 11–12, 35).

Effectiveness is the power or ability to bring about the desired results. A nursing home that sets a goal of achieving excellence in patient care and then does so can be said to be effective (Pfeffer & Salancik, pp. 10–11, 33).

It may not, however, be achieving excellence of patient care efficiently. The home may, for example, be employing a very large number of nurses and aides to accomplish excellence in patient care. Studies in personnel reveal, however, that when more people are placed on a workshift than are needed, the quality of care is not necessarily improved. The staff may simply divide the work up to lighten the load for everyone, or take more frequent breaks and not actually give additional attention to the patients. In this case, the too heavy staff/patient ratio may lead to both inefficiency and ineffectiveness (Robey, p. 10).

The solution is to assign the optimum number of staff known to be needed to provide excellence in care to a specified number of patients and then manage their time so that the work amount and quality are optimized. In this way, the manager achieves both efficiency (the desired effect with a minimum of effort, expense, or waste) and effectiveness (the desired results). Given enough resources and appropriate consultation, almost any nursing home administrator can achieve effectiveness. What is essential today is to be both effective *and* efficient.

1.7 Innovating

The effective manager is always an innovator. *Innovating is the process of bringing new ideas into the way an organization accomplishes its purposes.*

The process of innovating is the result of the administrator's study of the changes that are constantly occurring in the organization itself and the environment in which it functions. Innovating is an act of leadership. It is the manager's role to be the sensor of the organization for those external and internal changes that will have an impact on its well-being.

The manager is not necessarily the innovater but does have the task of assuring that innovation occurs within the organization. To achieve this, the manager can develop new ideas, combine old ideas into new ones, borrow and adapt ideas from other fields, or stimulate others to develop innovations (Dale, p. 7).

MAINTAINING OPENNESS TO INNOVATIONS

We have discussed the importance of carefully formulated policies that the administrator can implement through detailed plans of action. Edward Wrapp observed that "Good managers don't make policy decisions; rather, they give a sense of direction and are masters at developing opportunities" (Wrapp, p. 8).

Wrapp addressed the question of why the good manager shies away from very precise statements of his objectives for the organization. According to Wrapp, the effective manager finds it impossible to set down specific objectives that will be relevant for any extended period of time. The external environment changes continually, he observes, and the organization's strategies have to be continually revised to take these changes into account. He concludes that the more explicit the statement of strategy, the more difficult it is to persuade the employees to turn to different goals when needs and conditions change.

Wrapp believes that goals or objectives are communicated over time through a consistent pattern of operating decisions. We also advise guarding against the degree of specificity in goal and policy statements that discourages changes.

All of the forces that tend to lead to organizational resistance to change are formidable enemies of the manager who must introduce changes to keep the facility in tune with the environment. The nursing home facility administrator must keep policies precise enough to guide employee decisions and at the same time continually introduce change into the facility—not an easy task.

1.8 Representing

The administrator is the official, formally designated representative of the nursing facility to the community, to the outside world (Dale, p. 7). But in practice, all staff members of the facility represent the facility through their performance within and occasionally outside the facility. Members of the staff or patients/clients may be asked or appointed to represent it on stated occasions. Nevertheless, the administrator is the ultimate spokesperson. The board of directors or the owners assign this responsibility to the administrator, who is expected to perform in that capacity and to monitor and control all representation of the facility by other staff members.

We have now reviewed the basic management functions and some of the theories in the management literature. To the extent a consensus exists today about the functions of management, it has evolved over a period of time, with various individuals and schools of thought each contributing to the current views.

1.9 History of the Concept of Management

Administrators have been managing organizations, large and small, for thousands of years.

It is believed that some 5,000 years ago the Sumerian civilization (Iran and Iraq of today) developed a script to control business accounts (George, p. 143). Clay tablets recording business transactions of that ancient time have been found by archaeologists. We have records of Cheops, an Egyptian king who built the Great Pyramid about 2900 B.C. We know that this monument covered 13 acres and employed 100,000 laborers for 20 years and that 8,368 lower-, middle-, and upper-level managers administered the project (George, p. 5). In ancient Greece music was used to govern motions in the production lines. In the 5th century B.C., *The Republic* by Plato reports a dialogue between Socrates and a Greek general about the extent to which management is a transferable skill. The general, it seems, was incensed that the Athenian Assembly had just appointed as the commander-in-chief of the army the manager of the Athenian chorus, who had shown himself to be an excellent fund raiser and chorus director. Socrates argued that if the man could run the chorus well and raise the necessary revenue, then he could also be a good general (George, p. 16). Fifteen upper-level executives of General Motors recently expressed the same view of their own abilities to manage almost anything, during a 15-month study of their skills conducted by a Harvard Business School professor (Kotter, p. 8). Managers' opinions of their capabilities have not changed much over the last 5,000 years.

By the 1800s the early scientific management movement was underway in England as an outgrowth of the industrial revolution. The managers at Soho Foundry of Boulton, Watt and Co. were concerned with market research and forecasting, planned site location, machine layout study, production standards and planning, standard components, cost controls, cost accounting, employee training, work study and incentives, and employee welfare (George, p. 59).

During that epoch a management literature began to appear, but there was little recognition of the principles of management we have discussed. Current management philosophy in the West seems to have evolved from four schools of thought, although various writers refine these even further (Levey & Loomba, p. 495).

At the end of the 19th century a group of writers who believed management could be an exact science emerged. They focused on the physical activities involved in production (Drucker, p. 278; George, p. 89). Frederic Taylor conducted research in a Philadelphia machine shop, demonstrating with time and motion studies that work then done by as many as 450 shovelers at Bethlehem Steel could be accomplished by as few as 150 persons, provided they received instructions to improve their effort. Frank Gilbreth's time and motion studies are well known. Henry Gantt developed his now famous Gantt Chart with its task and bonus plan and standard hour concept.

Early in the 20th century Henri Fayol identified management "universals" as: to plan, to organize, to command (tell others), and to coordinate (control). Fayol thus developed one of the earliest formulations of a general theory of management. The Process School members, such as Fayol and James Mooney, focused on departmentalization, coordination, and organizational form—the issues we have discussed under "organizing."

During the 1920s and 1930s a group of theorists led by Elton Mayo described management as consisting primarily of human relations skills. According to them, successful organizations fulfill not only the employees' economic needs but also their social and psychological needs.

Sponsored by the National Research Council, Mayo conducted several experiments at the Hawthorne manufacturing plant to determine the effect of illumination on output. He found that production rose for the experimental group when illumination was increased. But the control group also produced more, although it had no increase in illumination. Illumination was then reduced to the barest minimum in both groups, yet their production continued to rise, the apparent reason being the increased attention they were given by the managers (George, pp. 136–137). His experiments convinced Mayo that human factors exercise the most powerful influence on employee behavior because of the worker's need to participate in social groups. Work arrangements, he concluded, besides meeting production requirements, must meet the employee's need for social satisfaction on the job. Unfortunately, the Behavioral School experienced a low predictability rate (Barnard, p. viii; Dale, pp. 200–202).

Various names are applied to management theory emerging after World War II (Levey & Loomba, p. 495). Its major thrust has been *systems theory*—our approach here. Mathematical quantification is the hallmark of these theories. This is made possible by the development of computers capable of processing enormous quantities of intricate data. Some members of the management science schools believe that almost everything can be quantified. This may be so. However, the problem remains that people assign the mathematical weights to each factor quantified, and then others must interpret for themselves the meaning they attach to the quantified results (Demski, p. 29).

Whatever one's personal views about quantification, it is clear that computers are affording managers access to much information previously too laborious, too expensive, or too slow to obtain on a timely basis (Miller & Barry, pp. 379–380). Computers are already a major management tool at regional and national offices of nursing home chains. It is expected that they will eventually become indispensable in every nursing home, no matter how small that facility. (See Keen for a discussion of the use of microcomputers in the small business setting.)

Managing is an exceptionally complex, multidimensional task not yet fully understood by the social sciences. Much has been learned, however, that can be useful to the nursing home administrator in his/her efforts to assure a caring environment while running the nursing facility as a good business operation.

1.10 Organization of the Nursing Facility

1.10.1 Two Administrative Models

Two basic administrative models appear in the nursing facility management literature: *the administrator-centered model* and *the medical director–centered model* (see Miller & Barry, pp. 15, 58; Miller, 1982, p. 3013; Davis, p. 33; Gordon & Stryker, pp. 83–84; Boling et al., p. 41).

The administrator-centered model is more frequently cited (Buttaro, pp. 1–39; Miller, 1982, p. 3013; Hogstel, p. 8; Boling et al., p. 41; Gordon & Stryker, pp. 83, 135). Here the administrator is invested with full control and responsibility for the successful functioning of the facility (see Figures 1-4 and 1-6).

The medical director-centered model gives the medical director original line authority over all functions except business, maintenance, housekeeping, laundry, and social activities. This model is based on the typical hospital organization pattern (see Figure 1-5).

ADMINISTRATOR-CENTERED MODEL

Figure 1-4 depicts the functions essential for the operation of a skilled nursing facility. The headings within Figure 1-4 are derived from those

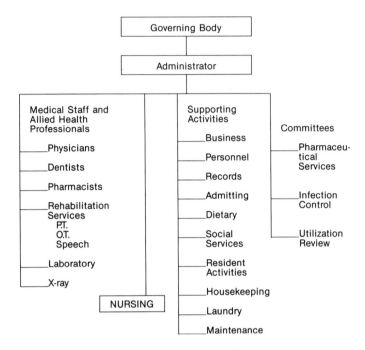

FIGURE 1-4. Federally required functions.

functions required by the federal Conditions of Participation and from the 17 departments recommended in the 1970 federal regulations establishing state licensure boards. In the federal Conditions of Participation model, the administrator has direct line authority for all operations of the facility.

Who Is Managing the Facility?

In Figures 1-4 and 1-6 the administrator manages the facility but is not permitted to make any medical decision, even if he/she is a physician. This is one of the more important and subtle distinctions of nursing facility administration.

Who Makes Medical Decisions?

All medical decisions are made by a doctor managing a patient's care, whether he/she is the medical director of the facility, a staff member, or the patient's attending physician.

Medical decisions are judgments covering most aspects of the

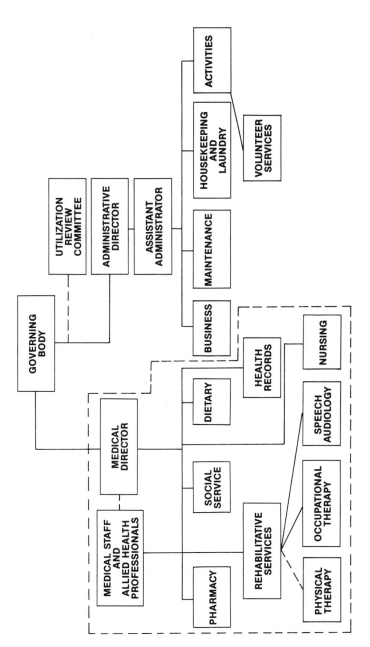

FIGURE 1-5. Medical director–centered organizational model for a skilled nursing facility.

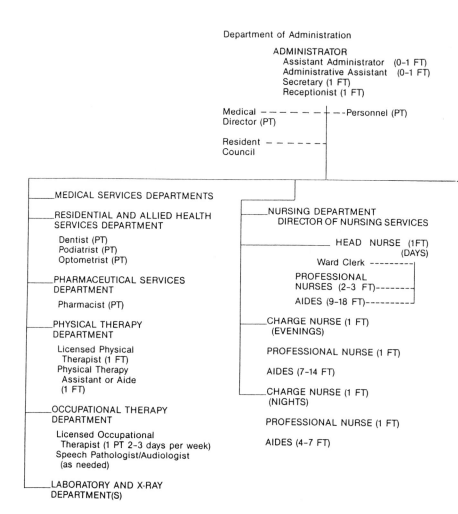

FIGURE 1-6. Organizational pattern for a 100-bed skilled nursing facility based on

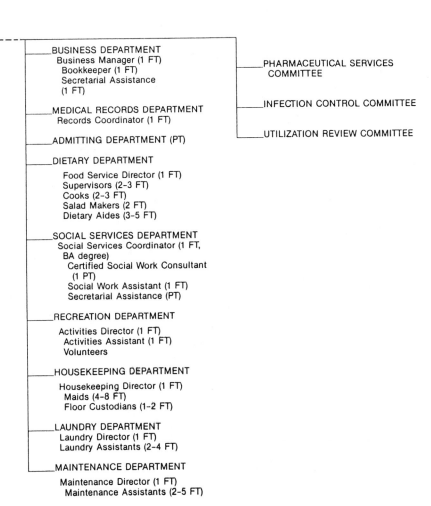

BUSINESS DEPARTMENT
    Business Manager (1 FT)
    Bookkeeper (1 FT)
    Secretarial Assistance
    (1 FT)

MEDICAL RECORDS DEPARTMENT
    Records Coordinator (1 FT)

ADMITTING DEPARTMENT (PT)

DIETARY DEPARTMENT
    Food Service Director (1 FT)
    Supervisors (2-3 FT)
    Cooks (2-3 FT)
    Salad Makers (2 FT)
    Dietary Aides (3-5 FT)

SOCIAL SERVICES DEPARTMENT
    Social Services Coordinator (1 FT,
    BA degree)
        Certified Social Work Consultant
        (1 PT)
        Social Work Assistant (1 FT)
        Secretarial Assistance (PT)

RECREATION DEPARTMENT
    Activities Director (1 FT)
    Activities Assistant (1 FT)
    Volunteers

HOUSEKEEPING DEPARTMENT
    Housekeeping Director (1 FT)
    Maids (4-8 FT)
    Floor Custodians (1-2 FT)

LAUNDRY DEPARTMENT
    Laundry Director (1 FT)
    Laundry Assistants (2-4 FT)

MAINTENANCE DEPARTMENT
    Maintenance Director (1 FT)
    Maintenance Assistants (2-5 FT)

PHARMACEUTICAL SERVICES
COMMITTEE

INFECTION CONTROL COMMITTEE

UTILIZATION REVIEW COMMITTEE

the 17 federally recommended departments.

resident's life in the facility. The more obvious are those most directly related to diagnosing patient illness and prescribing medicines. However, nearly all of the patient's activities are ultimately governed by the physician's judgments.

Medical orders must be obtained for the following:

- all rehabilitative services, including physical occupational, speech, and hearing therapies, or work with practitioners in other related fields such as podiatry
- all laboratory, X-ray and related procedures
- nursing procedures
- diet, whether regular or special
- range and level of activities permitted
- patient access to his/her medical record
- visits outside the facility

In short, all patient care, including admission and discharge, is given at the direction of the attending physician.

Having said this, one might conclude that the attending physicians and any medical staff in the facility are actually operating the facility, but this is not at all the case. The administrator is still responsible for assuring that the facility functions in conformity with the Conditions of Participation established by the federal government, with all state and local regulations, and with other laws.

State Licensing Boards

State licensing boards hold the administrator, not the medical director, responsible for assuring that every aspect of operating the facility is achieved at least at the required minimum levels. It is for this reason that Figure 1-5 portrays an administrative arrangement that is difficult to implement.

MEDICAL DIRECTOR–CENTERED MODEL

In Figure 1-5, the medical director has direct line control of all operations except the business office, maintenance, housekeeping, laundry, and activities (Miller & Barry, p. 15). This is similar to the traditional hospital division of authority, in which the medical staff report to the board of directors, rather than to the hospital administrator (Wilson, pp. 22–24; McGibony, p. 204).

Problems: Equals Coordinating Equals

The primary problem is that two persons are directing at the same level: the medical director has the final word in the first departments shown at left in Figure 1-5, and the administrator in those on the right. In this situation the administrator cannot tell the medical director how to deal with the social worker, and by the same token the medical director is not involved with supervision of the head of housekeeping (Levey & Loomba, pp. 257).

In other words two persons have the last word. For the facility to function, all 11 departments must choose to cooperate (Dale, p. 91). If the medical director and the administrator disagree, the governing body must settle the disputes. It is impractical for the governing body to spend its time settling disputes between two separate and equal administrators. No organization whose success depends on equals cooperating over a period of months and years can function long.

Who Should Hold the License?

As long as both the administrative director and the medical director are managers at the same level, it remains unclear in the medical director-centered model as to who should hold the license to operate the facility (Levey & Loomba, p. 258). It could appear that the medical director should be the administrator of record. Directing the laundry personnel, the housekeepers, the volunteers, and the repair staff is not perceived as the more important of the facility functions. Finally, the administrator is held legally responsible for the conduct of the facility but has no control over its more important decisions. This model, therefore, seems to us to be much less appropriate to the skilled nursing facility than the administrator-centered model.

SHIFTS OF POWER IN THE HOSPITAL MODEL

The hospital model itself is undergoing a power shift away from the medical director and toward the organizational design we advocate as more suitable for a nursing facility.

Decreasing Medical Staff Influence

As long as third-party payers, including the government, agreed to pay hospitals for any and all bills submitted for Medicare patients, there was no reason not to allow the medical staff to control the allocations of the hospitals resources (Starr, pp. 428–433, 444–449). Under this liberal policy, ordering more procedures generated more income for the hospital and reduced the chance of successful malpractice suits. The physicians retained most of the power under these circumstances.

With the advent in the early 1980s of the Diagnostically Related Groups (DRGs), for the first time hospitals were paid only a preset fee for each Medicare admission, no matter how many procedures, both necessary and unnecessary, the medical staff ordered for each patient.

Up to that point more was better. After the introduction of DRGs (discussed later) more efficient was better. With the present direct economic loss, if unnecessary or excessive expenses are incurred in caring for Medicare patients, the hospital administrator is now being seen to intervene, becoming more powerful, as he/she seeks to mitigate the losses.

1.11 Organizational Pattern for a 100-Bed Skilled Nursing Facility Based on the 17 Federally Recommended Departments

Figure 1-6 shows the organizational pattern for a 100-bed skilled nursing facility recommended in the federal government regulations published in July 1970. This listing of the essential functional areas is still valid.

VARIOUS CONFIGURATIONS

In actual practice, these 17 departmental areas can be, and routinely are, given different titles and combined variously. Nevertheless, however configured, these areas must be accounted for in the typical nursing facility organizational plan.

Descriptions of the work each department is expected to accomplish are given in the federal Conditions of Participation, reproduced on pages 379 through 412. *These are federal requirements with which every nursing facility administrator must be thoroughly familiar.*

In Figure 1-6 (which we will call the Old Well Nursing Home) each position within the 17 departments is depicted, along with the number of persons who might occupy it and whether it is full-time (FT) or part-time (PT).

18 FEDERAL CONDITIONS

The federal Conditions of Participation are organized around 18 conditions, each setting forth requirements for a separate area (see page 379 for a list of these Conditions). The Conditions are numbered 405.1120 to 405.1137, the last two digits representing the Condition number.

At this point it would be useful for the reader to turn to Part 4 to review all of the Conditions of Participation (pages 379 through 412) in order to have a frame of reference for the discussion that follows. One additional section, 405.1101 (see page 375), gives an extensive set of definitions used in the Conditions themselves.

17 DEPARTMENTS

Figure 1-6 shows the 17 departments recommended in the 1970 federal regulations. The *upper area* reflects the Department of Administration, the immediate staff, and advisory roles (indicated by the dotted lines) of the Medical Director and the Resident Council. The *first column* includes the medical and allied health professionals essential to the facility, e.g., the physicians, dentists, pharmacist, occupational and physical therapists. The nursing service with its three shifts is the *second column*. The *third column* contains areas also essential to the functioning of a facility, e.g., business operations, dietary, social services, social activities, housekeeping, and maintenance. The *last column* indicates the three committees mandated by the Conditions of Participation: the pharmaceutical services, infection control, and utilization review committees.

WORKABLE VARIATIONS

Numerous workable variations on this model exist. In this one, line authority is given to the administrator leading directly to each functional area or department. The administrator has responsibility and control, directly or indirectly, over all functions of the facility.

A common variant of this model is grouping several of these functions under middle-level managers who report to the administrator. One such arrangement, recommended by Dr. James Suver (Miller, 1982, p. 3013), is to appoint six middle-level managers:

- Director of Resident Services (e.g., volunteers, transportation, barbers, beauticians)

- Director of Administrative Services (admissions, business office, clerical, and personnel)
- Director of Therapy Services (e.g., physical therapy, occupational therapy, speech pathology)
- Director of Nursing Services (all nursing activities)
- Director of Supportive Services (housekeeping, laundry, and maintenance)
- Director of Dietary Services

In this organizational approach the number of persons reporting directly to the administrator is reduced from some 20 or more managers to six middle-level managers. In addition are individuals who serve on the Advisory Committee, consultants, and a chaplain.

Other organizational designs exist, with fewer or more persons reporting directly to the administrator. In a small facility the administrator may combine several functions. In a larger nursing home the number of middle or other managers may be greater. No matter what the model used, the 17 functions that constitute the essential work of the facility must be accomplished by its personnel.

Under each of the departments shown in Figure 1-6 we will consider up to seven issues:

1. Work responsibility of a particular department—what does it do?
2. Organizational interdependencies—how does that department interact with the rest of the facility?
3. Typical staffing pattern.
4. Equipment and supplies.
5. Information processed.
6. Management information needs.
7. Management control considerations.

For most departments, only selected topics from the above seven will be discussed.

1. DEPARTMENT OF ADMINISTRATION

Condition of Participation 405.1121 (see page 380) deals with administration and several relevant topics. The administrator is responsible for assuring that all of the necessary work is accomplished according to policy and at an acceptable level of quality.

Of all of the functions, administration has the greatest amount of interface with the rest of the facility (Miller, 1982, p. 4021). The administrator has either direct supervisory responsibility for each department and function, or indirect supervisory responsibility through a middle-level manager he/she has appointed. The director of nurses is such an appointee.

Staffing in the administrator's office depends on the size of the facility. In a 100-bed facility such as Old Well the administrator may or may not choose to have an assistant administrator and/or an administrative assistant.

Assistant Administrators and Administrative Assistants

An assistant administrator has line authority to represent the administrator, can make decisions on his/her behalf, and is usually assigned some area to oversee. An administrative assistant, on the other hand, has no line authority, cannot make decisions for the facility and does not represent the administrator except in an information gathering, or processing manner. The administrative assistant is a staff position.

In practice, the administrator of a 100-bed facility is more likely to appoint several middle-level managers than an assistant administrator. There tends not to be enough "organizational room" for two administrators in a facility of that size or smaller; 300 or more beds would call for an assistant administrator. In short, it depends on both the personality of the chief administrator and the division of work in the facility.

Secretary and Advisory Functions

Generally, the facility secretary works in the administrator's office, in an area shared with the receptionist/telephone operator. As a rule, the administrator has several advisory persons or groups, represented in Figure 1-6 by dotted lines. The medical director and resident council often fit into this slot. Other consultants and any other advisory committees might appear here.

Equipment and supplies for the proper functioning of any office—e.g., copying equipment, secretarial and desk supplies—are included here. The administrator's office is responsible for keeping on file the original of several types of information, e.g., reports of the state facility inspection teams, department reports, and any other important documents.

2. MEDICAL SERVICES DEPARTMENT

Condition of Participation 405.1122 (see page 385) sets requirements for the appointment and responsibilities of a medical director. Condition of Participation 405.1123 (see page 387) sets out requirements for physician services. How this is to be interpreted is another matter altogether.

Patterns of Medical Care

As a rule, the typical 100-bed facility does not require the services of a full time medical director. Even if it did, there appear to be an insufficient number of physicians who would choose this as their full-time occupation (Williams & Torrens, p. 182). In any case, their salary demands would make a full-time medical director for a 100-bed facility prohibitively costly.

The Open Medical Staff

The typical facility maintains an open medical staff. Under this arrangement, *any physician who is licensed to practice in a state is entitled to admit patients to the facility and to provide their medical care while they reside there.* Under this model the medical director ordinarily is a part-time staff member and tries to assure that the medical care needs of the patients are met as they arise and as specified in the Conditions of Participation. The medical director often substitutes for the personal physician who fails to visit the patient every 30 days as required by law, or to perform the annual physical examination. The duties of the medical director are stipulated in Condition of Participation 405.1122 (see page 385).

The Closed Medical Staff

A second model of medical direction is the closed medical staff. This means that *only physicians who have been approved by the organized medical staff of the facility may admit or treat its patients.* An organized medical staff is the closed group of physicians who provide all of the primary care to the patients in that facility. Initially, the board of trustees or governing body appoints one or more physicians to organize a medical staff, elect a medical director from their group, and write by-laws to govern the medical care given in that facility. Normally, this staff, through the medical director, reports directly to the governing body.

Closed medical staffs are more feasible for larger facilities of 300 to 600 patients. In a closed panel or staff situation, the physicians, usually 5 or 6 for a facility of 500 to 600 patients, divide care for the patients among themselves. Numerous variations are possible. A closed medical staff has several advantages. One of the staff is on duty at all times and can be given a list of all patients needing medical care, but whose assigned physician is not immediately available. The most obvious advantage is the availability of a staff of physicians who will provide continuous care and who have enough economic dependency on income from the facility to conform to all Conditions of Participation physician services requirements. This can greatly ease the strain on the facility administrator, who normally devotes considerable energy under the open staff arrangement to gain conformity of medical services on the timely basis required by the Conditions of Participation (Hogstel, pp. 27–28).

3. DENTAL AND ALLIED HEALTH SERVICES DEPARTMENT

Condition of Participation 405.1130 (see page 398) requires an agreement with an advisory dentist who is expected to recommend oral hygiene care for the facility. In addition, the facility is to make satisfactory arrangements for patients to receive dental care. Good communication policies would lead to reporting the need for dental care to a patient's physician to inform him/her and to obtain the physician's agreement to the appropriateness and/or safety of the proposed care in light of the patient's medical condition.

Administrative Observations

By walking around the facility, the administrator can gain an impression of the adequacy of daily dental hygiene being performed. In casual conversations the administrator can ask patients about their teeth and gums or whether their dentures are bothering them. The extent to which patients' dental appliances are kept in their mouths instead of soaking in water can easily be observed.

Foot and Eye Care

If the patient is alert, fully responsible for him/herself, and seeks to arrange for foot or eye care, this may be a matter between him/her and the attending physician. Even in this case, however, it would be prudent for the facility administrators, as a courtesy to the attending physician, to inform the doctor of the patient's intentions to obtain foot, eye, or similar care. A conservative policy would dictate that *all* appointments for care be on order of the attending physician *only*.

If the patient is not alert and is dependent on the facility staff to make any arrangements, such appointments are made only at the direction of the patient's attending physician.

4. PHARMACEUTICAL SERVICES DEPARTMENT

Condition of Participation 405.1127 (see page 396) mandates facility responsibility for providing drugs ordered for Medicare or Medicaid patients under its care. Supervision of services by a pharmacist is required.

The consulting pharmacist or the facility pharmacist is responsible at the minimum for assuring that

- all medications are available as ordered
- all medications are within expiration date and properly labeled and handled
- all reorders and stop orders are implemented
- each patient's medications are reviewed for possible adverse reactions and/or interactions
- appropriate pharmacy policy and procedures are followed

Contracting with a Local Pharmacy

A facility of 100 or fewer beds would normally contract with a local pharmacy to provide drugs and, ideally, with another pharmacist to perform the required supervision of services. These persons are responsible for meeting all drug needs of the facility and for compliance with all regulations and laws governing the handling and storing of drugs.

Administrative Monitoring

Besides reading the required reports from the facility pharmacist or pharmacy consultant, the administrator can talk with the pharmacist, the nurses, the physicians, and the patients to learn in greater depth how the system is functioning.

If drug reorders are not arriving on time, the nurses will be ready to share this information with the administrator. If the patients are not getting the pills they believe they depend on, they will be quite willing to report it. But in this, as every such case, both the resident and staff must be queried.

5. PHYSICAL THERAPY DEPARTMENT
AND
6. OCCUPATIONAL THERAPY DEPARTMENT

Condition of Participation 405.1126 (see page 394) mandates physical, speech, and occupational therapy as needed. On a physician's order, the services may be provided on the premises or on a contract basis.

The "work" achieved by the therapists is to provide services as ordered. A therapist's work is not fully accomplished unless the nursing and other staff are involved in the process of helping the patient achieve the desired level of function in that patient's activities of daily living and not merely during the therapy period. This implies cooperation between the specialized rehabilitative staff and the regular staff who, in effect, are doing "habilitative" therapy for patients all the time.

Staffing

A facility of 100 beds would probably employ one full-time physical therapist, one-full time occupational therapist, and a part-time speech therapist. In this situation adequate equipment, such as whirlpools, parallel bars, and other apparatus, must be furnished.

Administrative Observations

The administrator will want to observe whether a rehabilitative team approach is being pursued. This can be accomplished by studying one or two patients' rehabilitation plans, then casually observing the extent to which they are being implemented by the involved staff members.

7. LABORATORY AND X-RAY DEPARTMENTS

Condition of Participation 405.1128 (see page 397) requires that, on a physician's order, laboratory and X-ray services be provided. These may be on the premises or contracted for in a local hospital or private office.

Delayed or inaccurate lab work is often a concern among nursing and medical staff. Telephone calls placed by frustrated nurses inquiring about lab results that should have been received may indicate need for examining the current procedures and contracts.

8. NURSING DEPARTMENT

Condition of Participation 405.1124 (see page 389) covers nursing services in great detail. Nursing is at the heart of the facility.

Nursing Department Tasks

The nursing service has the following responsibilities:

- providing nursing care to patients as ordered by the physicians
- administering medications to the patients
- keeping patient records
- monitoring patients for changes in condition and notifying the responsible physician—in short, serving as the physician's eyes and ears on a 24—hour basis

- maintaining good-quality patient care
- making certain that each patient is functioning at the highest reasonable level (Freymann, p. 262)
- playing a coordinative role with other staff, e.g., assuring that planned physical therapy takes place.

Quality of Patient Life

This list could be extended (Hogstel, pp. 88–106). There are unwritten dimensions to caring performed by the nursing service. It is not possible, and perhaps not desirable, to set them all down, for many of the nursing acts that increase the quality of patient life cannot be fully spelled out in policy statements.

The quality of life enjoyed by the patients is directly proportional to the quality of care given by the nursing service.

Quality of Medical Care

The quality of medical care received by the patients is also, to an important degree, dependent on the nursing service. There is not enough physician time available in today's medical marketplace to provide extensive hours of medical care to each nursing facility patient.

Doctors typically develop a relationship of trust with the nursing service, depending on the quality of nursing care perceived as being provided. Just as the administrator is expected to use his/her skills as an organizational diagnostician, the nursing service normally uses its skills as diagnosticians of medical signs in the care of patients. When a relationship of trust and mutual respect exists between the nurses and the attending physicians, patients are most likely to receive good care.

Organizational Interdependencies

Organizational interdependencies between nursing and virtually every other department exist within the facility. Nursing is dependent on the dietary, housekeeper, laundry, and maintenance departments, the business office, the social worker, and the allied health professionals. In sum, for nursing to do its tasks properly, nearly every other department and functional area within the organization must also be doing its tasks in a cooperative manner.

Staffing

Three nursing shifts, 24 hours a day, 365 days a year offer a staffing challenge. The number of aides is dependent on the number of professional nurses employed and on the intensity of care the facility seeks, or can afford to provide.

In most states, a facility that is supported solely by Medicaid funds cannot afford to provide as many aides per shift as one in which nearly all the residents are private patients. Some states reimburse costs for Medicaid patients at a rate that does not allow for employment of as many nursing personnel as the director of nursing services and the administrator might wish (Wilson & Neuhauser, p. 174).

The majority of states mandate a minimum number of nursing hours per patient day. However, this minimum is usually too low to provide quality care, so most facilities staff above these levels.

Provision for nursing service should include sufficient physical space and adequately equipped nursing stations, lounge areas, locker space, and kitchenettes.

Administrative Observations

Just as the director of nursing services is expected to make daily patient rounds, the administrator may decide to emulate nursing. The administrator will receive daily reports on admissions, discharges, changes in patient conditions, accidents, transfers, and the like. These reports are not a satisfactory substitute for the administrator's personal observation, on a daily basis, to learn by wandering around what is actually taking place in the facility.

9. BUSINESS DEPARTMENT

All of Part 3 of this text is devoted to budgeting and finance, in which functions, personnel, and organizational interfaces of the business components of facility management are discussed in detail. The reader is referred to Part 3 for the discussion of this aspect of facility management.

10. MEDICAL RECORDS DEPARTMENT

Condition of Participation 405.1132 (see page 400) specifies that a full-time employee be assigned to keep the medical record service up to date. Usually this person is called the ward clerk (see the nursing services in Figure 1-6).

There are those who believe, with some justification, that if facilities were required to keep fewer records, more patient care time would be available from the nursing, physical therapy, and other staffs (Jonas,

p. 224). In any case, facilities are required to keep a great number of records. If they are not current on inspection, the facility is given citations (called deficiencies) by state inspectors for failure to meet some aspect of a Condition of Participation or a state or other recordkeeping regulation, with a directive that it be corrected within a specified period of time.

Recommendation for a Full-time Person

Dulcy Miller recommends that a full-time staff person assist the facility in its overall record-keeping effort (Miller & Barry, p. 386). This is reasonable, since there are often more than 100 forms being kept in the typical facility.

Because state inspectors have so strongly emphasized records, it is a common belief among administrators of nursing facilities that as far as the inspectors are concerned, "If it wasn't recorded, it wasn't done." Documentation is considered proof.

11. THE ADMITTING DEPARTMENT

Admitting is a function not formally addressed by the Conditions of Participation, yet it is of some importance within the facility.

Determining the Case Mix

The person(s) in charge of admissions determine the case mix of the facility. Case mix refers to such measures as the proportion of heavy-care patients to medium- and light-care patients, the proportion of private paying patients to publicly supported patients (Vogel & Palmer, p. 571), the ratio of old-old patients (aged 85 and older) to young-old patients (65 to 75), and so forth (U.S. DHHS, p. 43).

The mix of patients admitted dramatically affects the work load of nursing and other services, the income at the disposal of the facility for patient care, and even the general atmosphere of the facility. A nursing home where the entire resident population is in great pain or out of contact with reality is very different from one with a variety of patient orientations (Miller, 1982, p. 6021).

The staff member who handles admissions varies from one facility to another. Perhaps the most common pattern is for the social worker, together with the director of nursing, to admit new residents. Sometimes admissions are entirely the responsibility of the director of nursing services. In some facilities, the administrator may assume that function alone or in consultation with the nursing service.

12. DIETARY DEPARTMENT

Condition of Participation 405.1124 (see page 389) covers dietary requirements and are somewhat general. Most states, however, are highly specific about food sanitation.

The Food Standard

Food is an essential ingredient in the quality of patient life. Satisfaction with the facility is as often influenced by the food as by the quality of nursing care.

Some families feel they may not have enough medical background to judge the adequacy of nursing care, but most do consider themselves experts in the matter of food. Tasty food goes a long way toward maintaining a high quality of patient life in a nursing facility. Hospital food, eaten for a relatively short period, can be tolerated. Nursing home food, consumed for much longer periods, sometimes forever, is subject to much greater scrutiny by both patients and their families.

Dietary Department's Roles

The Dietary Department's influence extends 24 hours a day. The availability of midnight snacks for insomniac patients is as much a part of the ambience of the facility as the availability of continuous nursing services. This department is heavily interactive with nursing services (e.g., refreshments at social activities) and with most other departments. The food service depends on most other departments as well: housekeeping for sanitation, laundry for linens.

Food services may be provided in-house—many small facilities run their own food service—or contracted. Most chains and large facilities have food service contracts with major food vendors. Appropriate and adequate food preparation facilities are important to the facility's ability to provide an acceptable quality of life for its residents. Types of individual diets are discussed in Part 5 under "Nutrition."

Administrator Attention

The Dietary Department is an area demanding the attention of the administrator. Besides meeting the many sanitation and other code requirements, dietary costs need to be monitored, as does quality control over foodstuffs purchased. The administrator can monitor food services in a number of ways. Daily, randomly timed walks through the kitchen, eating with residents in the dining hall, and similar activities, are productive management behaviors. Much can be learned by getting a tray and eating its contents under circumstances similar to those of the resident.

13. SOCIAL SERVICES DEPARTMENT

Condition of Participation 405.1130 (see page 398) describes required social services, either by facility staff or through a written procedure referring patients.

Scope of Responsibilities

Social services is concerned not only with the patient's initial adjustment to the facility but also his/her continuing accommodation to the environment. The social worker is also responsible for monitoring each patient's sociopsychological experiences and orientation in the facility (U.S. DHHS, p. 29; Gordon & Stryker, p. 178). This will be discussed further under the heading of institutionalization in Part 5.

It is the social worker who is most directly in contact with the residents' family or sponsor (Williams & Torrens, p.191). This staff member is the one involved in assisting patients who have current or approaching financial needs that will be met by a public agency. In short, the social worker functions in the nursing home in a manner similar to social workers employed by the local Department of Social Services (Germain, pp. 207–209). Maintaining the quality of each patient's social well-being in a facility is a complex function (Britton & Britton, p. 99; Spicker & Ingman, pp. 194–195).

Typical staff for a 100-bed nursing facility would consist of one full-time social worker, help from a social work consultant, and one full-time social work assistant.

Administrative Monitoring

The administrator can monitor constantly for clues to the level of satisfaction among patients, their families, or sponsors and to the quality of the social interactions in the daily environment of the facility. "Chance" conversations in the hallways can yield invaluable feedback for the alert administrator.

14. RECREATION DEPARTMENT

Although short, Condition of Participation 405.1131 (see page 399) speaks eloquently to the need for each patient to participate in an activity program designed to meet his/her particular needs. Nursing services addresses the medical needs of the patients, and in that process partially meets their social and interpersonal requirements.

The activities coordinator's task is to assure that a plan is developed and implemented to enhance the physical, social and mental well-being of each patient. For the nearly comatose, disoriented, or agitated patients, this assignment is indeed a challenge. The activities director and the social service worker are assigned responsibility for the quality of psychosocial life that exists within a facility (Gordon & Stryker, pp. 185–187). It is difficult to imagine a more complicated undertaking in shaping the quality of patient life in the nursing facility.

The Conditions of Participation also assign patient care planning to the nursing department. This is one of the few areas in which the Conditions of Participation are not precise in assignment or responsibilities.

Administrative Participation

Personal participation in various patient activities is essential for the administrator who is to judge the activities program. Chatting with patients about what they have been doing can reveal a lot about the quality of the activities program.

15. HOUSEKEEPING DEPARTMENT

Housekeeping is indirectly addressed in Condition of Participation 405.1134 (see page 402) entitled "Physical Environment" and directly addressed in Condition of Participation 405.1135 point C (see page 406).

Two points worth noting are that a full-time employee must be designated responsible and that nursing personnel may not be assigned housekeeping duties.

Importance of "Good Housekeeping"

Not only do the state inspectors make intuitive value judgments about a facility based on its cleanliness and physical appearance, so also will most of the patients' relatives and sponsors. Dirty floors and walls, empty toilet paper holders, yellowing toilets and lavatories and the offensive odors associated with them communicate a message to the patients, staff, and the visitors revealing what the facility thinks about itself. Inattention to housekeeping details leads inspectors and the public alike to wonder to what extent it carries over into patient care, sanitation in food preparation, and cleanliness of the patients themselves.

The head housekeeper may have excellently designed job assignments for the four to eight maids and the one or two floor custodians. The administrator can tell how effective these schedules are simply by walking around the facility. On these tours the administrator must be able to "see" dirt.

16. LAUNDRY DEPARTMENT

Laundry is indirectly addressed in Condition of Participation 405.1135 (see page 406) under the subject of clean linen.

Clean linens, clean patient clothes, the availability of linens and clothes when needed, safe and sanitary handling techniques for both soiled and clean linen are areas of responsibility of the head of laundry. Whether it is better to do laundry in-house or to contract with a linen service is a subject of continuing debate. Whatever the decision, there will be procedures for handling linens that the administrator can observe for conformity to regulations and to facility policies. Contaminated linen policies and handling procedures are addressed in the Infection Control Procedures section of the Conditions of Participation.

17. MAINTENANCE DEPARTMENT

Maintenance is briefly mentioned in Condition of Participation 405.1134, point I (see page 402).

Distinguishing between Maintenance and Housekeeping

If a wall has a hole in it, it is clearly maintenance's job to fix the hole. If that same wall is only dirty and needs washing, it is probably house-keeping's job. Each facility must designate through established policies the respective responsibilities of these two functions. The repair and upkeep of physical systems is clearly the responsibility of maintenance. Preventive maintenance, anticipating when a machine will need servicing or risk ceasing to function, is a complex task requiring experienced judgment. A well-trained maintenance director can do much to anticipate troublesome, unnecessary breakdowns of equipment.

The administrator can participate in the maintenance process by occasionally assuming a "maintenance mind-set," then walking through the facility touching, feeling, judging the state of repair of all he/she encounters.

FEDERALLY REQUIRED COMMITTEES

Conditions of Participation 405.1127 (page 396), 405.1135 (page 406), and 405.1137 (page 407), respectively, mandate that a Pharmaceutical Services Committee, an Infection Control Committtee, and a Utilization Review Committee be established, and they clearly set out membership, purposes, and reporting requirements.

1.12 Legal and Business Terminology

In the course of operating a long-term care facility, the administrator will encounter numerous legal and business-related terms. In this section the major relevant sources of laws are cited, and the structure of the court system is described. Several terms related to law, risk management, and wills are broadly defined. The precise meaning of each term may vary from state to state.

1.12.1 Sources of Law

Constitution. The Constitution is the written agreement establishing the fundamental law of the United States of America, setting forth the conditions, mutual obligations, and rights of the federal and state governments and laying basic principles of government. The Bill of Rights fixed specific individual rights.

Statutes. Statutes are the laws under which we live. In the United States, they are the acts passed by the federal and state legislatures. Lesser governmental bodies, such as county commissioners, adopt ordinances; administrative agencies function by means of regulations.

Common Law. Common law is the accumulation of opinion handed down by judges. It is an outgrowth of court decisions over hundreds of years. Our common law originated in England, where judges followed unwritten principles of common sense in addition to statutory laws. Common law principles change over time with the changing values and needs of society.

Regulations. To implement statutes passed by legislative bodies, the executive branch of government, through its administrative agencies, writes regulations. These regulations are the official interpretations of the intent of each statute. As a consequence, regulations become, in effect, part of the law. One may challenge a regulation on the grounds that the "official interpretation" is unconstitutional or inconsistent with the legislative intent of the statute the regulation implements.

The Conditions of Participation for Skilled Nursing Facilities (see Part 4) are an example of regulations. These Conditions were written by the executive branch of the federal government during the process of spelling out the details of the Title 18 (Medicare) amendment to the Social Security Act of 1935. Until successfully challenged, the Conditions have the effect of law for nursing facility operations.

The Conditions of Participation, along with other federal administrative agency regulations, are published in the *Code of Federal Regulations* (often referred to as C.F.R.).

The President of the United States has the prerogative of issuing executive orders under the various statutes. Executive orders also have the effect of law.

Code. A code is a compilation of statutes and regulations. The statutes, together with the regulations written by the administrative agency implementing each statute, are systematically collected and placed into codes of law. *The United States Code*, often referred to as U.S.C., is an example.

1.12.2 The Court Systems

Federal Courts. The U.S. Constitution authorizes the creation of the Supreme Court and any additional courts Congress chooses to establish. Currently, entry into the federal court system is at the level of federal district courts (general courts of original jurisdiction). Jurisdiction is the power to hear and decide a case. Situated between these and the federal Supreme Court are twelve courts of appeal, which hear cases in the event a party is dissatisfied with the judgment of the federal district court.

The federal government also operates other courts, such as a Court of Claims, the Court of Customs and Patent Appeals, the Tax Court, and federal bankruptcy courts.

State Courts. The court systems vary from state to state. The lowest level of the state system is the magistrate court, which deals with misdemeanor cases, traffic violations, and small claims. Above the magistrate courts are the state circuit courts, or district courts, where more serious cases are tried.

Circuit or district courts have original jurisdiction over both civil and criminal cases. Most states have state courts of appeal, which normally do not have original jurisdiction and therefore limit themselves to appeals from lower courts in the state. Finally, each state has a state supreme court. This is the court of final appeal in all matters except those that involve a federal issue appealable to the U.S. Supreme Court.

1.12.3 Legal Terminology*

Accuse—to directly charge a person with committing an offense that is recognized as being against a law. The accused person becomes the defendant and must answer the complaint or accusation through the legal process.

Acquit—to set a person or corporation free of accusation(s). Acquittal is a decision (verdict) of not guilty and is rendered either by a jury or a judge (in nonjury trials). Under the principle of double jeopardy, a person or corporation cannot be tried again for the same accusation after a verdict of not guilty.

Actionable—conduct giving rise to a cause for legal action. For example, actionable negligence occurs only when a person unreasonably fails to perform a legal duty, resulting in damage or injury to another person. If there is no resulting damage, there may not be actionable negligence even though the person made a mistake.

Adjudication—decision or disposition of a case by the announcement of a judgment or decision by the court or other body.

Admission—the acknowledgment of certain facts by a party in a civil or criminal case. An admission does not necessarily constitute a confession of guilt. For example, the defendant may admit that he/she was driving the automobile but deny running a red light. The term "confession" is generally restricted to an acknowledgment of guilt.

Affidavit—a written statement given under oath before an officer having authority to administer oaths. A notary public is such a public officer and is authorized to signify by his/her signature that he/she witnessed the

---

* Sources for following terminology are given on page 106.

execution (signing) of certain documents, such as affidavits, deeds, and wills.

Aggrieved party—one whose legal rights have been invaded or who has suffered a loss or injury. "Aggrieved party" is frequently used in connection with proceedings by administrative agencies. For example, a person contesting the revocation of his/her nursing home administrator's license in an administrative proceeding is an aggrieved party.

Amicus curiae—literally, a friend (amicus) of the court (curiae). An amicus curiae brief is a written document that provides the court with information that might otherwise escape attention. A long-term care ombudsman might, for example, appear in a court case on behalf of a patient. The "friend of the court" has no absolute right to appear in the proceeding, so must obtain the court's permission prior to intervening.

Appeal—the request by a party to a lawsuit for a higher court to review a lower court's decision when he/she believes the lower court committed error.

Appearance—the coming into court of a person on being summoned to do so. Appearance without receiving a summons is a voluntary appearance. Appearance in court after papers have been served is an involuntary appearance.

Arbitrator—an impartial person chosen by the parties to an argument to decide the issue between them. Arbitration is used to avoid unnecessary and costly court actions.

Arraignment—an early step in a criminal proceeding at which the defendant is formally charged with an offense.

Assault—see Torts.

Battery—see Torts.

Burden of proof or **burden of persuasion**—the obligation of the person bringing an action to prove facts in dispute. In criminal cases the state must prove its case beyond a reasonable doubt. In civil cases the burden of proof is met by a "preponderance" of the evidence, i.e., at least 51%.

Civil law—pertains to suits outside of criminal law. Civil law deals with rights and duties between individuals in areas such as contracts and torts. The party complaining of the invasion of rights (plaintiff) brings the civil action against the alleged wrongdoer (defendant). Certain wrongs can be the subject of both a civil action and a criminal proceeding.

Criminal law—pertains to a crime—any act the government has deemed to be injurious to the public and actionable in a criminal proceeding. The criminal acts may be felonies (serious crimes such as murder, arson, rape, armed robbery) or misdemeanors (less serious crimes such as minor traffic violations). Criminal violations are prosecuted by the public's representative, the district attorney. A criminal violation may result in either a jail sentence, a fine or both.

To picture the interaction of civil and criminal law, assume an employee intentionally runs over a patient in the facility parking lot. The employee may be sued by the patient for money damages in a civil action and may also be brought to trial on criminal charges by the district attorney for the same act. (The nursing facility probably will be sued civilly by the patient, too, particularly if the employee has very little money).

Consent, informed—consent given after full information regarding the matter has been provided to the person consenting. In the nursing facility context, patients must understand the nature and risks of certain treatments before the facility can claim exemption from responsibility for resulting complications.

A diabetic patient may, for example, volunteer to participate in an experimental diet program. Unless the patient fully understands the risks involved, the facility may be held liable for subsequent complications. The facility should require the patient to sign a properly prepared consent form.

Consent to one treatment or procedure is not necessarily consent to another treatment or procedure, even if such treatment or procedure is beneficial. If a patient consented to a tonsillectomy, but the surgeon also removed the appendix, the surgeon may have committed a battery.

Counterclaim—a counterdemand by a defendant against a plaintiff (accuser), not merely responding to the accuser but asserting an independent cause of action against the accuser. For example, if the patient in the knitting needle illustration (see Torts) sued the orderly for damages for assault or battery, the orderly might counterclaim with a demand for damages for assault or battery.

Damages—money awarded by a court (or jury) to a person who has been wronged by the action of another. The meaning of the terms used to describe the various types of damages available differs from state to state, and depends on the type of case. Generally, actual damages, consequential damages and incidental damages are designed to compensate the person wronged.

Nominal damages are an award of a small sum of money in recognition of the invasion of some legal right of the plaintiff, which results in no actual injury or pecuniary loss to the plaintiff. Punitive damages are designed to punish the defendant for particularly bad conduct, and to deter the defendant from such conduct in the future. Punitive damages are also sometimes called exemplary damages. Double and treble damages are a type of punitive damages sometimes provided for by particular statutes.

Defendant—in criminal cases, the accused. In civil cases, the one who is sued and who must "defend" against a claim of wrongdoing brought by another.

Defamation—the communication to a third person of that which is injurious to the reputation or good name of the victim. Oral defamation is slander. Written defamation is libel.

Libel is written publication that exposes someone to public scorn, hatred, contempt, or ridicule, especially if related to an individual's profession or livelihood.

Slander, because it is spoken, is more difficult to establish. The action for slander has been restricted because of the right of free speech and to avoid overloading the courts with trivial cases. Only if slanderous statements lead to actual damages (e.g., loss of employment) can they be actionable, unless the words imply crime, unchastity, or relate to a person's profession or business.

In the cases of both libel and slander, there must be communication to a third party, e.g., showing a third party written words or speaking slanderous words in the presence of a third party.

Deposition—a statement given under oath, reduced to writing, and authenticated by a notary public. A deposition gives the attorneys for both sides an opportunity to find out what the person deposed (deponent) knows about the relevant event.

Directed verdict—a verdict given by a jury at the direction of a judge. If, for example, a plaintiff fails to make a reasonable case, or a defendant fails to make a necessary defense, the judge may direct the jury to render a specified verdict.

Discovery—pretrial devices used by the parties' lawyers to gather information or knowledge about the case. Discovery devices include depositions, interrogatories to parties, and requests for documents and articles. The purpose of the discovery devices is to facilitate pretrial settlements and to reduce surprises at trial in order that cases might be decided on their merit (rather than by ambush).

False imprisonment—see Torts.

Fraud—intentional deception that results in injury to another.

Indictment—a formal, written accusation by a public prosecutor, submitted to a grand jury and charging a crime. The grand jury is a body authorized to investigate crimes and accuse, i.e., indict, persons within its jurisdiction when it decides a trial ought to be undertaken.

Injunction—a judicial direction to a party to do or to refrain from doing some act. Injunctions guard against future acts but do not remedy past acts. When the court issues an injunction, the party to whom it is issued is said to be "enjoined."

Litigants—the parties to a lawsuit, i.e., the plaintiff and defendant.

Malice—the intentional doing of a wrongful act, without just cause or excuse, with the intent to inflict injury. Under some circumstances the law will imply evil intent. Therefore, malice (in law) does not necessarily mean personal hate or ill will. The law will imply malice to an act done with reckless disregard for another's safety, even though the actor did not dislike the party he/she injured. For example, the law may imply malice to the act of one who shoots a rifle into a crowd of strangers.

Motion—an application to the court asking for an action favorable to one's side.

Negligence—the failure to exercise the degree of care a reasonable person would exercise under the same circumstances, which results in injury to another. Negligent conduct falls below the standard established by society (a jury) for the protection of others from an unreasonable risk of harm. Negligence may arise from either an overt act or from a failure to act.

The term "negligence" is used in several different ways:

1. *Comparative negligence.* In some states one can recover damages even though he/she was negligent him/herself. For example, a patient slips and injures him/herself partly as a result of the unreasonably slippery floors in the facility and partly because the patient had chosen very slippery shoes. The facility is negligent because it failed to warn the patient that the floors were unusually slippery. But the patient was also negligent because he/she wore shoes that had slippery soles. In states that have comparative negligence, the jury determines how much of the patient's injury should be blamed on the facility's negligence and how much the patient is to blame. The jury then apportions the damages (money) accordingly.

2. *Contributory negligence.* Contributory negligence is similar to comparative negligence in that the victim is partly responsible for his/her own injury. However, in states where the doctrine of contributory negligence applies, all recovery by the victim is barred. "Contrib" is a favorite of defendants because they can win the case by convincing the jury that the victim was just the least bit to blame for his/her own injury.

3. *Negligence per se.* Conduct treated as negligence without proof. It is usually necessary to show failure to exercise a reasonable degree of care. Negligence per se is found where the act complained of is in violation of a safety statute. Negligence per se also includes acts that are so clearly harmful to others that it is plain to any reasonable person that negligence must have occurred.

4. *Criminal negligence.* Recklessness or carelessness resulting in injury or death punishable as a crime. Criminal negligence implies reckless disregard or indifference to the safety or rights of others.

Risk, assumption of—the principle that a person may not recover for an injury he/she received when he/she voluntarily exposed him/herself to a known danger. Although hockey players and race car drivers might be said to assume the risks of their occupations, it is difficult to imagine circumstances where the doctrine of assumption of risk could be used successfully by the defendant in a lawsuit against a nursing facility.

Res ipsa loquitur—a Latin phrase that literally means "the thing speaks for itself." The defendant's negligence is inferred from the mere fact that the event happened and that the instrumentality causing the injury was under the exclusive control of the defendant. *Res ipsa loquitur* could apply to an otherwise unexplained boiler explosion in a nursing facility.

Prosecutor—a public official, either elected or appointed, who conducts cases on behalf of the government against persons accused of crimes.

Res judicata—Latin for "a thing decided." Once a court of competent jurisdiction has decided a matter, that decision continues to bind those parties in any future litigation on the same issue.

Retainer—a fee paid an attorney in advance for services on a case. In exchange, the attorney must refuse employment as the client's adversary in the case.

Search warrant—a written order from a judge permitting certain law enforcement officers to conduct a search for and seize specified things or persons. Warrants are issued on sworn testimony or affidavits supporting probable cause. Law enforcement officers may not search or seize items or persons not within the scope of the search warrant.

Stare decisis—a Latin phrase meaning "to stand by that which was decided earlier." The doctrine of *stare decisis* means that once a court has laid down a principle of law as applicable to a certain set of facts, it will adhere to that principle in all future cases in which the facts are substantially the same. *Stare decisis* gives the law a measure of predictability. However, a court will reverse itself occasionally where considerations of public policy demand it. For example, nonprofit health care institutions were once immune from lawsuits. Public policy has demanded that such immunity no longer apply.

Subpoena—a written order issued by a court to require the appearance of a person in court. A person failing to appear may be held in contempt of court.

Subpoena duces tecum—a written court order for a person to bring to a judicial proceeding certain objects or documents in his/her possession. The court may, for example, require a nursing facility administrator to bring patient records to a court proceeding.

Summons—a written instrument notifying a defendant that a lawsuit has commenced against him/her. Failure to appear may result in a **default judgment**, wherein the defendant has a judgment entered against him/her for failure to appear.

Tort—a wrong. Literally, tort means "twisted." A tort exists when (a) a legal duty is owed by a defendant to a plaintiff, (b) that duty is breached, and (c) the plaintiff is harmed as a direct result of the breach of duty.

For example, the duty to provide care to patients is imposed on the nursing facility by virtue of holding itself out as a health care provider. If the facility breaches its duty to provide care for a patient, and the patient is harmed as a direct result of the breach of duty, a tort has occurred. The general term "tort" includes several specific types of bad or wrongful conduct. Assault, battery, false imprisonment, and negligence are among the types of conduct labeled by the law as torts.

An *assault* is an attempt to inflict bodily harm on another person that creates well-founded fear of imminent peril. An assault does not require actual touching. An assault can be the basis for a civil action (actions outside criminal practice) and/or a criminal action (violation of criminal laws). In the civil action for assault, the person assaulted brings the action seeking to be awarded money. In the criminal action for assault, the district attorney brings assault charges for the purpose of punishment.

The tort of assault is closely linked to, and often confused with, the tort of *battery*. Battery is the unlawful touching or application of force to another human being without his/her consent. For battery to occur there must be an intent to touch, actual touching, and a lack of consent. If the touching is knowingly consented to, it is not battery.

Assault has been defined as a "failed battery," because an assault must cause apprehension of immediate harmful contact, without actual contact. For example, if the doctor ordered pills, and the nurse approaches the patient with a 12-inch needle, causing apprehension in the patient of immediate contact, it is an assault. When the nurse actually uses the needle (the touching), it becomes a battery (unless the patient has consented).

To illustrate the differences between assault and battery, a lawyer used the following illustration. An orderly bumps into a female patient's breast. If it is purely accidental, no battery has occurred. If the orderly intended to bump into the patient's breast, it may be battery. The angry patient retaliates by throwing a knitting needle at the orderly. If the knitting needle misses, but the orderly is apprehensive of immediate harmful contact, the patient has committed an assault. If the knitting needle hits the orderly, it is battery (even if the orderly was not apprehensive of the contact). The orderly then throws a towel at the patient. If it hits the patient, it is a battery. If it misses the patient, but the patient apprehends immediate harmful contact, it is an assault.

False imprisonment is another tort occasionally related to assault and battery; it is the confining of another human being within fixed boundaries against his/her will. Numerous circumstances within the nursing facility can give rise to false imprisonment. If a competent patient refuses side rails, but the nurse raises the side rails anyway, false imprisonment has occurred.

If a physician leaves orders to tie a competent patient in a wheelchair, but that patient refuses, tying the patient in the wheelchair will constitute false imprisonment. (Tying the patient in the wheelchair may also be a battery.) Another common example of false imprisonment occurs when the competent patient demands to be released from the facility, but the facility will not allow the patient to leave.

Tort-feasor—the person who commits a tort.

Warrant, arrest—a written order for the arrest of a person from a judge having authority in that jurisdiction.

Witness—a person who gives sworn testimony in a court proceeding.

1.12.4 Risks Assumed by the Operation of a Long-Term Care Facility

The act of obtaining a license to operate, and operating, a long-term care facility automatically brings a set of risks to the facility. Some of these are defined below.

EMPLOYER'S LIABILITY ACTS

Various states have statutes that set forth the extent to which employers are liable to their employees for injuries to the employees. Generally, the employer is held responsible only for injuries to employees occurring in the course of employment. Workers' compensation acts and the federal Employer's Liability Act are examples. Employer's liability acts usually pay for physician and hospital costs. These statutes removed the earlier claims by employers that the employee knew the hazards of a job and accepted those hazards when agreeing to work for the employer.

Often these statutes also hold the employer responsible for negligent acts of fellow employees within the zone of employment. The zone of employment is the physical area within which employers are liable (legally responsible) under workers' compensation acts. This usually includes the parking areas, entryways, and other areas under the control of the employer.

STRICT LIABILITY

An employer held strictly liable is subject to liability without fault, i.e., without the employee having to show employer fault. Strict liability also applies to ultrahazardous enterprises such as making explosives.

VICARIOUS OR IMPUTED LIABILITY (*RESPONDEAT SUPERIOR*)

The employer is held responsible for the acts of employees within the scope of their employment. For example, if a nurse's aide carelessly dumps a patient from a wheelchair, causing injuries to the patient, the employer is normally held liable for the patient's injuries. *Respondeat superior* is Latin term literally meaning "let the master answer for the acts of his/her servants," or "let the employer answer for the acts of his/her employees."

SCOPE OF EMPLOYMENT

The range of employee activities held by the courts to be the legal responsibility of the employer is called the scope of employment. Basically, it includes any acts performed in the process of carrying out one's duties. Ascertaining the scope of employment is important when determining the master's (employer's) liability for the acts of his/her servants (employees).

The nurse's aide who, in the process of hurrying down the hall to aid another patient, knocks down and injures a patient on crutches, is likely to be found to be acting as a servant within the scope of employment, resulting in employer liability for the accident. An employee may be found to be acting within the scope of employment even though the employee is doing his/her job contrary to the instructions of the employer.

BORROWED SERVANT

A borrowed servant is a person under the temporary employ of another person. In a nursing facility, a nurse employed by the local community college as a nursing instructor but temporarily working under the direction of the nursing facility's director of nurses might be found to be a borrowed servant. Using the concept of *respondeat superior*, the nursing facility might be found liable for the wrongful acts of the "borrowed" nurse.

INDEPENDENT CONTRACTOR

An independent contractor agrees with another person to perform a certain job and remains in control of the means and methods of performing the job. Because an independent contractor is not an employee, the doctrine of *respondeat superior* has no application to independent contractors. Therefore, the nursing facility would not be liable ordinarily for the negligence of an independent contractor.

Determining whether a person is acting as an employee, with the facility liable for the employee's negligence, or as an independent contractor, without this liability, depends on a number of factors:

- the extent to which the facility controls the details of the work
- whether the person is engaged in a distinct occupation or profession
- whether the work is usually done under the direction of the employer or by a specialist without supervision
- the skill required
- the portion of time the person is employed
- who supplies the equipment used
- whether the work is part of the regular business of the facility
- whether the facility and worker believe they have formed an employer–employee relationship
- whether or not the person is in business

Depending on the circumstances, physical therapists under contract to the nursing facility and private duty nurses may (or may not) be found to be independent contractors. Because facilities would obviously attempt to have everyone employed as an independent contractor in order to minimize liability, courts do not give great weight to the label the facility places on the worker.

1.12.5 Business-Related Concepts and Terms

Agency—a relationship in which one persons acts on behalf of and under the control of another. The acts of the agent are binding on the person or business the agent represents. The nursing home administrator is the agent of the facility, thus the facility is bound by the agreements the administrator makes on behalf of the facility.

Article of incorporation—the instrument that creates a corporation under the laws of a state.

Attachment—a legal procedure in which a defendant's property is seized by court order pending the outcome of a claim against the defendant. The purpose is to gain control over property that may be used to satisfy payment of a judgment if the plaintiff's suit is successful.

Bad faith—generally implies a design to mislead or deceive another. Good faith means being truthful and faithful to one's obligations in business dealings.

Bankruptcy—inability to pay one's debts, insolvency. Also refers to the legal process of Chapter 7 of the federal Bankruptcy Code, under which the assets of the business or individual(s) are liquidated, creditors paid, and the debtor given a fresh start. In a Chapter 11 reorganization under the Bankruptcy Code, the debtor's assets are not liquidated. Instead, the debt structure and business are rearranged, creditors are paid some or all of what they are owed under a "plan," and the business continues to function without serious interruption.

Caveat emptor—Latin expression for "let the buyer beware." The purchaser buys at his/her own risk. In recent years consumer protection laws and the Uniform Commercial Code have implied certain warranties in most purchases, unless the goods are bought "as is."

Charter—a document issued by a state or other sovereign government establishing a corporate entity (same as article of incorporation).

Contract—an agreement between two or more persons that creates legally enforceable rights and remedies. Contracts must have the following elements:

- *competent parties* (of majority age and of sound mind). In the case of many nursing home patients, the courts decide on their competence to enter into a contract.

- *consideration*—something of value given in return for performance of an act or the promise to perform an act. A promise to refrain from an act, that is, giving up a legal right, may qualify as consideration.

- *mutuality of agreement*—the parties must agree willingly. Often stated as "a meeting of the minds."

- *mutuality of obligation*—all parties must be bound to some reciprocal performance. A promise by one person to do something at the will of another person without any consideration (benefit) to the first person is not a contract.

An *oral contract* is an enforceable agreement that is not in writing or signed by the parties. Oral contracts are enforceable but are subject to limitations. Various state statutes impose monetary limits on oral contracts for the purchase of goods, and almost every agreement dealing with real estate must be in writing to be enforceable.

Normally, no punitive damages are available for breach of contract. A person or facility suing for breach of contract can recover only what would have been received had the contract been fulfilled. Generally, the non-breaching party can recover money damages but cannot command performance of actual work. Ordinarily, attorney's fees cannot be recovered by the successful party.

Contractor—one who agrees to do work for another and retains control over the means, method, and manner in which the work is done. A physical therapist may be an independent contractor in a nursing facility, depending on the terms of the contract. Concerning building, a *general contractor* is one who contracts with the owner of a property to accomplish agreed-on construction. A *subcontractor* is one who deals only with the general contractor for performance of some portion of the work to be accomplished by the general contractor.

Corporation—an association of shareholder(s) (even one shareholder) created by statute and treated by the law as a "person." In effect, it is an artificial person with a legal existence entirely separate from the individuals who compose it. A corporation may have perpetual existence: buy, own, and dispose of property; sue and be sued; and exercise any other powers conferred on it by statute.

Normally, a stockholder's liability is limited to the assets of the corporation; thus, stockholders avoid personal liability for their corporation's acts. Corporations are taxed at special rates, but normally stockholders must pay an additional tax on any profits received from the corporation (dividends).

A small corporation earning a modest profit may elect to be taxed as a partnership (see Partnership below). Stockholders, in this case, avoid personal liability for the acts of the corporation, and avoid double taxation. A corporation choosing to pay federal taxes as a partnership is called an "S" corporation.

Each state enacts its own corporation laws. Some states, such as Delaware, give the officers and board of directors more freedom from minority shareholder controls and thereby attract unusually large numbers of groups to incorporate under their state's laws.

De facto corporations are those that exist de facto (in fact) without actual authorization by the law. Three conditions must be met: (a) a statute exists under which it *could* be incorporated; (b) it behaves in such a way as to *appear* to be functioning as a corporation; and (c) it assumes some corporate privileges.

Public corporations are created by authorization of the federal government and the states to accomplish certain purposes. They include towns, counties, water and sewage districts, and radio and television stations. The U.S. Postal Service and the Corporation for Public Broadcasting are two such entities.

Private corporations are corporations created by private individuals for nongovernmental purposes.

Professional corporations are professional associations of one or more physicians or other professionals who form themselves into a corporation.

Courts may choose to ignore the protection provided to stockholders from personal liability, typically when it can be shown that the purported corporation is found to be the "alter ego" of a principal (person). When, for example, it can be shown that the purported corporation does not hold stockholder meetings or generally ignores the duties and activities associated with operating a corporation, and neglects other corporate formalities, the courts may ignore the stockholders' usual immunity from personal liability and assign personal liability to the stockholders for acts of the corporation. If the incorporation itself was undertaken to defraud, the courts may hold the stockholders and officers personally liable for acts of the corporation.

Default—a failure to perform an act or obligation. A common example is default on mortgage payments due.

Garnishment—a legal process through which a plaintiff can obtain goods or money belonging to a defendant, held by a third party, that are due or will become due to the plaintiff. Garnishment is similar to attachment.

A person who receives notice to retain assets belonging to a defendant is the garnishee. Thus, the nursing home may be the garnishee when a court directs the nursing home to pay over a portion of an employee's salary to a plaintiff to repay a portion of an employee's debt.

Grandfather clause—provision whereby persons already engaged in a business or profession receive a license or entitlement without meeting all of the conditions new entrants would have to meet. Nursing home administrators already operating homes prior to the nursing home administrator licensure laws are "grandfathered."

Lien—a claim on the property of another person(s) as security for a debt owed. A lien does not give any title (ownership) to the property; it is a right of the person holding the lien to have a debt satisfied out of the property to which the lien applies. If a general contractor building a nursing home is not paid money due under the terms of the contract, he/she may seek to have a lien placed on the facility until the indebtedness is satisfied. Similarly, regular creditors of the nursing facility, if not paid within a specified period of time, might seek to have a lien placed against the facility.

Partnership—a contract between two or more persons to pool resources and efforts for the purposes of conducting a business operation. Normally, partnership status requires an agreement to divide profits and assume indebtedness in some proportionate share. Unlike stockholders in a corporation, the partners do not have limited liability, unless it is a *limited partnership*—an entity in which one or more persons are designated general partners (who assume unlimited personal liability for the acts of the partnership) and one or more persons are designated limited partners (whose liability is limited to their investment). Limited partners do not share in the management of the partnership.

Joint venture—a business undertaking similar to a partnership but usually more limited in purpose, e.g., to buy and hold a single piece of land.

Sole proprietorship—ownership of a business by one individual. Before incorporation became popular among physicians, most physicians were the sole proprietors of their office practices.

Product liability—the liability of manufacturers and sellers for products they place on the market that cause harm to a person because of defects.

1.12.6 Insurance Terms

Actuary—a person who computes insurance costs, usually for the purpose of determining rates to be charged.

Annuity—a fixed amount of money payable periodically by an insurer under the terms of an insurance contract. Normally, the annuitant (the person receiving the payments) has no rights other than entitlement to payments for a fixed period of time.

Beneficiary—the person named in an insurance policy to receive the proceeds or benefits under the policy.

Binder—a contract for temporary insurance until a permanent policy can be issued.

Co-insurance—a division of responsibility for losses or risks between the insurer and the insured. The insured individual might agree to pay, for example, the first $50 in costs of any claim.

Life insurance—insurance that may be one of several types. *Whole life* insurance policies can build cash value (i.e., can be turned in by the insured for cash) and normally pay dividends (i.e., interest on the cash value). *Term insurance*, on the other hand, has no cash value; hence, no dividends. When term insurance expires, no value is left. Whole life insurance costs more than term insurance. An almost infinite variety of types of policies exist as variations on these two basic forms of life insurance.

Medical malpractice or professional liability insurance—insurance that provides for protection against lawsuits by patients alleging negligence in the care provided by the health care provider.

General liability insurance—insurance that protects against lawsuits arising out of day-to-day activities carried on in the facility.

The nursing facility normally purchases numerous additional types of insurance against casualties such as fire, lightning, and hail and to cover damage to automobiles and buildings.

1.12.7 Terms Associated with Wills and Estates

Administrator—a person appointed to transfer the property of one who dies *intestate* to those who succeed in ownership. To die intestate is to die without leaving a will. The estate (or property) of persons who die testate (with a will) is administered by an *executor* of the estate, usually named in the will.

Codicil—see Will.

Decedent—the person who has died.

Competence—the capability of a person to make a will. A person is judged capable or competent if he/she understands the nature and extent of his/her property, the identity of the property owned, and the consequences of the act of making a will.

Incompetency—inability to function within limits judged normal by a court of law. A *guardian* must be appointed if a person is found to be incompetent. The guardian must handle the incompetent person's affairs until the court determines that competency has returned, in which case the guardian is discharged.

Estate—a term that originally referred to ownership of land but now refers broadly to all real and personal property a person owns or leaves at death.

Probate—the process of proving that an instrument presented as a will is in fact the valid and duly executed will of the deceased person. Some states have special courts, called probate courts, to conduct these procedures.

Will—a person's declaration as to how he/she wishes his/her real and personal property to be disposed of after death. A will may call for actions desired by the decedent (testator) but must dispose of some property, real or personal, to be valid. Originally "will" referred to real estate and "testament" to personal property. "Last will and testament" refers to the most recent valid will left by the decedent.

Some nursing facility residents make "living wills," which govern the type(s) of treatment to be given the patient in the event the patient becomes comatose or a similar condition. A living will has nothing to do with the disposition of property.

A *holographic will* is an entirely handwritten will. In some states a will may be handwritten and need not be witnessed to be valid. A *codicil* is a supplement or amendment to a will. "Codicil" literally means "to say along with." A codicil must meet the same formal requirements as the will.

SOURCES

Black, H.C. (1979). *Black's law dictionary* (5th ed.). St. Paul, MN: West Publishing.

Burton, W.C. (1980). *Legal thesaurus.* New York: Macmillan.

Buttaro, P.J. *Home study program in principles of long term health care administration.* Aberdeen, SD: Health Care Facility Consultants.

Davis, W.E. (1985). *Introduction to health care administration.* Bossier City, LA: Publicare Press.

Dobbs, D.B. (1971). *Law of remedies* (4th ed.). St. Paul, MN: West Publishing.

Gifis, S.H. (1975). *Law dictionary.* Woodbury, NY: Barron's Educational Series.

Miller, D.B. (Ed.). (1982). *Long term care administrator's desk manual.* Greenvale, NY: Panel Publishers.

Prosser, W.L. (1973). *Law of torts.* St. Paul, MN: West Publishing.

1.13 Origins of the Nursing Home Industry

1.13.1 Long-Term Care: A 400-Year Tradition

Long-term care administration is not a new phenomenon. It did not, as currently perceived, spring suddenly into existence after the 1965 passage of Titles 18 and 19 amending the Social Security Act.

Every country has its own tradition of providing care for the aged, chronically ill, and disabled that reflects the demands of the particular culture. Like other American institutions, the U.S. health care system was modeled on the English, just as our legal system has its foundation in English common law.

EARLY NURSING HOME ADMINISTRATION

Throughout most of English and American history, until about 1850, there was little distinction made between the long-term care facility and the hospital. The long-term care facilities in England were called hospitals, but their functions were much more nearly what is now considered those of a nursing home. From the 12th through the 15th centuries nearly 700 shelters for the aged, the destitute, and pilgrims were built in England (Dainton,

p. 21). These institutions housed populations similar to those in today's nursing homes: the aged, those without means of support in their own homes, and the disabled.

State Medicaid officials today are concerned about inappropriate and/or unnecessary placement of persons in nursing homes. This has probably been the complaint of many a community that has found it necessary to look after those who cannot do so for themselves. Before 1453 all of these facilities were associated with monasteries, in theory, but were administered by men appointed jointly by the king and the local bishop (Freymann, p. 21). Did administrators receive training for their jobs in those days? Probably so, in an apprenticeship system not unlike our administrator-in-training programs of today.

In 1536 King Henry VIII, in a dispute with the Catholic Church, closed all of the monasteries and their health care facilities simultaneously. One of the most famous, St. Bartholomew's "hospital" in London, had been operating since 1123 A.D. There are no records, however, that St. Bart's had any medical staff during those first 400 years. Pressures to provide care for the poor forced the king to allow St. Bart's to be reopened 10 years later (1546). He took responsibility for management from the bishops and appointed local citizens to direct such facilities throughout England. In this process of removing health care from the Church's charge the king appointed what is believed to be the first recorded board of citizen directors of a public hospital, consisting of 30 leading citizens. This board decided that the reopened St. Bart's could accommodate 400 aged, 650 decayed householders (Medicaid-eligible persons?), 200 idle vagabonds, 350 poor men overburdened with children (no mention of the women!), 20 sore and sick persons (Freymann, pp. 21, 22).

In sum, the board viewed the hospital as providing 99% long-term care and 1% acute care. The shift from chronic to acute care slowly evolved over the next 400 years.

During those years, physicians had little or no contact with what were being called hospitals. Medical care, such as it was, was provided on a solo practitioner basis to those who could afford to pay. In essence, physicians served the upper classes in the patients' homes or in their private clinics. Times have not changed much. The majority of nursing home patients today are recipients of Medicaid assistance; they are aged, chronically ill, and poor; and they have lost the ability to earn an income to support themselves or have not accumulated enough during their working lives to sustain them in old age. The well-to-do typically remain in their own homes or move to a continuing-care retirement community that admits only persons who have ample means to pay.

Nursing homes, like the hospitals, gained the ability to "cure" or offer effective restorative care to patients in the same way as hospitals did during the late 19th and early 20th centuries.

1.13.2 Home Health Care versus Institutional Care: A 400-year-old Debate

For the average person in most societies, to live to be very old or to be chronically ill is to eventually be without means of a steady income. These conditions are becoming ever more closely linked. It is as much an economic condition as one of health.

An issue hotly debated in the U.S. Congress and the state legislatures is nursing home versus home health care. Which is better, less expensive for the state? Is health care provided to older and chronically ill persons in their own homes better and less costly? Or, is it more frugal and at least as desirable to institutionalize them in a long-term facility and pay for their care where economies of scale prevail?

This controversy has its roots in the Elizabethan Poor Law of 1601. The first Queen Elizabeth required each local community to care for its poor through providing them cash and in-kind help to enable them to remain in their own homes. In the century that followed, the major mode of assistance to the elderly and chronically ill and disabled was a program to allow them to stay in their own homes as long as possible in England and in its colonies in the New World.

Our present-day state legislatures and the Congress are now warning that the projected increases in the number of older and chronically ill Americans by the end of this century may bankrupt Medicaid funds and state treasuries. The English government and our colonial predecessors, when faced with the same issue early in the 18th century, decided to provide public welfare and health assistance only in institutional settings. In 1722 England enacted a new Poor Law that established almshouses, or workhouses, where it was hoped the aged, chronically ill, and disabled, as well as other persons receiving assistance, could be cared for less expensively (Hunter, p. 27). This was emulated in Philadelphia (1722), New York City (1734), and Charleston, South Carolina (1735).

1830 TO 1930: NURSING HOME CARE IS OUT; HOME HEALTH CARE IS IN

During the early 19th century the pendulum swung back toward provision of in-home assistance to the aged, chronically ill, and the poor. In England this was known as the Speenhamland System (Freymann, p. 30), in which a minimum annual income was guaranteed to everyone—what our Democratic Party has called the "minimum annual income" and our Republican party has called the "safety net," below which or through which no one should be allowed to fall. But these programs are expensive and suspected by many to be abused by persons who are not truly needy. As a result, the pendulum swung back toward a requirement that persons needing assistance move into institutional settings, where care was believed to be less expensive and less subject to abuse.

Between 1830 and 1930, when America was a land of great economic opportunity for all, the predominant mood was to insist that aid to the aged, chronically ill, and disabled be available only in what were called public workhouses.

These institutions fostered two trends that are important in the history of long-term care in the United States. First, they had infirmaries for the ill among their population that were the origins of the early public hospitals in this country. Second, as care for subpopulations in the workhouses moved steadily toward specialization, the basis for the current nursing home population was established.

1.13.3 Separating Long-Term Care from Acute Care: Precursors of the 20th-Century Nursing Home in the United States

To understand the process by which long-term care facilities and acute care hospitals evolved from the same institution, let us consider the Philadelphia Almshouse and the Publick Workhouse of New York City (1734). Their operations included an infirmary from its inception. It was not until 19 years later that the first American private or voluntary hospital, the Pennsylvania Hospital, was opened in the same city. By 1795, 114 of the 301 patients/residents of the Philadelphia Almshouse were classified as sick (Freymann, p. 28). Its medical functions were finally recognized in 1835. At that time a reorganization was undertaken and the name changed to Philadelphia Hospital and Almshouse (read: long-term care facility). In 1903 the hospital section became the Philadelphia General Hospital.

By 1920 the Philadelphia Almshouse and the Philadelphia General Hospital were officially separated (Freymann, p. 28). From the original combined facility, two separate institutions had emerged: an acute-care hospital and a long term-care organization.

EMERGENCE OF SPECIALIZATION

The Publick Workhouse of New York City illustrates the slow emergence of health care services specialization from an early nonspecialized long-term care facility. It had been established in 1734, thus predating the New York Hospital, which opened in 1769. By 1825 the medical functions of the workhouse infirmary, until then without medical personnel, had been given administrative recognition when the first resident physician was appointed to its staff. The name was simultaneously changed to Bellevue Hospital (Freymann, pp. 28–29). Then began a process of specialization of care leading to the current structuring of our nursing home populations. In 1831 the blind were removed to specialized care; in 1848 the hospital assumed care of the acutely ill in addition to responsibility for the mentally retarded, children, the insane, epileptics, the infirm, the aged, and the chronically ill.

Subsequent removal of certain categories of patients to facilities delivering specialized care occurred in the second half of the century, so that by 1900 the Bellevue Hospital had evolved into an institution providing care to persons with infectious diseases, the aged, the chronically ill, the infirm (disabled) (Carlisle, pp. 32–33).

20TH CENTURY

The dual functions of (a) short-term acute care and (b) long-term care for the aged and chronically ill had evolved as the primary functions remaining from what had begun nearly two centuries earlier as the public almshouse. This process laid the groundwork for the dual development of short-term acute-care hospitals and of long-term care institutions in the 20th century. This was a response to the great strides in clinical medicine in the early years of the 20th century. When physicians were actually able to cure their patients of many diseases, separation of short-term acute care and long-term care into distinct facilities seemed indicated.

The first specific remedy in the pharmacopaea of modern 20th-century chemotherapy—Salversan, for an infection, syphilis—was discovered by Paul Ehrlich in 1907. In 1912 L.J. Henderson observed that "a random patient, encountering a random physician with a random disease has, for

the first time, a better than even chance of profiting from the encounter"
(Blake, p. 13). Astonishing progress was to be made over the next 40
years.

1.13.4 Separating Long-Term from Short-Term Care

From 1900 to 1954 the age-adjusted death rate in the United States fell by
57%. This occurred in three identifiable stages: from 1900 to 1919
engineering and preventive measures accounted for a 1% drop per year;
from 1920 to 1935 mortality decreased 0.7% per year; and between 1936
and 1954, with the introduction of sulfonamides and antibiotics, the rate of
decline became 1.5% per year.

With the capacity to cure many common diseases, the typical hospital
rapidly evolved into an institution focused primarily, if not exclusively,
on short-term acute care. Some of them specialized in long-term care, and
some assigned a wing to long-term care, but the time had come for a fuller
separation of the long-term care functions.

During these years deaths due to infection were reduced from 33% to
4% (Freymann, p. 13), with dramatic implications for channels of health
care delivery.

1.13.5 Genesis of the Current Nursing Home Industry: Federal Government Reimbursement

With hospitals focusing more and more exclusively on short-term acute
care, pressures mounted for long-term support to the aged, the chronically
ill, and the disabled. In response the United States once more tried giving
financial support to persons in their home instead of having them occupy a
nursing home or other institutional bed. It began when the New York Old
Age Security Act of 1930 was enacted.

Like its federal successor, which would not appear until 1935, the New York Act provided cash income to persons in need of economic support in their old age. But it excluded those who were in public and private institutions. Similarly, its health care provisions emphasized short-term acute episodic care to the exclusion of direct payments for long-term care in institutions. Persons needing such care were expected to pay for this out of direct cash assistance made to them through the Act. This was a step in the right direction, but these cash payments were typically not large enough to support the patient in a full-time institutional-care setting. In any case, few institutions at the time were able to deal with this population.

Short-term hospital beds were far more available than long-term ones. More and more acute-care beds were being built to match the ever-increasing capacity of the medical profession to effect cures. Not much thought was given to the needs of patients with chronic diseases.

Their care had traditionally been the responsibility of the states and of the cities and counties within those states. As life expectancy increased, so did pressures to develop a care system for this burgeoning sector of the population.

The states, cities, and counties were unwilling to assume the economic burden generated by this development and searched for sources other than their own tax bases to meet the cost of this care. A partial solution was to come through judicial interpretations of a seemingly minor provision of the federal Social Security Act passed in 1935.

THE SOCIAL SECURITY ACT OF 1935

As a response to the growing numbers of aged persons who could not afford to pay the costs of living out of their savings, Congress passed the Social Security Act of 1935. It amounted to an old-age insurance policy. Old people then were able, if they chose, to use the cash to pay for the first small nursing homes that sprang up. Today this legislation, primarily through the 1965 Title 18 and Title 19 amendments, provides a substantial proportion of the cash flow that supports the modern nursing home industry.

Like the New York Old Age Security Act after which it was in part patterned, the U.S. Social Security Act sought to enable the aged, and subsequently the chronically ill and disabled, to stay in their homes through funding to support them. It also enabled them to choose to enter the small "mom and pop" type of nursing home that became available. In its earliest form the Act was almost entirely a cash assistance program. The monthly Social Security check was to be the extent of federal governmental participation. This explains why, like the New York legislation, the framers of the federal Act excluded payments to persons who were institutionalized. Similarly, no home health program, such as exists currently, was set up or envisioned.

LEGISLATIVE AND JUDICIAL ORIGINS OF TODAY'S NURSING HOME INDUSTRY

By limiting Social Security payments to noninstitutionalized persons, the federal Social Security Act left to the states, counties, and cities the onus of paying for long-term institutional care for the aged, chronically ill, and disabled. This seems to have been the intention of the Congress. However, the Act did make federal dollars available for up to half of costs for noninstitutionalized care for the long-term care population. Local officials, under pressure to provide assistance for institutional care, sought ways of making this sector of the community eligible for federal dollars, despite the original intent of the federal lawmakers.

BACKING INTO THE CURRENT SOLUTION

The solution (for the state and local officials) came in a series of court cases concerning persons in need of long-term institutionalization, who had been placed by local officials in private homes for care. Often these were the homes of retired nurses or other persons seeking supplemental income. The courts ruled that these private homes/boarding houses were "nonpublic" institutions and therefore eligible for federal dollar reimbursement. In this way state and local officials were successful in shifting a significant portion of the costs of long-term care from the local and state governments to the federal government. Once the federal government began systematically paying for long-term institutionalized care through the Social Security Act, the nursing home industry began an expansion phase that appears likely to last through the rest of this century.

1.14 Federal Legislation that Shapes the Nursing Home Industry

1.14.1 Social Security Act

The nursing home industry is molded by the Social Security Act and owes the large scale of its economic existence to this legislation. This one Act is mainly responsible for generating the financial support for older persons that has enabled the nursing home industry to become one of the most influential components in the U.S. health care complex.

ORIGINS OF THE ACT

The Social Security Act came into existence in 1935. It was a response to a fundamental societal change in American life: our evolution from an agrarian to a highly industrialized form of society. Growing old suddenly became visible nationally during the shift from an agricultural form of society in which the aged were normally cared for by the family in the home to a society where the workplace was a factory. In industrialized societies workers are controlled by economic conditions beyond their influence. Urbanization and industrialization brought increased problems to the aged, such as unemployment and economic survivorship of the dependents when the wage earner died.

The event that brought these problems to the attention of America in dramatic terms was the Great Depression of the 1930s. By 1935, 50% of the aged were indigent. Within 5 years, the proportion had grown to 66% (Clement, p. 21).

IMPACTS OF THE ACT

Although additional factors are involved, a comparison of the number of aged persons receiving Social Security checks and the percentage of aged persons living at the poverty level reveals a clear association. By 1959 the proportion of aged Americans who were indigent had fallen to 35%. Although this reflected some improvement, it still constituted a major social problem. As Social Security benefits during the 1950s and 1960s continued to expand, the percentage of aged living in poverty declined to 14% of older persons by 1978 (Kaplan, p. 5). According to the U.S. Census Bureau, during the inflation and recession period from 1979 to 1982, the elderly receiving Social Security checks based on Cost of Living Adjustments (COLAs), which began in 1975, were the only group studied whose poverty rate did not increase.

In 1985 the President's Council of Economic Advisors declared that older Americans were no longer disproportionately poor, that the percentage of the general population in poverty (15.2%) was slightly higher than that of the same segment of the elderly population (Kaplan, p. 7). Today nearly all Americans are covered by Social Security. In 1950 this was true for only 1 of every 4 older persons; by 1977 9 of 10 received Social Security checks.

In 1980 nearly 7 of every 10 older persons relied on Social Security for at least half of their income. In 1981 1 of every 5 older persons relied almost exclusively on Social Security for their entire income (Kaplan, p. 5). Many factors, such as the political activism of the aged, general improvements in the economy, the Older Americans Act of 1965, and related actions have led to general improvement in the economic condition of the aged. Even so, while direct measurement is not feasible, it appears that the now nearly universal benefits of the Social Security Act play a central role in these improvements.

ASPECTS AFFECTING THE NURSING HOME INDUSTRY

The nursing home industry, on the scale we know it, would not be possible without Social Security checks and reimbursement of Medicare and Medicaid bills for patients.

The Original Social Security Act and its Amendments

The original Social Security Act, as passed in 1935, consisted of 11 titles enacting the program, authorizing the necessary taxes, and establishing the administrative mechanisms of the Act. Numerous amendments have been added to the Social Security Act over the years. Only those more directly affecting the nursing home industry are mentioned here.

In 1950 permanently and totally disabled persons, who might at some time need nursing home care, were added as beneficiaries. In that same year, federal matching money was made available to states to pay for medical care for persons on public assistance—a precursor of Medicaid, which was to come in 1965 and today supports the largest category of patients in nursing facilities.

By 1956 the Social Security program was known as OASDI—old age (OA), survivors (S), and disabled (D) insurance (I). It was not until 1960 that the H (for health) was added, and it became OASDHI. The next step toward the Medicaid program, so critical to the nursing home industry, came in 1960 with the Kerr-Mills Act, which amended the Social Security Act to provide Medical Assistance to the Aged (MAA). This amendment offered 50% to 83% in matching funds to states, depending on the per capita income of each state. However, during the following 5 years only 25 states implemented this program to assist their aged.

The major amendments affecting the nursing home industry were added in 1965, with the passage of Title 18, known as Medicare, and 1 year later, Title 19, known as Medicaid. These are discussed below.

Amendments in 1967 called for the licensure of nursing home administrators and recognized the category of "intermediate care facility." The 1972 amendments established the current definition of the skilled nursing facility (SNF) and dropped the term "extended care facility" (ECF), which had been causing some confusion.

Title 20 was added in 1974, supporting, among other things, in-home services to the elderly. In 1977 antifraud amendments were passed to minimize abuse of the program. Numerous additional amendments have been passed during the 1980s. Their primary focus has been containment of costs, rather than expansion of services.

In general, it appears that from 1935 to about 1975 the federal government sought to expand benefits under the Social Security Act, whereas since 1975 the thrust has been reduction of the rate of cost increases and the units of service for which payment is made.

Both the federal and most state governments have been seeking ways to reduce expenditures under Medicare and Medicaid. Consequently, details of the payment plans described below are subject to change. The reader should obtain a current copy of *Your Medicare Handbook* and check with the local Medicaid office for the latest coverages and payment mechanisms.

MEDICARE

In its first full year of operation, 1967, Medicare spent $4.7 billion (3% of the federal budget) to cover 19 million people. By 1984 Medicare was spending $65 billion (7% of the federal budget) to cover 30 million people (27 million persons 65 and over, plus 3 million disabled persons) (Califano, p. 140). In 1985 Medicare spent $70.5 billion, a 12% increase over 1984.

Plan A

Everyone receiving Social Security is automatically covered under Plan A.

Hospital Costs. Covered hospital-related costs are paid on the following basis: during the first 60 days of hospitalization for each period of illness (defined below), the patient pays for the equivalent of the first day, and Medicare pays for the other 59.

During Days 61 to 90 of hospitalization, the patient pays for about 25% of the daily rate. Medicare picks up the remaining costs. Inpatient services are covered only during the first 90 days of any spell of illness (defined below). Each Medicare recipient has a lifetime reserve of 60 days, which may be used after the 90th day of hospitalization. During Days 91 to 150 the patient pays for about 50% of the daily rate. In addition, each Medicare recipient is eligible for up to 190 days of inpatient psychiatric care during his/her lifetime.

Prospective Payment: the Era of DRG's. Beginning with federal fiscal year 1984, the federal government began paying hospitals for Medicare patient costs on the basis of 467 diagnostic/reimbursement categories (Prospective Payment, pp. 1–6). Each year, Medicare officials prospectively (ahead of time) decide how much will be paid for each Medicare hospital admission based on the principal diagnosis, i.e., the condition established after study to be chiefly responsible for admission of the patient to the hospital.

DRG stands for Diagnostically Related Group (of diseases). There are 9,000 disease codes listed in a book called *International Classification of Diseases*. Using the 9th edition's clinical modifications (called ICD 9 CM), the federal government has identified 467 diseases. It reimburses hospitals for care of Medicare patients based on the principal diagnosis *and* the severity level of the disease for which the Medicare patient was admitted.

The theory is that some patients' length of stay will be shorter than average and some longer than average. Medicare reimburses on the *average* length of stay for each disease, based on the level of severity experienced by the patient. At the end of each year Medicare makes adjustments, using up to approximately 6% of its total funds to reimburse hospitals for especially expensive cases (called outliers).

Payments vary for each of the nine U.S. geographical regions established by Medicare and by whether the hospital is rural or urban. For example, an urban hospital in New York City would be reimbursed at a higher rate than a rural Georgia hospital for treating a patient with the same principal diagnosis. Each hospital's reimbursement rate is based 25% on whether it is rural or urban and 75% on the cost experience of that hospital during the first year it was in the program, called the base year.

One impact for the long-term care industry is that since payment is by disease, no matter how long the length of stay of each patient, hospitals are seeking to place Medicare patients in nursing facilities for care that has traditionally been given in the hospitals. The Health Care Financing Administration is considering reimbursing nursing homes on prospective pricing beginning in 1988 or 1989 (Rudensky, p. 36).

Skilled Nursing Facility Costs. For each spell of illness, Medicare pays 100% of "reasonable costs" during the first 20 days. During Days 21 to 100 the patient co-pays a required amount, set typically at over half the daily cost. Medicare will pay nothing beyond 100 days of skilled-nursing-facility care during any one spell of illness.

Home Health Care Costs. Medicare will pay 100% of all home health care costs associated with any one spell of illness.

Spell of Illness. Spell of illness, or benefit period, is an important and a complicated concept. A spell of illness begins the first day of hospitalization and ends when the participant has been out of a hospital or other facility providing skilled nursing or rehabilitation services—whether or not it participates in Medicare—for 60 days in a row, including the day of discharge (U.S. DHHS, 1985, p. 10).

The length of time that services are received under a spell of illness can vary greatly. The length of time covered by the 100 skilled-nursing-facility days is not fixed from the first day of admission to a skilled nursing facility. A Medicare patient can reenter a skilled nursing facility several times as long as it is within 30 days of discharge from that facility and is for the same diagnosis, until 100 days have been used up. Readmission to a hospital for 3 days is not required for readmission to a skilled nursing facility for the same diagnosis during a single spell of illness.

Complicated Calculations and Trade-offs. For the Medicare beneficiary, an uncovered hospitalization of any length can be economically disastrous. Because of this, it is important for each Medicare beneficiary to realize that until he/she has been out of a hospital or skilled nursing facility for 60 days, he/she cannot qualify for another benefit period or spell of illness. After 60 days the patient can even be covered for the same type of illness and is eligible for another 90 days of hospital coverage—but only if he/she has not been in a skilled nursing facility for 60 days.

Medicare will count days in an intermediate-care facility toward the 60 required days necessary for eligibility for coverage for a new spell of illness. There is no limit to the number of spells of illness that Medicare will cover, except in the case of hospice care, which is discussed below.

A factor with extremely critical implications for the nursing home industry is that once having entered a skilled nursing facility for an extended period of time, eligibility for a new spell of illness virtually ceases to exist for a Medicare participant. It is important to realize that Medicare is intended to cover brief periods of illness. Medicare is short-term acute care. It does not cover long-term care of patients. Medicaid is the vehicle for covering long periods of illness, but only after the individual has spent all but about $1,000 of his/her total resources.

Eligibility for Skilled Nursing Facility Care.   To be eligible for inpatient skilled-nursing-facility care, five conditions must be met by the Medicare patient. He/she must

- have spent three consecutive days in a hospital (not including the day of discharge)
- be transferred to a skilled nursing facility because treatment for the original cause of hospitalization is required
- be admitted within 14 days of hospital discharge (leeway is generally allowed up to 30)
- be certified by a physician to be in need of and receiving skilled nursing care or skilled rehabilitation services on a *daily* basis
- have approval for the stay by the skilled nursing facility utilization review committee (or Professional Review Committee)

Plan B

Plan B is voluntary. The Medicare recipient must pay a small monthly premium—determined every 2 years and based on the benefits paid and administration costs of Plan B. General funds from the U.S. Treasury pay one-half of the costs of Plan B and the participants pay the other half.

Three major expenses are covered under Plan B:

1. Medical expenses (including physicians services, inpatient and out-patient medical services, and supplies, physical and speech therapy, ambulance, diagnostic X-ray, laboratory and other tests, dressings, splints, medical equipment used in the home).
2. Outpatient hospital treatment.
3. Home health care.

Payments under Plan B.   After the recipient pays an annual deductible amount, Medicare Plan B pays 80% of Medicare-determined reasonable charges for medical expenses, outpatient hospital treatment, and home health care. If home health care qualifies under Plan A posthospital care, 100% of home health care costs are paid under Plan A.

Excluded from Coverage. Many health care costs associated with the elderly are excluded from payment by Medicare plans A and B. Neither plan will pay for

- routine physical and related tests
- eyeglasses or eye examinations
- hearing examinations or hearing aids
- immunizations (except for pneumococcal shots)
- routine foot care
- orthopedic shoes or other supportive devices for the feet
- custodial care
- preventive care, filling, removal, or replacement of teeth

Some Definitions

Intermediaries and carriers. Medicare payments are actually made by private insurance organizations that have contracted with the federal government to do so. Organizations handling claims from skilled nursing facilities, hospitals, and home health agencies are called *intermediaries.* Organizations dealing with claims from doctors and other medical suppliers covered under the medical insurance (Plan B) are called *carriers.*

Approved charges. Under Plan B, approved charges are determined as follows: the carrier in each geographic area annually reviews the charges made by doctors and suppliers during the previous year. Suppliers are persons or organizations other than physicians who furnish equipment or services, such as ambulance transportation, laboratory tests, and medical equipment, e.g., wheelchairs.

To calculate an approved charge, the carrier determines the customary charge, the one most frequently made by each physician and supplier during the previous year. Then the carrier finds the prevailing charge for each service and material supplied during that year. The prevailing charge is a sufficient amount to pay for the customary charges in three out of every four bills that were submitted in the previous year for each service and supply (limited by an economic index ceiling). When a claim is received from a physician or supplier, the carrier compares the actual charge with the customary and prevailing charges for that service or supply and pays 80% of the lowest of the three. The Medicare recipient pays the remaining 20%, either out of pocket or through a small insurance policy (called Medigap insurance), which is designed to pay the remaining 20%.

Assignment. When a physician or supplier accepts an assignment of the medical insurance payment under Plan B, he/she agrees that the total charge to the patient will be the one approved by the carrier. In this case, Medicare pays the physician or supplier directly, after subtracting any part of the annual deductible not met.

Assignment is voluntary and must be agreed to by both the provider and the patient. It guarantees that the physician or supplier will not charge the patient more than the 20% of approved charges not paid by the carrier. After pressure from the federal government, more than half of Medicare physicians have agreed to accept assignment.

TITLE 19: MEDICAID

Medicaid and Medicare were both passed as amendments to the Social Security Act in 1965. Medicare is essentially an insurance program for recipients of Social Security benefits. Medicaid is not insurance. Medicaid is, literally, medical aid for persons receiving welfare and for comparable groups of persons who are defined as medically indigent.

Whereas Medicare is a federally run program, Medicaid is a program of federal grants to the states to enable them to provide medical assistance to four categories of persons: (a) families with dependent children (AFDC); (b) the aged—persons receiving Old Age Assistance (OAA); (c) the blind—Aid to the Blind (AB); (d) persons permanently and totally disabled (that is, to persons receiving federally aided public assistance); and to comparable groups of medically indigent persons, not currently on welfare but who fall into the same preceding four categories. Such persons are categorized as medically needy when medical expenses reduce their income below the Medicaid eligibility level, set typically at approximately 133% of poverty. This is called "spend down."

The federal share ranges from 50% to 83% of costs, depending on the state's per capita income. All states except Arizona have elected to participate in Medicaid. Each state determines its coverage above a basic minimum of at least some of each of the following services: inpatient hospital, outpatient hospital, other laboratory and X-ray, skilled nursing, and medical. In 1985 Medicaid payments amounted to $40 billion. They covered 22 million Americans, some 6 million of whom were aged, blind or disabled (Califano, p. 151).

In addition to these basic services, a state may include any medical care recognized under state law if it chooses. No residency requirements may be established for eligibility for services. Medicaid recipients are not subject to deductible payments, as in the case of Medicare, but states are allowed to require some co-payments from recipients for care. Some states, for example, charge co-payments for prescriptions, typically 50 cents per prescription; dental visits, eye visits, and similar services, charging a $1 to $2 co-payment fee per visit (Muse & Sawyer, p. 96).

Changing Congressional Goals. Originally the federal government set July 1, 1975, as the date by which all participating states were to be offering comprehensive services to all eligible persons. As costs soared under the program, Congress scaled down this goal and in the 1980s is moving toward containing Medicaid costs rather than expanding its services. Congress is concerned because neither Medicare nor Medicaid have ceilings on annual expenditures, and the federal government is committed to pay all Medicare costs and its share of services the states provide Medicaid recipients.

Buy-in Agreements. To maximize the contribution of federal dollars to state programs, all but 5 of the 49 participating states have signed "buy-in agreements" under which the state pays for Plan B costs for Medicaid recipients. The buy-in obligates the federal government to pay entirely for medical costs that might have been cost-shared by the states' Medicaid programs, thus reducing the total dollar costs to the states (Muse & Sawyer, p. 115).

States themselves have become concerned about the outflow of Medicaid dollars. To contain costs, some states have obligated county governments to use county funds to pay for a portion (usually about 4%) of Medicaid costs. Medicaid dollars, initially committed by county social workers, are thus more carefully supervised by the county governments.

Eligibility for Medicaid is generally determined at the county level by a social worker, and the program is usually administered by the local Department of Social Services, which assigns recipients as part of the case load of its social workers.

As mentioned elsewhere, the elderly have traditionally benefited to a great extent under the Medicaid program; they represent approximately 15% of all recipients but receive slightly more than one-third of the benefits paid out (Muse & Sawyer, p. 8).

1.14.2 Older Americans Act of 1965

The Older Americans Act (OAA) can be characterized as Congress's response to the *noninstitutional* needs of the elderly. Medicare and Medicaid provide their *institutional* care. Title 20 of the Social Security Act is a response to the noninstitutional needs of this segment of our population.

The OAA deals with those not yet institutionalized. Under the legislation, payment is authorized for almost any activity that may lead to an improved quality of life for persons over 60 years of age. The funds and agencies authorized and generated by the OAA play major roles in shaping the long term-care industry in the United States. For this reason some of its more important features are explored below.

PRECURSORS OF THE OAA

Events that laid the foundation for the passage of the OAA in 1965 began about 1945, when the first state, Connecticut, set up a commission concerned with the needs of older individuals. By 1961 all states had established similar commissions or aging units. That same year a White House Conference on Aging was held, at which heavy pressure for a federal role in addressing the needs of the elderly was brought to bear by lobbyists. Two years later President John F. Kennedy sent a message to Congress entitled "Elderly Citizens of Our Nation." He recommended federal help for older individuals who do not need institutional care but are encountering the expected increase in difficulty of successfully performing the activities of daily living. Continued lobbying for federal aid for the functional elderly led to the passage of the OAA in 1965.

GRAND OBJECTIVES: TITLE 1

Title 1 states the goals of the OAA: equal opportunity of every older individual to the full and free enjoyment of

- adequate income
- the best possible physical and mental health science can offer, without regard to economic status
- affordable, suitable housing
- full restorative services for those needing institutional care
- employment
- retirement in health and dignity
- pursuit of the widest civic, cultural, educational, and recreational opportunities
- efficient community services: low-cost transportation, choices in living arrangements, coordinated social service assistance
- immediate benefit of technological developments
- freedom, independence, and the free exercise of individual initiative in planning and managing his/her own life

Other portions of the OAA authorize the Commissioner on Aging, administrator of the OAA, to pay for virtually any service or activity that will foster these broadly stated goals. The goals and authorizations are sweeping; however, the economic realities of the level of funding have prevented implementing large-scale programs to achieve these goals.

OTHER TITLES

Title 2 establishes the Administration on Aging (AOA) within the Office of Human Development Services (OHDS) which is in the federal Department of Health and Human Services (DHHS). A Commissioner on Aging, appointed by the President and confirmed by the Senate, is empowered to administer the OAA and report directly to the Secretary of Health and Human Services.

Title 3 authorizes grants to the states to create Planning and Service Areas within which the local Area Agencies on Aging (AAAs) function. Title 3b is concerned with social services, Title 3c1 with congregate nutrition services for those 60 or over as well as their spouses, and Title 3c2 with home delivered meals. Title 4 deals with research and training. Title 5 creates the Senior Community Services Employment Program (SCSEP) for those 55 or older with limited incomes (usually 125% of poverty). Title 6 addresses grants to American Indian tribes. Title 7, passed in 1984, authorizes a health education and training program for older individuals.

PROFILE OF A RECENT YEAR

In 1982, OAA's 17th year of operation, $913 million was appropriated by the federal government for activities under the Act. At that time there were 682 Planning and Service Areas (PSAs) (Title 3a) served by the local Area Agencies on Aging; 6,674 multipurpose senior centers; 13,200 congregate nutrition sites (Title 3c1). Nine million older individuals participated in the social and community services (Title 3a) and nearly 3 million in the nutrition site meal program (Title 3c1) (*Developments in Aging*, p. 448). In 1986, $671 million was appropriated—down nearly $250 million from four years earlier.

AMENDMENTS

The OAA was amended in 1967 and 1969, annually from 1972 to 1975, in 1977, 1978, 1981, and 1984. Most of the amendments focus on expanding and repositioning the various programs, especially those under Title 3. The amendments of 1978 are of special interest to the nursing home industry. They require state plans to include a long-term care ombudsman program that will

- investigate and resolve complaints by or on behalf of long-term care patients
- monitor, develop, and assure implementation of federal, state, and local laws governing long-term care facilities
- give public agencies information about problems of older individuals residing in long-term care facilities
- train volunteers and enlist and develop community citizen organizations.

To accomplish these goals the states must set up procedures so that ombudsmen can have access to any long-term care facility records and patient records without disclosing the identity of the person bringing the complaint, without that person's written consent, and without a court order. Further, the state is to establish a statewide complaint recording system to spot problems over time and report them to the state agency that licenses and certifies the long-term care facilities, and to report complaints to the federal Commissioner on Aging.

Finally, under the 1978 amendments, the state is to assure that the ombudsmen's files are secure, meaning accessible only to the ombudsmen themselves unless the inquiring person, such as a concerned nursing home administrator, has written permission from the person who lodged the complaint or has a court order. In short, the state agency is to serve as a watchdog over the nursing facilities, and although the state agency cannot take legal action against a facility, it is expected to go to the state licensing and certification agency, which is empowered to do so.

Beyond the ombudsman program itself, the state agency and the local Area Agencies on Aging are authorized to serve as advocates for the elderly in their area. This is interpreted to mean that they assure that the nursing facilities observe the laws and give good quality patient care.

Comprehensive Service Systems

Another major assignment to the states and their local Area Agencies on Aging is to foster the development of comprehensive and coordinated service systems for all of the elderly. This is to be accomplished primarily through establishing numerous supportive services, nutrition programs, and multipurpose senior centers.

Definition of Supportive Services

The local Area Agency on Aging has legislative approval to engage in all of the following very broad range of activities:

health services, including education, training, welfare, information, recreation, homemaker, counseling, and referral to specialists.

transportation to and from supportive services.

services to encourage the elderly to use supportive services.

housing to help older persons obtain housing, repair and renovate to minimum housing standards, adapt homes to individual's disabilities, and introduce modifications to prevent unlawful entry.

services to avoid institutionalization, including preinstitution evaluation and screening, home health, homemaker, shopping, escort, reader, letter writing, and similar services.

legal services, including tax and financial counseling.

physical exercise services

health screening

career counseling

ombudsman services for long-term-care complaints.

unique disabilities services

job counseling

other services necessary for the welfare of older individuals.

In sum, the local Area Agency on Aging is empowered to engage in a wide variety of activities on behalf of older persons in the community. Generally, however, funding has been at a modest level.

Funding

Nationally, supportive services and senior centers (Part b of Title 3) have received between $300 million and $400 million per year. This amounts to about $13 per year per older adult or $91 for each older adult in poverty. There are about 25 million Americans aged 65 and older; about 14% of these live in poverty (Older Americans Act, Section 303). Similar funding exists for congregate meals. For home-delivered meals, somewhere between $60 million and $100 million has been made available, resulting in a national government expenditure per year of about $2.50 for each person, $15.50 per older adult living in poverty (Older Americans Act, Section 303).

To summarize, under the OAA, on average about $28.50 per year is spent per older adult, about $200 per year per older adult in poverty. All persons over 60 are eligible for all programs under OAA regardless of income. There is no means test for services. However, local Area Agencies on Aging target their services to the economically needy.

Effectiveness of the Act

The extent to which the OAA has achieved its goals is debatable. Clearly, the local Area Agencies on Aging have been given a mandate that could cost billions of dollars if fully implemented, and awarded a shoestring budget to accomplish the task. Two hundred dollars per year per impoverished adult cannot go far toward achieving the goals set forth in Title 1. Whether the services under the OAA should be available without a means test to every elderly person is also in question. Of the group who received social and community services in 1982, 52% were considered in greatest economic need, according to estimates submitted nationally by the local Area Agencies on Aging (Developments in Aging, p. 448). That year these agencies also found that approximately 61% of the nutrition service participants were among the most economically needy.

One of the greatest burdens of growing old is the loneliness resulting from loss of friends and family members of the same generation. Participating in the congregate meal is, for many individuals, regardless of their income level, a primary source of social contact with other people.

Have the Area Agencies on Aging been successful in establishing a coordinated service system for long-term care in their communities? No. They have neither the funds nor the organizational authority to bring together and organize the long-term care providers in their communities. Despite the meager funding levels and lack of authority, however, there is a network of services in place for all older Americans who need assistance in remaining outside an institution. This is a major improvement over the decades before the 1960s, when such services did not exist at all. This network and the nutritional assistance to all older Americans has become integral to the long-term care system in which nursing facilities are active participants.

1.14.3 Overview of the Long-Term Care Continuum

The American long-term care system, to the extent that it can be called a system, is loosely interconnected. Each of the agencies and programs is separately authorized by various pieces of legislation. No single agency or program is authorized, or indeed able, to coordinate the various efforts on behalf of the elderly. Although the Older Americans Act calls for and authorizes coordination, in reality officials of the Older Americans Act have not been empowered to bring this about.

The result has been that the elderly must fend for themselves in seeking services. One proposed remedy for this situation is called case management, which is the assignment of each elderly person needing an assistance program to a specific caseworker, who will help that individual plan and carry out a care program composed of services from a number of different agencies (Steinberg, pp. 1–10). This is, in fact, what employees in the departments of social services and the Area Agencies on Aging attempt to do. However, funds are insufficient to employ enough staff to assist all older Americans who need this type of assistance, and most of them are left to fend for themselves. In any event, case management can occur only if the clients can get to an agency in the first place.

Figure 1-7 presents the major sources of services available to older Americans.

The skilled nursing facility (SNF) plays *at least* two major roles in this continuum. First, the SNF may be simultaneously providing rehabilitative services to almost anyone receiving a combination of long-term services. It is estimated that 25% of all older persons use the services of an SNF at some point. Second, the SNF is the major provider of intensive services for persons no longer able to care for themselves and in need of nursing care on a 24-hour basis. It is estimated that at any one point in time, 5% of all the elderly are patients in SNFs.

Following are some additional comments on the various service options illustrated in Figure 1-7. As will be noted, certain SNFs are beginning to offer some of these services.

HOME-BASED LONG-TERM CARE OPTIONS

Friendly Visiting

Both the Area Agency on Aging and local volunteer groups arrange for regular visits to the elderly living alone. This offers both needed social contact and continuous monitoring of these individuals.

Meals on Wheels

Title 3c of the Older Americans Act pays for home-delivered meals. To qualify, an organization must deliver meals on each of 5 days or more per week and meet certain standards, including providing one-third of daily nutritional requirements. Normally, the Area Agency on Aging contracts with groups to provide these meals. SNFs frequently offer meals on wheels, both as a public service and as a contact mechanism with potential patients. The dietary department of the SNF automatically meets the various requirements of the program through preparing food for its residents.

Choreworker—Homemaker

Area Agency on Aging subcontractors offer the services of persons who will come into older persons' homes to perform specific tasks. Chore-

HOME BASED LONG-TERM CARE

- FRIENDLY VISITING   AAA
- MEALS ON WHEELS   AAA
- CHOREWORKER   AAA
- HOMEMAKER   AAA
- HOME HEALTH AIDE
                    MEDICARE OR MEDICAID
- SOCIAL WORKER VISITS   DSS
- PROTECTIVE SERVICES   AAA
- HOME REHABILITATION   AAA
- HOME HEALTH AGENCY
            MEDICARE OR MEDICAID-DSS
- HOSPICE CARE   MEDICARE

COMMUNITY BASED LONG-TERM CARE

- CONGREGATE MEALS   AAA
- SENIOR CITIZENS CENTER   AAA
- COMMUNITY MENTAL
    HEALTH   MENH
- ADULT DAY CARE   MEDICAID
- GERIATRIC DAY HOSPITAL
- RESPITE CARE
        MEDICARE, IF HOSPICE CARE

INSTITUTION BASED LONG-TERM CARE

- **LOW INTENSITY** — VARIOUS HOUSING
    ARRANGEMENTS — GROUP PERSONAL
    CARE, FOSTER CARE, DOMICILIARY CARE,
    REST HOME   DSS AND OTHERS
        CONGREGATE HOUSING   DSS, AAA, HUD
        WITH MEALS
            WITH SOCIAL SERVICES
            WITH MEDICAL SERVICES
            WITH HOUSEKEEPING
    LIFE OR CONTINUING CARE
    COMMUNITIES
            NO PUBLIC PROGRAM SUPPORT

- **MODERATE INTENSITY:** INTERMEDIATE
    NURSING FACILITY   DSS - MEDICAID

- **HIGH INTENSITY:** SKILLED NURSING FACILITY
                        DSS - MEDICAID

AAA = AREA AGENCY ON AGING
        (OLDER AMERICANS ACT)

DSS = DEPARTMENT OF SOCIAL SERVICES
        (ADMINISTERS MEDICAID)

MENH = DEPARTMENT OF MENTAL HEALTH

HUD = DEPARTMENT OF HOUSING & URBAN
        DEVELOPMENT

LEAST RESTRICTIVE →

MOST RESTRICTIVE ↑

FIGURE 1-7. Overview of the long-term care continuum.

workers typically do window washing or other less routine tasks. The homemaker visits on a more regular basis and performs housekeeping tasks such as dusting, dishwashing, and laundry.

Home Health Aide

The home health aide, in contrast to the homemaker and choreworker, is expected to perform only health-specific tasks, such as administering medicines, changing bandages, and the like. The home health aide is paid from Medicaid or Medicare funds, not by the Area Agency on Aging. A home health agency, discussed below, can send such an aide if the older person is receiving Medicare services in the home for a specific illness or injury. Over the past few years local Medicaid offices have increasingly been permitted to use Medicaid funds to pay for services designed to prevent or postpone institutionalizing older persons. Originally, these were called Title 19 waivers, for which states had to apply.

In 1984 the federal Department of Health and Human Services authorized all Medicaid programs to offer a variety of services similar to those available under the Older Americans Act if they were conducive to postponement or prevention of institutionalization. Typically, these services would be funded up to three-quarters of the costs of institutionalizing the client.

Social Worker Visits

The local department of social services, under Title 20 or other authorizations, is permitted to pay for social worker visits to the homes of the elderly. This is similar to a social worker or a caseworker visiting any other client.

Protective Services—Home Rehabilitation Services

The Area Agency on Aging is authorized to assist elderly persons to bring their homes up to minimum standards and to provide added security measures to reduce the possibility of break-ins.

Home Health Care

An older person is entitled to receive home health care through any one of three programs, all under the Social Security Act: Medicare Plan A, Medicare Plan B, and Medicaid.

Services under Medicare Plan A. Unlimited home health visits at no cost are available to any Medicare recipient hospitalized under Plan A and determined to need posthospital home health care.

Services under Medicare Plan B. Unlimited visits, at 80% of cost, are available to persons covered by Medicare Plan B who are found to need part-time skilled health care in their home for the treatment of an illness or injury. No prior hospitalization is required, but four conditions must be met: (a) the care must include part-time skilled nursing care, physical therapy, or speech therapy; (b) the client must be confined to his/her home; (c) a doctor must diagnose the need and design the plan; (d) the agency must participate in Medicare.

Medicare does not cover general household services, meal preparation, shopping, assistance in bathing or dressing, or other home assistance to meet personal, family, or domestic needs (U.S. DHHS, 1985, p. 41). Thus, to keep an ailing older adult who requires various types of home assistance functioning, several agencies, with separate priorities and interests, must be coordinated by that client or by a friend or a caseworker acting in his/her behalf. During the two decades from 1966 (the year Congress authorized Medicare to pay for home care) to 1986 the number of home health care agencies rose from 1,000 in 1966 to 6,000 in 1986. In 1982, 1.1 million Americans were receiving home health care; by 1985 the number had risen to 1.6 million (FactSheet, National Association for Home Care, p. 1). About half (608,000) of the recipients of home health care paid some of the monthly costs (about $164) out-of-pocket (Liu, p. 54). Total 1986 U.S. spending on home health care is estimated to be $9 billion (Califano, p. 61). Total spending is expected to reach $15 billion by 1995 (FactSheet, National Association for Home Care, p. 2).

Medicaid Services. *If* a Medicaid recipient is found likely to need full-time institutional care, such as a nursing facility, Medicaid can pay for nearly any of the types of in-home services available through either Medicare or the Area Agency on Aging.

The economic rationale of this program is to reduce public expenditures by offering services that allow people to function in their own home where they, or often their family, will be sharing the financial burden, thus reducing public costs. The care rationale is to allow persons to function in their own homes as long as they have the capacity when assisted.

HOSPICE CARE

Hospice care is care given a person usually believed to have 6 months or less to live, who primarily seeks alleviation from pain rather than intensive technological medical treatment. Hospice care is typically provided in the home, although there are also both freestanding hospice centers for inpatients and patient wards in hospitals designated as hospice units.

Medicare Plan A pays for hospice care provided the following three conditions are met: (a) medical certification that patient is terminally ill;

(b) patient's choice to receive care from a hospice instead of the standard Medicare benefits; (c) program provided by a Medicare-certified hospice.

The Health Care Financing Administration, which administers Medicare and Medicaid, defines hospice as a public agency or private organization that is primarily engaged in providing pain relief, symptom management, and supportive services to terminally ill people and their families (U.S. DHHS, 1985, p. 19). Medicare pays 100% of all hospice services except for 5% of outpatient drugs and respite care (see below). A special benefit period definition applies: the patient is entitled to a maximum of two 90-day benefit periods and one 30-day benefit period.

COMMUNITY-BASED LONG-TERM CARE

Congregate Meals at Nutrition Sites and Senior Citizens Centers

Under Title 3c of the Older Americans Act, an effort has been made to make congregate meal sites available to as many as possible of the elderly in both urban and rural areas.

To accomplish this the Area Agencies on Aging give subcontracts to many thousands of groups who serve such meals 5 or more days a week, offering one-third of the daily nutritional needs of the participants. Often these nutrition sites, as they are called, are rural churches or schools that are usually centrally located. Transportation is typically provided as well as counseling, nutrition education, recreation, and referral services at the same site and time.

Senior Citizen Centers Activities and In-Center Services

The Area Agencies on Aging offer a variety of activities and services at these centers, and usually congregate meals as well.

Community Mental Health Centers

Mental health legislation over the past two decades has resulted in the establishment of an extensive network of community mental health centers to which older persons may refer themselves or be referred. However, the utilization rate of these centers has tended to be disproportionately low among this age group.

Adult Day Care

An adult day-care program is a community organization providing daytime health and/or recreational services to groups of impaired older adults in a centralized protective environment, often over long periods of time.

Skilled nursing facilities are uniquely positioned to offer adult day-care programs, and many do. Payments for adult day care can come from a variety of sources, including the Model Cities Program, the federal revenue-sharing program, Title 4 of the Older Americans Act, Title 6 of the Social Security Act, and Medicaid (Trans Century Corporation, Table 1-1).

Persons enter an adult day-care program for a variety of reasons, such as need for the caregiver to be at work during the day. Its primary function is to allow older persons with various kinds of disabilities to remain in the home setting longer.

Often the adult day-care participant in a skilled nursing facility eventually becomes a patient there. The earlier exposure to the environment serves to reduce the trauma typically involved in the transition to institutional care. This trauma is discussed at length in Part 5: Patient Care.

Geriatric day rehabilitation hospitals are a medical model of the adult day-care program. Adult day-care programs range from entirely recreational with no health care to nearly full health services similar in intensity to those of the SNF.

Respite Care

Respite care is a relatively new program under Medicare Plan A, where it is defined as a short-term inpatient stay that provides temporary relief to the person who regularly assists with home care (U.S. DHHS, 1985, p. 20).

Under Medicare, respite care is available only to caregivers of hospice patients. Medicare will pay 95% of the costs and 100% of the costs after the patient has paid a specified number of dollars of coinsurance. Medicare limits inpatient respite care to stays of no more than 5 consecutive days.

Depending on occupancy level, skilled- and intermediate-care nursing facilities have offered respite care over the years. Some organizational obstacles to their ability to do so are (a) costs involved in the extensive paperwork required at each admission and discharge, regardless of whether the ICF or SNF patient is a regular or a hospice patient; and (b) costs associated with keeping beds empty for hospice-type admissions, which by definition are of short duration and therefore incur higher administrative costs to the facility.

INSTITUTION-BASED CARE

Low-Intensity Institution-Based Arrangements: Housing

An almost infinite range of housing options faces the elderly attempting to decide where and how to live out their final years. Numerous group housing arrangements exist. These are variously called group homes, personal care homes, foster care homes, domiciliary care homes, or often rest homes. The number of older adults involved varies from three or four in a group or foster home to as many as several hundred in rest homes. The major source of public support for these housing arrangements is the local department of social services that administers the Medicaid program.

Congregate-care housing arrangements exist in many forms. These typically are publicly supported housing sites for elderly and disabled persons. Support can come from numerous public sources, including local tax monies.

These housing arrangements range from no services to a progressive array that includes meals, social services, housekeeping, and medical care. Frequently, they are high-rise buildings or small complexes that offer the low-income person an approximate equivalent to the services offered to middle- and upper-income Americans in what are called life-care or continuing-care communities.

Life- or continuing-care retirement communities are a relatively new phenomenon, at least on the scale on which they are now being offered. These are discussed more extensively elsewhere in this text. This type of setting can be a microcosm of the community at large with its diverse services. In a life-care community the resident typically moves progressively from a detached apartment, to a single room, to a low-care health facility, and finally to an intensive-care facility (SNF equivalent), depending on his/her health needs.

Moderate-Intensity Institution-Based Arrangements: Intermediate-Care Facility

Individuals eligible for intermediate care are no longer able to function in the home or group-housing setting where health assistance is available on a part-time basis only.

Intermediate nursing usually involves counseling, teaching, and implementing prescribed treatment for persons needing continuous care, who are in a stable condition but suffering from a combination of chronic diseases.

An intermediate-care facility differs from an SNF mainly in the intensity of services for its residents, who are expected to be more ambulatory and capable of more self-care, thus requiring fewer nursing hours per patient day than those in an SNF.

High-Intensity Institution-Based Arrangements: SNF

Skilled nursing care is prescribed for persons in a stable or unstable condition who require continuing medical supervision and services of licensed nursing personnel around the clock.

The decision as to whether a publicly supported patient needs intermediate- or skilled-level care is the responsibility of the utilization review committees. The purpose is to assure the most responsible stewardship of public monies, since SNF care routinely costs more than intermediate care. Medicare does not pay for intermediate nursing care.

A privately paying patient, at the physician's direction, may be admitted to either a skilled- or intermediate-level facility.

The Most Intense Level of Care: Hospital

In 1984 there were 6,965 short-term general hospitals in the U.S., which is 93 hospitals fewer than existed in 1980 ("The Health Care Cost Squeeze," p. 23). These hospitals operated a total of 1.1 million beds. This compares to 23,000 nursing homes with 1.5 million beds in 1984 (Califano, p. 169).

Short-term general hospitals provided 5 beds per 1,000 Americans. In comparison, nursing homes provided 56 beds per 1,000 Americans 65 years and older (U.S. DHHS, 1981, p. 193). The average length of stay in hospitals was 7.6 days, and their average rate of occupancy had dropped to approximately 63% in 1985.

For the sake of efficiency, about 80% to 85% occupancy is necessary. The present low occupancy rate is leading numerous hospitals to consider competing with nursing homes by converting unused acute care beds into skilled-nursing beds.

Differences in the level of intensity of care between short-term general hospitals and nursing homes can be seen in the following statistics: short-term general hospital, 390 staff per 100 patients; nursing homes, 50 staff per 100 patients.

ROLES OF THE SNF IN THE LONG-TERM CARE CONTINUUM

The SNF has roles to play in each type of long-term care: home-based, community-based, and institutional care. For persons receiving care from a home health agency, the SNF serves primarily as a facility for restorative care after strokes or other debilitating experiences from which the patient can recover and return home. The SNF plays a similar role for participants in community-based programs, and for persons seeking respite care. For persons already in other long-term care institutions, such as congregate housing, the SNF plays a similar role. The SNF offers the continuation of long-term care for those persons, maintaining them at their highest functional levels.

Under the Diagnostically Related Groups approach to hospital reimbursement, the SNF is increasingly interacting with hospitals seeking placement of Medicare patients still needing skilled nursing but not at the acute-care level of the hospital.

1.14.4 Additional Resources of the SNF: Churches, Community Groups, and Volunteers

Besides its association with the other caregivers in the long-term care continuum, the nursing facility has special relationships with several organizations in the community. Churches, schools, and other community groups, along with individual volunteers, are typically associated with caregiving in local SNFs.

Outliving one's peers is one of the more difficult adjustments in old age. For persons living to the age of 80 and beyond, the deaths of most of one's friends and family members is a sad reality. In every SNF facility there is a portion of the patient population with no one left who is interested in their welfare.

There is simply not enough money in the average nursing home budget to staff at a level sufficient to provide all of the human contact and caring that is needed by the patients. Even in those few instances where there are funds, such as the more expensive life-care communities or individual SNFs serving only privately paying patients, there is a qualitative difference between care offered by a paid staff member and what a volunteer from the community can bring to the situation. If the nursing home experience is to be fully humanized, this will occur only when there is sufficient contact between the patients and concerned community volunteers.

1.15 Profile of the Nursing Home Industry

Every day 5,000 Americans celebrate their 65th birthday and join the elderly sector of the population. In 1900, 4% of the population were aged 65 or older. In 1980, 11% of the population were in that group. In 2030, 18% of the population is expected to be 65 years or older. See Table 1-1.

TABLE 1-1. U.S. Population 65 Years of Age or Over
and Percentage of Total Population: Selected Years and
Projections 1950–2030

Year	No. 65 or over in thousands	% of U.S. population
1950	12,397	8.1
1970	20,087	9.9
1980	24,927	11.2
2000	31,822	12.2
2010	34,837	12.7
2020	45,102	15.5
2030	55,024	18.3

Source: U.S. Bureau of the Census as referenced in Doty, P., Korbin, L. and Wiener, J. "An Overview of Long Term Care," HEALTH CARE FINANCING REVIEW Spring, 1985, Vol. 6, No. 3, p. 69.

INCREASED LIFE EXPECTANCY

Increased life expectancy accounts for much of the change in the elderly population. Since 1900 life expectancy has increased from 46 years to 73.7 years (Waldo & Lazenby, p. 1). Greater numbers of people are reaching age 65.

Increased Proportions of the "Old-Old"

As a group the elderly are growing older all the time. The 64-to-74 cohort (the "young-olds") will continue to increase at approximately the rate of the general population during the 1980s, but those 74 to 84 and those 85 and older will increase at twice the rate of the general population (Liu, Manton, & Allston, p. 84). Thus, by the year 2000, a full quarter of the elderly are predicted to be old-old. See Table 1-2.

TABLE 1-2. Percent Increases in U.S. Population for 10-Year Intervals, by Age Groups: Selected Years and Projections 1950–2010

Year	All ages	65–74 years	75–84 years	85 years or over
1950–1960	18.7	30.1	41.2	59.3
1960–1970	13.4	13.0	31.7	52.3
1970–1980	8.7	23.4	14.2	44.6
1980–1990	10.0	13.8	26.6	20.1
1990–2000	7.1	−2.6	15.6	29.4
2000–2010	6.2	13.3	−2.4	19.4

Source: U.S. Bureau of the Census as referenced in Doty, P., Korbin, L. and Wiener, J. "An Overview of Long Term Care" HEALTH CARE FINANCING REVIEW Spring, 1985, Vol. 6, No. 3, page 69.

Fewer Men, More Women

As the elderly grow older, their age group becomes more and more dominated by women. In 1900, men in all age groups outnumbered women 102 to 100, but by 1975 the ratio had reversed, with men being outnumbered by women: 69 men for every 100 women. By 1990 this is expected to be further reduced to 66 men for every 100 women. This preponderance of women is even more pronounced in the 75 and older age group: the ratio of men to women for 1900 in this age group was 96 men for every 100 women; in 1975 this had decreased to 58 men per 100 women; and in 1990, even fewer—54 men—are expected to be alive for every 100 women.

PROPORTIONS IN INSTITUTIONS

Most of the elderly live outside institutions. About 1 out of 20 persons aged 65 and over reside in nursing homes at any one time. For those over 75, however, the proportion increases to 1 in 10 (Vladeck, p. 1). One of every five persons aged 65 and older will eventually spend time in a nursing home (Pegels, p. 82).

Projected Increases in Nursing Home Utilization

In Table 1-3, column 1 shows projections of nursing home utilization in the future. Thus, if these projections by the National Center for Health Statistics and the Social Security Administration are accurate, the number of persons in nursing homes will increase by over 300% during the years 1985 to 2040.

Table 1-3 also depicts an increasing need for assistance from spouses, offspring, other relatives, and even nonrelatives during this same time

TABLE 1-3. Projections of Daily Volume of Long-Term Care Assistance, by Source of Assistance: 1980–2040

Year	Source of assistance				
	Institution[1]	Spouse[2]	Offspring[2]	Other relative[2]	Non-relative[2]
	Number in thousands				
1980	1,187	1,442	1,436	1,213	655
1985	1,411	1,612	1,701	1,414	771
1990	1,623	1,801	1,950	1,610	880
1995	1,861	1,953	2,232	1,814	1,003
2000	2,081	2,049	2,484	1,989	1,110
2020	2,805	2,976	3,392	2,728	1,530
2040	4,354	3,900	5,172	4,028	2,298

[1]These projections refer to a full day of care in an institution.
[2]These projections refer to the number of episodes of caregiving on a given day.

SOURCE: Preliminary data from the Department of Health and Human Services, 1982 National Long-Term Care Survey, 1977 National Nursing Home Survey, National Center for Health Statistics, and Social Security Administration projections as referenced in Doty, P., Korbin, L. and Wiener, J. "An Overview of Long Term Care" HEALTH CARE FINANCING REVIEW Spring, 1985, Vol. 6, No. 3, p. 71.

span. To the extent these noninstitutional resources are unavailable, the number of persons needing institutional care may actually be larger than projected in Table 1-3.

INCREASING DEPENDENCY LEVELS AMONG THE AGED

As individuals age, they become susceptible to chronic conditions (explored in depth in Part 5). Therefore, it is no surprise to learn that aged Americans also dominate the dependent population. Of people dependent on others for bathing, dressing, toileting, feeding, or any combination of these activities (called the Activities of Daily Living), approximately 7 in every 10 are elderly (Weissert, p. 11).

The elderly have higher dependency rates than the non-aged population, and aged women are much more likely to have dependency in mobility and personal care than aged men. Old-old female nonwhites are especially hard hit. Their dependency rates are double those for white males and triple those of nonwhite males. The population at risk for institutionalization is most likely those elderly who need personal care assistance. Studies have shown that nearly 20 times as many nursing home residents need this type of assistance compared to those needing mobility assistance (Weissert, p. 13).

1.15.1 Nursing Homes

In the mid-1980s, the total number of nursing homes in the United States was approximately 23,000 with 1.5 million beds. A final and fully accurate figure is difficult to determine because of varying definitions of countable beds.

The National Center for Health Statistics (NCHS) has conducted the National Master Facility Inventory (NMFI) approximately every 2 years since 1963. The NCHS defines the nursing home as a home that maintains "three or more beds, and at a minimum, provides one or more personal care services" (Sirocco, p. 1). Thus, even though the NCHS statistics are accurate, they may not include homes counted or not counted by other surveys.

INCREASES IN NURSING HOMES

The number of nursing homes rose dramatically between 1939 (1,200) and 1961 (9,900), then growth slowed somewhat (Lane, p. 11). Table 1-4 illustrates the rise in number of facilities and beds. As indicated in the table, these numbers are approximate and will vary from survey to survey, depending on the definition of nursing facility.

The approximate percentages of market shares is shown in Table 1-5. These data suggest that for-profit homes may be smaller in size than not-for-profit homes and that government homes tend to be large in size. The

TABLE 1-4. Estimates of Number of Nursing Facilities and Beds: 1960–1984

	1960[a]	1973[b]	1977[c]	1980	1984[e]
Facilities	9,582	15,800	18,300	23,065[d]	23,000
Beds	331,000	1,175,000	1,385,600	1,400,000	1,500,000

Sources:
[a] From Pegels, p. 81.
[b] From U.S. Public Health Service, National Center for Health Statistics, *Selected Operating and Financial Characteristics of Nursing Homes, U.S.: 1973–1974* National Nursing Home Survey, Series 13, No. 22, Table 2, p. 11 (in Kart et al. p. 202.)
[c] From National Center for Health Statistics. "An Overview of Nursing Home Characteristics: Provisional Data from the 1977 National Nursing Home Survey." Advance Data, no. 35, DHEW (DHHS) Pub. No. (PHS 78-150). Hyattsville, MD. September 6, 1978. (Table 13-2 in Kart, p. 293.)
[d] From Sirocco, A. (in preparation).
[e] From Califano (1986) p. 169. The number of nursing homes and beds varies among surveys due to changes in the definition of a nursing facility. The 23,065 figure includes a number of smaller "residential type" facilities that were previously not counted, thus changes in the figures do not necessarily represent new construction.

TABLE 1-5. Sponsorship of Nursing Facilities, 1984 by Percent

	% Facilities	% Beds
For profit	77	70
Not for profit	18	22
Governmental	5	8

Califano, (1986). p. 169.

percentage of facilities and beds owned by the for-profit sector of the industry is expected to increase as the chains continue a policy of purchasing additional freestanding facilities.

Restricting the Supply of New Beds

Various factors have contributed to a slowdown in construction of nursing facilities. This has, however, strengthened the financial picture of the industry. A 9-year low in the ratios of debt to net worth was reported in 1981. Profit margins for 1982 were the third highest in 15 years of tracking data (Morton Research as reported in Lane, p. 12). This deceleration in the production of new beds combined with the increasing number of elderly in need of nursing home beds has resulted in a high occupancy rate in nearly all states.

NURSING HOME EMPLOYMENT RATES

Nursing home employment has increased steadily over the past several years, due in part at least, to the combined effects of restrictions on the bed supply and the increasing proportion of Americans living to advanced age. Nursing home employment increased 3.8% in 1984, 5.4% in 1985 and at an annual rate of 6% in the first half of 1986. In contrast, hospital employment decreased 1.1% in 1984, .2% in 1985, perhaps due to the pressures of the Medicare DRG prospective fixed reimbursement rates regardless of length of hospital stay (Update Weekly, p. 2).

Other Effects of Restricting the Supply of New Beds

Building constraints have encouraged the larger proprietary nursing homes to purchase smaller ones in order to expand (Lane, p. 14). Thus, in recent years the number of beds held by larger nursing home chains has steadily increased.

Another trend possibly stimulated by the slowdown of nursing home construction is diversification of activities into other health care market areas. *Vertical integration*, the linking of services within the health care industry that provide care to different categories of patients, became an attractive alternative. Thus, nursing homes have begun continuing-care retirement communities, adult day-care centers, and programs linked to nutrition programs under the Older Americans Act (Lane, p. 14; Hill Haven/Brim to Build 22 New Retirement Centers, p. 1).

Other nursing homes have moved into areas outside long-term care and have begun to purchase acute-care hospitals or to establish health maintenance organizations for the elderly, which are called Social Health Maintenance Organizations (SHMOS). Some of the proprietary chains (usually the smaller companies) have moved into other fields, such as housing for special groups (Lane, p. 14).

NURSING HOME BED RATES

Nursing home bed rates, i.e., the number of nursing home beds per 1,000 persons aged 65 and over, vary geographically. The West North Central states have a bed rate of nearly double that of the South Atlantic region. These rates vary greatly among individual states from a low of 22 in Florida to a high of 94 in Wisconsin (Lane, p. 10).

A study of the map reveals that states having severe cold conditions tend to provide more beds per 1,000 persons aged 65 and over than the more southern states, where the climate is less threatening to survival of elderly persons.

Other analyses suggest that states may also utilize their nursing home beds differently. California, for example, appears to use SNF beds predominantly for short-term restorative nursing care, whereas the northern states assign them for longer-term care of older persons.

FACILITY SIZES AND OCCUPANCY RATES

Two-thirds of all nursing homes in this country have fewer than 75 beds. Occupancy rates tend to be high overall, with an average of 90% across the nation with only a small fluctuation. A few states—Texas, for example— have lower occupancy rates. This is probably due to the absence of any restrictions on building nursing homes, resulting in apparent overbuilding in that state.

MEDICAID–MEDICARE PARTICIPATION RATES

Three-quarters of all nursing homes are certified to accept Medicaid. Of these, 19% are SNFs, 24% give combined skilled and intermediate care, and 32% intermediate care only (Lloyd & Greenspan, p. 136).

TURNOVER

The number of admissions per year per 10 beds is a measure of turnover. Turnover appears to be highest in proprietary homes and in medium-size facilities (75–200 beds). Turnover varies considerably across geographic regions, with the highest ratio of admission per 10 beds in the West, reflecting a preference for short-term-stay patients.

Turnover rate may also vary with the admissions philosophy of the administrator. Some nursing homes, primarily those near hospitals, may specialize in providing rehabilitative care and value a high turnover rate of, say, 20% to 30% of patients per month. Other nursing homes may, by policy, seek a more stable patient population through admitting primarily longer-term care patients, thus experiencing a turnover rate of 5% to 8% per month.

Location can affect the policy options available to the administrator. In highly urbanized areas the administrator typically can, through admission policies, determine the relative turnover rate. In primarily rural areas, the administrator may experience a low turnover rate regardless of her/his preferences.

1.15.2 Who Pays?

In 1985, 10.7% of the gross national product was spent for health care. This amounted to $425 billion or $1,721 per person ("Health-care Spending Rises 8.9%," p. 12a). This percentage has climbed steadily from approximately 6% of the gross national product in 1965. In 1960 Americans paid $500 million for nursing home care. In 1984 Americans paid $32 billion for nursing home care. In 1990 Americans may pay $60 billion for nursing home care (Califano, p. 168).

Part of the growth is due to rapid expansion in intermediate-care facilities for the mentally retarded (ICFMR). Medicaid benefits for these facilities began in 1972, and since that time there has been an average increase in this type of facility of 40% per year (Gibson et al., p. 9).

Medicaid pays approximately half of all nursing home expenditures, while Medicare pays less than 2% (Harrington & Swan, p. 39). Midway through the decade of the 1980s, nursing home costs were shared in approximately the following proportions: Medicaid, 48%; private individuals, 44%; insurance, 6%; Medicare, 2% (Harrington & Swan, pp. 39–49).

TABLE 1-6. U.S. Total Expenditures for Nursing Home Care and Annual Percentage Change: Calendar Years 1960–1990

Year	Expenditures ($ billions)	Annual % change
1960	.5	—
1965	2.1	64.0
1970	4.7	24.7
1971	5.6	19.1
1972	6.5	16.1
1973	7.1	9.2
1974	8.5	19.7
1975	10.1	18.8
1976	11.4	12.9
1977	13.2	15.8
1978	15.2	15.2
1979	17.6	15.8
1980	20.6	17.1
1981	24.2	17.5
1982	27.3	12.8
1984	32	—
1990	60 (estimate)	—

Source: Data for 1960–1982 referenced by Health Care Financing Administration Office of Financial and Actuarial Analysis, in Doty, Korbin, & Wiener (1985, p. 70). Data for 1984 and 1990 from Califano (1986, p. 168).

"SPENDING DOWN"

Nationally, the monthly bills for care for almost half of the patients in nursing homes are paid for by Medicaid. How does this come about? As an individual's health fails and his/her age advances, personal savings and other resources are used up at a faster and faster pace. Typically, a person enters a long-term care facility as a private paying patient. Monthly bills for care, which can range up to $4,000 and more per month, steadily reduce the financial resources of the patient. Approximately half of Medicaid nursing home recipients were not initially poor but "spent down" to Medicaid eligibility levels as a result of high medical costs (Washington Report on Medicine and Health, insert, p. 1). When patients have used up their financial resources on health care and have literally spent down to some figure—approximately $1,000 of assets remaining—they become eligible for Medicaid, and the shift is made from being a private paying patient to becoming a Medicaid patient.

REFERENCES TO PART ONE

Allport, F.H. (1962). A structuronomic conception of behavior. *Journal of Abnormal and Social Psychology.* pp. 3–30.

Barnard, C.I. (1938). *The functions of the executive.* Cambridge, MA: Harvard University Press.

Bertalanffy, von, L. (1967). Der Organismus als Physikalishes System Betrachtet. In D. Katz & R.L. Kahn, *The social psychology of organizations.* New York: John Wiley & Sons. (Reprinted from *Naturwissenschaften,* 1940, *28*).

Blake, J.B. (1959). *Public health in the town of Boston.* Cambridge, MA: Harvard University Press.

Boling, T.E. Vrooman, D.M., & Sommers, K.M. (1983). *Nursing home management.* Springfield IL: Charles C Thomas.

Bradley, D.F., & Calvin, M. (1956). Behavior: Imbalance in a network of chemical transformations. In *General systems yearbook of the Society for the Advancement of General Systems Theory* (Vol. 1), pp. 56–65.

Britton, J.H., & Britton, J.O. (1972). *Personality changes in aging.* New York: Springer Publishing Co.

Buttaro, P.J. (1980). *Home study program in principles of administration of long term care facilities.* Aberdeen, SD: Health Care Facility Consultants.

Califano, J.A., Jr. (1986). *America's health care revolution.* New York: Random House.

Childe, V.G. (1951). *Man makes himself.* New York: New American Library.

Christensen, C.R., Berg, N.A., & Salter, M.S. (1980). *Policy formulation and administration* (8th ed.). Homewood, IL: Richard D. Irwin.

Clement, P.F. (1985). History of U.S. aged's poverty shows welfare program changes. *Perspectives on Aging, 9*(2) 4–7.

Dainton, C. (1961). *The story of England's hospitals.* Springfield, IL: Charles C Thomas.

Dale, E. (1969). *Management: Theory and practice* (2nd ed.). New York: McGraw Hill.

Davis, W.E. (1985). *Introduction to health care administration.* Bossier City, LA: Publicare Press.

Dearden, J., & McFarlan, F.W. (1966). *Management information systems: Text and cases.* Homewood, IL: Richard D. Irwin.

DeGroot, M.H. (1970). *Optimal statistical decisions.* New York: McGraw Hill.

Demski, J.S. (1980). *Information analysis* (2nd ed.). Reading, MA: Addison-Wesley.

Doty, P., Korbin, L., & Wiener, J. (1985). An overview of long term care. *Health Care Financing Review, 6*(3), 69–71.

Drucker, P.F. (1954). *The practice of management.* New York: Harper and Row.

FactSheet. (1985). National Association of Home Care, Richmond Virginia, November 30–December 6, 12 pp.

Falek, J.I. (1986). "The Administrator Sets the Environment," *Provider, 12*(10), 8–10.

French, J.R.P., Jr., & Raven, B.H. (1960). The bases of social power. In D. Cartwright & A. Zander (Eds.), *Group dynamics: Research and Theory* (2nd. ed.). Evanston, IL: Row, Peterson.

Freymann, J.G. (1980). *The American health care system: Its genesis and trajectory.* Huntington, NY: Robert E. Krieger Publishing.

George, C.S., Jr. (1972). *The history of management thought* (2nd. ed.). Englewood Cliffs, NJ: Prentice Hall.

Germain, C.B. (1984). *Social work practice in health care.* New York: The Free Press.

Gibson, R.M., Levit, K.R., Lazenby, H., & Waldo, D.R. (1984). "National health expenditures, 1983." *Health Care Financing Review, 6*(2), 1–29.

Glueck, W.F. (1982). *Personnel: A diagnostic approach* (3rd ed., rev. by G.T. Milkovich). Plano, TX: Business Publishers.

Gordon, G.K., & Stryker, R. (1983). *Creative long term care administration.* Springfield, IL: Charles C Thomas.

Gulick, L., & Gulick, L. (eds.). (1937). *Papers on the science of administration.* New York: Institute of Public Administration.

Harrington, C., & Swan, J. (1984). Medicaid nursing home reimbursement policies, rates and expenditures. *Health Care Financing Review, 6*(1), 39–49.

Health-care Spending Rises 8.9%. (1986, July 30). *News and Observer,* p. 12a. Raleigh, NC.

The Health Care Cost Squeeze. (1986). *Medical Meetings, 13*(2), 20–29.

Hillhaven/Brim to Build 22 Retirement Centers. *Today's Nursing Home, 7*(10), 1–3.

Hogstel, M.O. (1983). *Management of personnel in long term care.* Bowie, MD: Robert J. Brady Co.

Hunter, R.J. (1955). *The origin of the Philadelphia General Hospital.* Philadelphia: Rittenhouse Press.

Jackson, J. (1960). The organization and its communication problems. In A. Grimshaw & J.W. Hennessey, Jr., *Organizational behavior: Cases and readings.* New York: McGraw Hill.

Jonas, S. (1981). *Health care delivery in the United States.* New York: Springer Publishing Co.

Kaplan, B. (1985). Social Security: 50 years later. *Perspectives on Aging, 9*(2), 4–7.

Kart, C.S. (1981). *The realities of aging.* Boston: Allyn and Bacon.

Kart, C.S., Metress, E.S., & Mettress, J.F. (1978). *Aging and health.* Menlo Park, CA: Addison-Wesley.

Katz, D., & Kahn, R.L. (1967). *The social psychology of organizations.* New York: John Wiley and Sons.

Keeler, E.B., Kane, R.L., & Solomon, D. (1981). Short and long term residents of nursing homes. *Medical Care, 19*(3), 363–369.

Keen, P.G.W., & Woodman, L.A. (1984). What to do with all those micros. *Harvard Business Review, 62*(5) 142–150.

Kotter, J.P. (1982). *The general managers.* New York: The Free Press.

Lane, L.F. (1984, January). Developments in facility-based services. Prepared for the National Institute of Medicine's Nursing Home Study Commission, unpublished paper.

Levey, S., & Loomba, N.P. (1973). *Health care administration: A managerial perspective.* Philadelphia: J.B. Lippincott.

Likert, R. (1961). *New patterns of management.* New York: McGraw Hill.

Likert, R. (1967). *The human organization: Its management and value.* New York: McGraw Hill.

Liu, K., Manton, K.G., & Liu, B. Mar Zetta, "Home Care Expenses for the Disabled Elderly" *Health Care Financing Review.* Washington, D.C., Volume 7, No. 2, Winter, 1985, pp. 51–58.

Liu, K., Manton, K., & Allston, W. (1982). Demographic and epidemiological determinants of expenditures. In R. Vogel & H. Palmer (Eds.), *Long term care*. (pp. 81–132). Washington, DC: Health Care Financing Administration, Department of Health and Human Services.

Lloyd, S., & Greenspan, N.T. (1987). Nursing homes, home health care, and adult day care. In R. Vogel & H. Palmer (Eds.), *Long term care*. Washington, DC: Health Care Financing Administration, Department of Health and Human Services.

Long term care insurance. (1985, April 22). *Washington Report on Medicine and Health, 39*(16), 4.

McGibony, J.R. (1969). *Principles of hospital administration* (2nd ed.) New York: G.P. Putnam's Sons.

Meal, H.C. (1984). Putting production decisions where they belong. *Harvard Business Review, 62*(2), 102–111.

Miller, D.B. (Ed.). (1982). *Long term care administrator's desk manual*. Greenvale, NY: Panel Publishers.

Miller, D.B., & Barry, J.T. (1979). *Nursing home organization and operation*. Boston: CBI Publishing.

Miller, J.G. (1955). Toward a general theory for the behavioral sciences. *American Psychologist, 10*, 513–531.

Mintzberg, H. (1979). *The structuring of organizations: A synthesis of the research*. Englewood Cliffs, NJ: Prentice Hall.

Muse, D.N., & Sawyer, D. (1982). *The Medicare and Medicaid databook*. Washington, DC: Department of Health and Human Services, Health Care Financing Administration.

National Association of Boards of Examiners for Nursing Home Administrators. (1986). *Mid-Year Meeting, November 11–12* (64 pp.). Park Suite Hotel, Oklahoma City, OK.

Pegels, C. (1981). *Health care and the elderly*. Rockville, MD: Aspen Books.

Pfeffer, J., & Salancik, G.R. (1978). *The external control of organizations*. New York: Harper and Row.

Pressman, J.L., & Wildavsky, A.B. (1974). *Implementation*. Berkeley, CA: University of California Press.

Prospective payment: DRG era dawns. (1983, September 5). *Medicine and health*.

Robey, D. (1982). *Designing organizations*. Homewood, IL: Richard D. Irwin, Inc.

Rogers, W.W. (1980). *General administration in the nursing home* (3rd ed.). Boston: CBI Publishing.

Rudensky, M. "SNF's may get prospective prices." *Modern Healthcare*, August 29, 1986, p. 36–37.

Shackle, G.L.S. (1957). *Uncertainty and business decisions: A symposium* (2nd ed.). Liverpool: Liverpool University Press.

Simon, H.A. (1960). *The new science of management decision*. New York: Harper and Row.

Sirocco, A. (in preparation). An overview of the 1980 national facility inventory survey of nursing and related care homes.

Spicker, S.F., & Ingman, S.R. (Eds.). (1984). *Vitalizing long term care: The teaching nursing home and other perspectives*. New York: Springer Publishing Co.

Starr, P. (1982). *The social transformation of American medicine*. New York:

Basic Books.

Steinberg, R.M., & Carter, G.W. (1983). *Case management and the elderly.* Lexington, MA: Lexington Books.

Swiss, J.E. (1983). Establishing a management system: The interaction of power shifts and personality under federal MBO. *Public Administration Review,* 43(3), 238–245.

Tannenbaum, R., Wechsler, I., & Massarik, F. (1961). *Leadership and organization.* New York: McGraw Hill.

Terry, G.R. (1969). *Principles of management.* Homewood, IL: Richard D. Irwin, Inc.

Thomas, W.C., Jr. (1969). *Nursing homes and public policy: Drift and decision in New York State.* Ithaca, NY: Cornell University Press.

TransCentury Corporation. (1975). *Adult day care in the U.S.: A comparative study.* Washington, DC: National Center for Health Services Research.

U.S. Department of Health, Education and Welfare. (1979). *Older Americans Act of 1965, as amended, history and related acts.* Washington, DC: Administration on Aging, Office of Human Development Services.

U.S. Department of Health and Human Services. (1981). *Long term care: Background and future directions.* Washington, DC: U.S. Department of Health and Human Services, Health Care Financing Aministration. (HCFA 81-20047).

U.S. Department of Health and Human Services. (1981). *Health U.S.: 1981.* Washington, DC: Public Health Service.

U.S. Department of Health and Human Services. (1981). *Need for long term care: Information and issues.* Washington, DC: Federal Council on the Aging, Office of Human Development Services. [DHHS Publication No. (OHDS) 81-20704]

U.S. Department of Health and Human Services. (1985). *Your Medicare Handbook.* Washington, DC: Health Care Financing Administration. (Publication No. HCFA-10050).

U.S. National Center for Health Statistics. (1979). *The national nursing home survey: 1977 summary for the United States.* Hyattsville, MD: DHEW (DHHS) Public Health Service, Office of Health Research, Statistics, and Technology. (Series 13, No. 43).

Update Weekly. (1986, October 23). North Carolina Health Care Facilities Association, Raleigh, NC. Issue 450, p. 2.

Vladeck, B. (1980). *Unloving care.* New York: Basic Books.

Vogel, R.J., & Palmer, H.C. (Eds.). (1982). *Long term care: Perspectives from research and demonstrations.* Washington, DC: U.S. Department of Health and Human Services, Health Care Financing Administration.

Waldo, D.R., & Lazenby, H.C. (1984). Demographic characteristics and health care use and expenditures by the aged in the U.S.: 1977–1984. *Health Care Financing Review,* 6(1), 1–29.

Washington Report on Medicine and Health. (April, 1985). *Long Term Care Insurance.*

Weissert, W. (April, 1985). *Estimating the Long Term Care Population: National Prevalence Rates and Selected Characteristics.* Report for the Office of the Assistant Secretary for Planning and Evaluation, U.S. Department of Health and Human Services.

Wrapp, H.E. (1984). Good managers don't make policy decisions. *Harvard*

Business Review, *84*(4) 6–120.

Zmud, R.W. (1983). *Information systems in organizations.* Dallas, TX: Scott Foresman.

PART TWO

Personnel

2.1 Identifying the Personnel Functions

Managers in organizations have always performed certain basic personnel functions.

PERSONNEL FUNCTIONS

Personnel functions are a range of activities that can include record keeping, employee recruitment and selection, training and development, compensation management, performance evaluation, and often labor relations (Chruden & Sherman, p. 23):

Record keeping—assuring that all necessary information is in the employee's file and that it is kept confidential

Recruitment—assisting department heads in finding employees for vacant positions

Selection—assisting department heads in interviewing and assessing job applicants

Training and retaining employees—assisting department heads in employee orientation, in-service training, and continuing education

Compensation management—assisting department heads and payroll office in administering salary and the other benefits offered by the facility

Performance evaluation—assisting managers in conducting employee appraisals in conformity with the facility personnel policies

Labor relations—assisting managers in creating a favorable work environment

PERSONNEL MANAGEMENT AS AN OCCUPATION

In his text *Personnel Management*, Chruden says that in its rudimentary state, personnel was the responsibility of each department supervisor. He speculates that as the department supervisor's job became more complex, the responsibility for certain personnel activities, e.g., hours worked and payroll, were taken over by a clerical assistant. From this initial record-keeping activity, the responsibilities were gradually broadened until individuals began making a full-time career in what is now called personnel administration.

Personnel managers do not "manage" employees except for those who work under them in the personnel department, if there is more than one employee in that unit. *Personnel management is a staff function; it has no line authority in the organization.* All of the employees in the organization are directly managed by their department supervisors, who hold line authority. It is the line managers who, in fact, are responsible for performing most of the personnel functions for the employees under them. The department heads do the actual hiring, require in-service training and development, give performance appraisals and promotions, award raises, and discipline, suspend, and fire their staff.

The role of the personnel manager and staff is to assist the line supervisors, e.g., the department heads in the nursing facility, to carry out their personnel responsibilities according to the personnel policies set by facility ownership. The personnel staff make an important contribution to overall employee satisfaction by making sure that personnel policies are carried out consistently from department to department.

2.2 Planning Employment Needs: Writing Job Descriptions

In Part 1 we indicated the need for each facility to break down all work to be accomplished into a set of activities that can be performed by one person. Several definitions provided by the U.S. Employment Service and the U.S. Office of Personnel Management may be useful to review at this point (Ivancevich et al., p. 98).

Job analysis—the process of defining a job in terms of tasks or behaviors required and specifying the qualifications of the employee to be placed in that job.

Job description—information about the job that results in a statement of the job to be done, usually including a list of duties and responsibilities of the job in order of importance. Typically, a job description includes (a) the title, (b) the qualifications, (c) to whom the worker is primarily responsible, and (d) the duties or specific expectations (Boling, p. 50).

Job specification—a statement of the skills, education and experience required to perform the work. This is derived from the job description.

Job titles (or job classifications)—that which distinguishes one job from all others. Job titles may also indicate the occupational level of the job (e.g., nurse supervisor indicates a higher position (administratively, at least) than registered nurse) or the level of authority or seniority of the job, e.g., registered nurse, levels 1, 2, and 3.

Task—a coordinated and aggregated series of work elements used to produce an output (e.g., making beds).

Position—the responsibilities and duties performed by one individual. There are as many positions as there are employees.

Job—a group of positions that are similar in their duties, e.g., laundry, housekeeping, and grounds.

Job family—a group of two or more jobs that have similar duties, e.g., the duties of the registered nurses and the licensed practical nurses. (Ivancevich et al., p. 98, p. 100).

All of the work to be accomplished in operating a nursing facility must be broken down into a series of tasks. Tasks are grouped together so that they can be performed by one individual.

Job analysis is the process of grouping a series of related tasks into a position. Each position can then be described in terms of the tasks and behaviors involved and of the education and training needed to perform the job successfully.

POTENTIAL PROBLEMS WITH JOB DESCRIPTIONS

The federal government examines job descriptions and specification for possible discriminatory effects. Each of the requirements for a job must be necessary for the adequate performance of that job. If, for example, a nursing facility in an area with an unusually large number of available job applicants required 2 years of college for applicants for the nurse's aide position, it must be able to demonstrate why this is essential to perform the job, that is, that the requirement has proven validity. This is a higher educational requirement than usual; therefore, the facility would be obliged to prove that it did not serve to discriminate against members of a particular group on the basis of sex or ethnic origins.

Once job descriptions have been written and the expected work load of the facility estimated, future employment needs can be forecast.

2.3 Forecasting Future Employment Needs

The planning process begins with a projection of the number of persons the facility expects to serve over a period of time, usually during the next 1 to 5 years. This forecast can then be translated into specific personnel requirements for the future period.

TAKING A MANPOWER INVENTORY

Numerous factors must be taken into account in projecting the present and future availability of qualified personnel in sufficient number. This is the process of taking a manpower inventory.

Several sources of employment information exist. The Employment Security Commission and the Department of Labor gather data that are useful in estimating the future availability of needed employees.

Identifying Trends

Data such as those mentioned help to identify trends. A number of trends are of potential importance.

Competition for Personnel. It is practical to take an inventory of present and planned health and related facilities that are or will be competing for similarly qualified personnel. For example, if no acute-care hospital exists in the geographic area, but a large for-profit hospital is expected to be constructed within 2 years, competition may increase dramatically. Or, similarly, if the local hospital is expected to close its doors within the next 2 years, the labor pool may be suddenly increased.

In-Migration or Out-Migration Patterns in the Labor Supply.   Knowledge of whether the worker pool from which employees must be chosen is shrinking or enlarging is important.

Wage Scale Movements in the Area.   An increasing worker pool may reduce wage scales, while a shrinking worker pool may cause the wage scale to rise.

Expected Impacts of Local Educational Institutions.   Educational institutions such as community colleges are becoming major sources of training for manpower needed by nursing facilities. Any expected increase or decrease in training activities, e.g., the addition or closing of a licensed practical nurse program in the local community college, could dramatically affect the availability of labor, especially trained nurse's aides.

Knowledge of these trends can assist planners to take action before an anticipated employment crisis. If, for example, a shortage is foreseen, the facility might join with other local facilities in a program to attract additional health-related personnel to the area.

2.4 Recruiting Employees

Once the forecast of persons expected to be served has been translated into specific personnel requirements for the facility, they become the basis for the recruitment and selection program. The forecast assists the facility in determining the number and types of employees it will need to recruit as well as the sources for recruitment.

Here we will consider only the process of locating and recruiting applicants for jobs in the facility. Interviewing and hiring will be discussed later.

INFLUENCE OF AFFIRMATIVE ACTION

Since the passage of the Civil Rights Act in 1964, the process of seeking new employees has become more public. Prior to 1964, facilities could choose employees without being examined by government agencies with regard to possible job discrimination based on age, sex, race, marital status, religion, national origin, or handicap (Miller, 1979, p. 31).

Today government agencies can review for possible legal violations by examining the following: (a) the facility's list of recruitment sources for each job category; (b) recruitment advertising; (c) statistics on the number of applicants processed by personal category (e.g., sex, age, race) and by job category and level (Ivancevich et al., p. 157).

The government may require a nursing home chain or an individual facility to recruit qualified employees whose group is not well represented in their present staff. If, for example, there are no black nurses on the staff and the government ascertains that the facility does not advertise its job openings at black nursing schools or in newspapers or other sources normally used by blacks seeking jobs, the government may require that a governmentally defined Equal Employment Opportunity program be used by that facility or chain.

Many employers are under governmental pressure to increase the number of minority members and women employed in the facility, especially at the higher levels from which these groups have traditionally been excluded (Chruden, p. 90). Requiring a facility to increase the proportion of women or minority persons is called *ratio hiring*.

INFLUENCE OF THE LABOR MARKET

The labor market is the geographic area from which applicants are to be recruited.

Recruitment for a new administrator or director of nurses may be national in scope. The new administrator may be willing to move across the country. When staffing for jobs requiring little skill, the scope of the labor market will tend to be a relatively small geographic area surrounding the facility. The new janitor or nurse's aide is unlikely to be willing, or economically able, to move to accept a position at the facility.

If there is a surplus of labor at recruiting time, the facility may be flooded with applications. If there is a shortage, on the other hand, it may take considerable initiative to find and hire well-trained staff.

Impacts of Transportation

The ease with which employees can commute to the facility will have a direct impact on the geographic area from which the facility can recruit. The absence of an efficient public transportation system, especially for evening and night workers, will oblige the facility to hire only persons who have access to automobiles, or can walk to work.

Nursing facilities in the central city face special problems in finding suitable employees. Population migration to the suburbs traditionally leaves less-qualified persons living in the central city, a place to which suburbanites are little inclined to commute. Some larger institutions have arranged special transportation to and from work for suburban employees in an effort to attract competent staff.

RECRUITMENT SOURCES

A number of sources for recruitment exist, both within and outside the facility. Present employees may be the best source.

Present Employees

The current employees of the facility can be the primary source for filling vacancies above the beginning level. Facility hiring policies will determine the extent to which present employees are viewed as the initial source of recruitment for those openings.

Hiring from among present employees is a policy decision to promote from within. There are a number of advantages to such a policy.

Career Ladders

Career ladders are paths along which the employee can hope to progress. They constitute a major source of employee incentive and satisfaction. Persons entering the facility are encouraged to stay if there is reasonable expectation that, when openings occur, there will be advancement possibilities from within the organization. This practice stimulates employees to develop skills that will be necessary to qualify for promotion.

Job Posting and Job Bidding

A job that becomes available is literally posted on appropriate bulletin boards, and employees are encouraged to bid, or apply. Through this device employees become more aware of the actual requirements of positions and the selection processes for filling vacancies. Advancement of present employees has the obvious advantage of recognizing and rewarding successful workers. It also has benefits for the facility by placing a person who already has some understanding of the organization and is loyal to its policies.

However, invariably hiring from within may measurably slow the process of introducing persons with new ideas and fresh approaches into the facility. There are times when the management may purposely seek to bring in an outsider who will be expected to reorganize or reshape a department or work area.

Outside Sources

Unless it is planned to reduce the size of the staff, every vacancy presents the organization with an option to promote from within or hire from without.

A promotion from within might trigger a series of promotions. If the nursing supervisor is promoted to director of nursing, the charge nurse may be moved up to nursing supervisor, and the senior registered nurse to charge nurse, thus creating an opportunity for several moves up in seniority or level and eventually opening a beginning registered nurse position. Any vacancy, if filled from within, will eventually result in hiring a new person from an outside source. Some of the more common outside sources are discussed below.

Referrals. Employees, patients, and relatives of patients are good sources of referrals. Satisfied employees, patients, and their relatives constitute a valuable asset for the recruiting effort.

Employee referrals can be especially beneficial. When a staff member's recommendation is accepted, he/she is receiving special recognition by the facility. In addition, the employee will have a vested interest in assisting the recruit to adjust to the environment and to be productive. However, the facility must be careful to avoid referrals that lead to nepotism (favoring one's family members) or to the formation of closely knit groups or cliques composed of persons who have close outside ties and tend to exclude others. Employee, patient, and family referrals are, in essence, word-of-mouth recommendations that reflect the reputation of the facility in the community.

Advertisements. Advertisement in appropriate media, such as newspapers and professional and trade journals, is one of the most common methods for contacting prospective applicants. For registered nurses, the professional journal may be the most appropriate medium. For nurse's aides and maintenance staff, the local newspaper will probably draw a better response.

Public Employment Agencies. The states operate local public employment agencies using federal payroll tax rebates from the U.S. Employment Service (USES). Public employment agencies can provide lists of individuals who are unemployed and currently drawing unemployment insurance benefits.

Private Employment Agencies. Agencies in the private sector offer specialized services, more closely matching the needs of the potential employer and employees. Fees are charged.

Most often the employee pays the agency. However, the employer sometimes shares in the fee and occasionally pays it altogether. The facility may also sign a contract with a private employment agency over a period of time. In this case, the contract should be carefully reviewed to avoid unwanted or unintended commitments, such as a fee to the agency for all new employees, whether found by the agency or the employer.

Search Firms. Search firms generally focus their efforts on middle- and upper-level management positions. Clients for search firms normally are employers who agree to pay the search firm for finding a suitable candidate. The search firm operates in a more far-flung geographic area than is normally possible for the employer, and it is able to offer a nationwide inventory. These firms can save employer time and energy by providing extensive screening before any candidate is recommended.

Educational Institutions. Accredited schools are an increasingly important source for nursing home personnel. Community colleges and technical institutes are training students not only for licensed practical nurse positions but also to be nurse's aides. This represents a valuable apprenticeship to several of the nursing facility's critical jobs.

Professional Organizations. Many professional organizations, such as nurses' associations, maintain rosters of their members who are seeking employment, which they publish in their journals and post at national or local meetings.

Unsolicited Applications. A number of unsolicited employment inquiries will arrive at the facility by mail or in person. Although the proportion of such applicants who are suitable may be low, there are nevertheless important reasons for careful attention to them. It is good public relations practice to extend courteous treatment to applicants who approach the facility on their own initiative and to deal with them candidly about the likelihood of employment with the organization.

Some administrators have noticed a tendency for long-term care employees to seek a change of job every few years. They may be entirely competent people who periodically look for a new work situation while remaining within the field of long-term care. Such individuals may submit unsolicited applications simply to let a facility know of their availability.

2.5 Hiring Employees

Recruitment is the process of locating prospective employees. Personnel selection is the process of deciding which of the applicants best fit the requirements of the job for which they are being considered (Owen, p. 14). Often, however, this prospective staff member is evaluated not only for one of several positions the organization has open at that moment, but simultaneously for anticipated slots expected in the near future.

Through experience, employers have learned that when individuals are carefully selected for clearly defined positions, the result is faster adjustment to the position, greater job satisfaction, and a minimum number of misfits between applicants and job needs in the organization (Chruden & Sherman, p. 114).

MEASURING THE IMPACTS OF LEGISLATION

Employers are directing greater attention to the job selection process. This is because of the often intense scrutiny given employers by the government enforcers of the Civil Rights Act of 1964, the Equal Employment Act of 1972, and other antidiscriminatory laws and regulations, such as the *Uniform Guidelines on Employee Selection Procedures* written by the Equal Employment Opportunity Commission.

The Civil Rights Act of 1964 prohibits discrimination in employment practices on the basis of race, color, religion, sex, or national origin. This act created the Equal Employment Opportunities Commission (EEOC) to implement the provisions of the Act. A later amendment, known as the Tower Amendment to Title 7, permitted the use of ability tests in employee selection procedures. Subsequently, the courts and the EEOC have made numerous rulings that determine the construction and uses of ability tests.

The Equal Employment Act of 1972 is an amendment to Title 7 of the Civil Rights Act of 1964 and is intended to cover all employers of 15 or more persons and numerous other groups, such as educational institutions. Enforcement machinery was authorized and subsequently set up. Today personnel policy is shaped by these acts as well as court decisions and regulations instituted by authorized governmental agencies. They affect such employment practices as retirement rules and treatment of pregnancy; they are discussed at greater length in Part 4 under the section "Management and Labor Legislation and Regulations."

In 1978 four federal agencies jointly published a far-reaching document entitled *Uniform Guidelines on Employee Selection Procedures* (EEOC, pp. 38295–38309), establishing the standards by which federal agencies determine the acceptability of validation procedures used for written tests and other selection devices (Chruden & Sherman, p. 122).

The guidelines require the employer to be able to demonstrate that the selection procedures used are valid in predicting or measuring employee performance in a specific job. They define discrimination as adverse impact:

> The use of any selection procedure which has an adverse impact on the hiring, promotion or other employment or membership opportunities of members of any race, sex, or ethnic group will be considered to be discriminatory and inconsistent with these guidelines, unless the procedure has been validated in accordance with these guidelines. (EEOC, Sec. 3A)

"Adverse impact" is defined as occurring whenever the selection rate for any racial, ethnic, or sex group is less than 80% of the rate of the group with the highest selection rate.

If 200 of 1,000 white applicants are selected (a selection rate of 20%), at least 16% of the minority applicants (80% of the 20) must be selected. Several court rulings, such as Griggs v. Duke Power Company (which we discuss in detail in Part 4), have clearly established the principle that all personnel tests and activities must avoid having any discriminatory effect, whether intended or unintended.

The "Uniform Guidelines" have, in effect, become a handbook for decision making in personnel matters. The personnel selection process must now be reported to state and federal compliance agencies, usually on EEOC forms that require accurate data on the actual hiring results of the nursing facility. As Chruden observes, what used to be the exclusive concern of the facility administrator and personnel officer can now be carried into the courtroom (Chruden & Sherman, p. 114).

MATCHING FACILITY PERSONNEL NEEDS AND APPLICANTS

Hiring the right employee for a position is a complex task. The employer understandably wants to find out as much about the applicant as possible to determine his/her likelihood of success if hired for a position in the facility (Matheny, p. 12).

Methods of Obtaining Information

Several methods are used to obtain information about applicants. Most organizations use written application forms, interviews, and background checks. The search for a new assistant administrator or director of nurses may involve appointing a committee, lengthy exploration, extensive interviewing, and final selection recommendations. Filling a vacancy for a nurse's aide is normally a much less involved process. In both cases it is important that all the information solicited be demonstrably job related or predictive of success in that position.

The "Can Do" and "Will Do" Factors

Using tests, interviews, and background checks, it may be possible to gain an accurate impression of what the applicant can do (Jensen, p. 22). *Can-do factors are knowledge, skills, and aptitudes that can be measured and established for the applicant.* The personnel officer can ascertain whether a particular applicant for a registered nurse vacancy has had suitable training, is licensed, and, from background checks, has demonstrated the use of skilled nursing techniques while working for previous employers.

What is much more difficult to measure are the will-do factors, such as motivation, interest in the facility, and other personality characteristics (Matheny, p. 14). To some degree it is possible to measure objectively how much an applicant can do. How much an applicant *will* do, if hired, can only be inferred by the interviewer.

Reliability and Validity of Information

Information that is valid and reliable is necessary for making an informed decision about an applicant's skills, knowledge, and aptitudes (the can-do factors), the applicant's level of motivation and the likely fit of the applicant's personality (the will-do factors). The EEOC's *Uniform Guidelines on Employee Selection Procedures*, together with the employer's need to evaluate applicants successfully, has resulted in greater attention to the reliability and validity of the information employers obtain from applicants.

Reliability of the tests, interviews, and other tools used in selecting among applicants refers to the consistency with which the same results are obtained over a period of time and when used by different testers (called interrater reliability).

In measuring applicants' abilities, reliability means that an applicant will achieve the same or nearly the same score or results when taking the test at different times, e.g., a week or two apart. If a test were to give differing results from week to week it would be unreliable, just as a set of scales used to weigh produce in a store must reliably give the same weight week after week every time produce of equal weight is placed on it. Reliability also requires that different applicants with the same skills score the same on the test. If typing skill is being measured, applicants with the same level of skill must score the same on the test. Just as the scales in a supermarket must give consistent weights week after week, the scales must accurately weigh the different types of produce.

A test or selection procedure provides *validity* when it actually measures what it is intended to measure and does it well. In essence, validity is a measure of how effectively an instrument does its job (Chruden & Sherman, p. 118).

Two Types of Validity. Personnel experts have relied on at least two types of validity for several years: content validity and construct validity. Content and construct validity are used by governmental agencies in judging the results of a facility's hiring program.

Content Validity. Content validity is the degree to which a test, interview procedure, or other selection tool measures the skills, knowledge, or performance requirements actually needed to fill the position for which the applicant is applying. If a nursing position requires the ability to administer drugs intravenously (IVs), a test establishing that the applicant can perform IVs skillfully has content validity.

Construct Validity. The extent to which a selection tool measures a trait or behavior perceived as important to functioning in a job is construct validity. Intelligence is an abstract construct that is established through putting together answers to a series of different questions that together yield a measure of the theoretical construct called intelligence.

The following is an example of construct validity: A nursing home administrator's requirement of a "friendly facial expression" toward patients is an example of a construct (trait) that the administrator believes is needed for the position.

To validate a friendly facial expression as a job requirement the administrator would have to identify the work behaviors required for the position; identify the constructs, e.g. smiling, that are required; and then show by empirical evidence that this selection requirement is truly related to the construct.

It is of real importance for a nursing facility to require that all staff treat patients in a cheerful or friendly manner, although this directive may be difficult to achieve. In July 1985 a federal judge in Fort Worth, Texas, ruled that American Airlines had the right to fire an otherwise good flight attendant because he did not smile enough. The flight attendant sued the company, contending that he was a good employee and met all requirements of the job except for the smile. The federal judge upheld American's policy of requiring a friendly facial expression as "essential in the competitive airline industry" ("Now We Know Why They're So Friendly," p. 120).

APPLICATION FORMS—PREEMPLOYMENT QUESTIONS

Employers must avoid questions that might be construed as violating the Civil Rights Act, Title 7. Before hiring a person, questions should be avoided that relate to age, sex, race, national origins, education, religion, arrest and conviction records, marital status, credit rating, or handicaps.

Table 2-1 gives a list of subject areas about which one is permitted, or not, to ask questions on application forms or in preemployment interviews.

INTERVIEWING APPLICANTS

Interviews are used extensively in evaluating job applicants. Each organization will develop its own style and identify its varying information needs as it conducts interviews.

Preliminary Interviews. The preliminary encounter generally consists of having the applicant fill out a short questionnaire, after which there is a brief conversation with him/her based on the questionnaire. This serves to screen out unsuitable candidates, using a minimum of time and organizational resources.

Interviewing Methods. Interviewing methods vary, but can be generally classified into three types according to the degree of structure used: the nondirective, the in-depth, and the patterned interview.

In the *nondirective interview* the interrogator refrains from influencing the applicant's remarks. This allows the applicant maximum freedom to ask questions and give information. The interviewer's task is to pay special attention to attitudes, values, or feelings that may be exhibited by the candidate.

This approach maximizes the amount of information the applicant may reveal and is often called an open-ended interview technique. The interviewer asks only broad general questions such as "Tell me about what you did and how you liked your last job," or "What is it about working in a

TABLE 2-1. Suggestions for Interviewers

INQUIRIES BEFORE HIRING	LAWFUL	UNLAWFUL*
1. NAME	Name	Inquiry into any title which indicates race, color, religion, sex, national origin, handicap, age or ancestry.
2. ADDRESS	Inquiry into place and length of current address.	Inquiry into foreign addresses which would indicate national origin.
3. AGE	Any inquiry limited to establishing that applicant meets any minimum age requirement that may be established by law.	A. Requiring birth certificate or baptismal record before hiring. B. Any other inquiry which may reveal whether applicant is at least 40 and less than 70 years of age.
4. BIRTHPLACE OR NATIONAL ORIGIN		A. Any inquiry into place of birth. B. Any inquiry into place of birth of grandparents or spouse. C. Any other inquiry into national origin.
5. RACE OR COLOR		Any inquiry which would indicate race or color.
6. SEX		A. Any inquiry which would indicate sex. B. Any inquiry made of members of one sex, but not the other.
7. RELIGION–CREED		A. Any inquiry which would indicate or identify religious denomination or custom. B. Applicant may not be told any religious identity or preference of the employer. C. Request pastor's recommendation or reference.
8. HANDICAP	Inquiries necessary to determine applicant's ability to substantially perform specific job without significant hazard.	Any other inquiry which would reveal handicap.
9. CITIZENSHIP	A. Whether a U.S. citizen B. If not, whether applicant intends to become one. C. If U.S. residence is legal. D. If spouse is citizen. E. Require proof of citizenship after being hired.	A. If native-born or naturalized. B. Proof of citizenship before hiring. C. Whether parents or spouse are native-born or naturalized.
10. PHOTOGRAPHS	May be required after hiring for identification purposes.	Require photograph before hiring.
11. ARRESTS AND CONVICTIONS	Inquiries into conviction of specific crimes related to qualifications for the job applied for.	Any inquiry which would reveal arrests without convictions.

TABLE 2-1. (continued)

INQUIRIES BEFORE HIRING	LAWFUL	UNLAWFUL*
12. EDUCATION	A. Inquiry into nature and extent of academic, professional or vocational training. B. Inquiry into language skills such as reading and writing of foreign languages.	A. Any inquiry which would reveal the nationality or religious affiliation of a school. B. Inquiry as to what mother tongue is or how foreign language ability was acquired.
13. RELATIVES	Inquiry into name, relationship and address of person to be notified in case of emergency.	Any inquiry about a relative which would be unlawful if made about the applicant.
14. ORGANIZATIONS	Inquiry into organization memberships and offices held, excluding any organization, the name or character of which indicates the race, color, religion, sex, national origin, handicap, age or ancestry of its members.	Inquiry into all clubs and organizations where membership is held.
15. MILITARY SERVICE	A. Inquiry into service in U.S. Armed Forces when such service is a qualification for the job. B. Require military discharge certificate after being hired.	A. Inquiry into military service in named service of any country but U.S. B. Request military service records. C. Inquiry into type of discharge.
16. WORK SCHEDULE	Inquiry into willingness to work required work schedule.	Any inquiry into willingness to work any particular religious holiday.
17. OTHER	Any question required to reveal qualifications for the job applied for.	Any non-job related inquiry which may reveal information permitting unlawful discrimination.
18. REFERENCES	General personal work references not relating to race, color, religion, sex, national origin, handicap, age or ancestry.	Request references specifically from clergymen or any other persons who might reflect race, color, religion, sex, national origin, handicap, age or ancestry of applicant.

I.   Employers acting under bona fide Affirmative Action Programs or acting under orders of Equal Employment law enforcement agencies of federal, state, or local governments may take some of the prohibited inquiries listed above to the extent that these inquiries are required by such programs or orders.

II. Employers having Federal defense contracts are exempt to the extent that otherwise prohibited inquiries are required by Federal law for security purposes.

III. Any inquiry is prohibited which, although not specifically listed above, elicits information as to, or which is not job related and may be used to discriminate on the basis of, race, color, religion, sex, national origin, handicap, age or ancestry in violation of law.

*   Unless bona fide occupational qualification is certified in advance by the State Civil Rights Commission.

Reprinted with Permission from Panel Publishers. Miller, Dulcy B, ed. LONG TERM CARE ADMINISTRATOR'S DESK MANUAL Greenvale,N.Y.: Panel Publishers, Inc., 1982, Exhibit 203.H, pp. 2059-2061.

long-term care facility that attracts you?" or "Where do you want to go in your career in the next five years?"

An *in-depth interview* provides more structure in the form of specific question areas to be covered. This is sometimes called a directed interview. Examples of questions appropriate to the in-depth interview:

What do you consider your most important skills for this job?
Tell me about your last job.
Under what type of supervision techniques do you function best?
What did you like most about your last job?

The *patterned interview* allows the least amount of freedom to both the interviewer and the applicant. All questions are sequential and highly detailed. Generally a summary sheet must be filled out by the interviewer interpreting the results of the encounter.

Research Findings on the Use of Interviews

A good deal of research has been conducted on the reliability and validity of interviews as a tool for judging job applicants. Chruden reports some of the major findings:

- structured interviews are more reliable than unstructured interviews.
- when there is a greater amount of information about a job, interrater reliability is increased, that is, several interviewers are more likely to come to the same decision.
- interviews can explain why a person would not be a good employee but cannot explain why they would be good.
- factual written data seem to be more important than physical appearance.
- interpersonal skills and level of applicant motivation are best evaluated by an interview.
- allowing the applicant time to talk provides a larger behavior sample.
- an interviewer's race affects the behavior of the person being interviewed. (Chruden & Sherman, p. 134)

BACKGROUND INVESTIGATIONS

If the interviewer decides the candidate is of interest to the organization, background information can be sought. If the nursing facility has a full-time staff member assigned to personnel, much of the background information may be obtained by that person. Both the department heads, and the administrator may assume responsibility for obtaining background information.

It is advisable to obtain a signed request for references from applicants. Many former employers refuse to give references without a signed statement from their former employee. Some employees, who subsequently discovered that poor recommendations were given by former employers, have sued them. All of this has led to an increasing reluctance by employers to put evaluations of former employees into writing.

The manager should also ask the candidate questions about the person providing the reference with regard to his/her identity and the basis of the person's acquaintance with the applicant (Matheny, p. 15).

The Privacy Act of 1974 (Public Law 93-579) gave federal employees the right to examine their personnel records, including letters of reference, unless they waived this right when they requested the letter. Although not mandated by federal law, the Privacy Act of 1974 seems to have led to a trend for employers to permit employees to review and challenge their personnel files (Chruden & Sherman, p. 128).

Credit Reports

Under the federal Fair Credit Reporting Act (Public Law 91-508), the employer must advise applicants if credit reports will be requested. If the candidate is rejected because of a poor credit report, he/she must be so informed and given the name and address of the reporting credit agency.

Physical Examination

Condition of Participation 405.1121, Standard G: "Personnel Policies and Procedures," instructs that all facility employees have periodic health examinations to ensure freedom from communicable disease. The practical impact of this stipulation is to require a preemployment physical to assure that this Standard is met by new employees.

There are several practical reasons for a physical exam. It establishes the physical capability of the applicant to meet the job requirements. It provides a baseline against which to assess their later periodic physical exams. The preemployment physical examination is especially valuable in determinations of claims of work-associated disabilities under Workman's Compensation laws (discussed at length in Part 4). The laboratory analyses that are part of the exam can detect the presence of drugs in the applicant.

THE DECISION TO HIRE

Who should decide which applicant to hire? Not the personnel staff. Generally, the final decision to hire is given to the head of the department in which the recruit will work. The administrator of the facility can define a role for him/herself in the final decision making or leave it entirely up to the department head.

Hiring Middle- and Upper-Level Persons

When selecting a new department head or filling other middle- and upper-level positions, the administrator normally plays a more active role in interviewing and in the hiring decision. The medical director could be invited to participate in the selection of a new director of nursing. This physician could also be valuable during negotiations to contract with physical therapists and related allied health personnel.

Two Approaches to the Hiring Decision

The hiring decision itself is complex. Two basic approaches have been identified in the literature: the clinical and the statistical.

In the *clinical approach* the decision maker reviews all the information in hand about the match of the applicant and the job, and then decides.

In the *statistical approach* the decision maker identifies the most valid predictors, then weighs them according to complicated formulas. This method has been shown to be superior to the clinical approach (Meehl, pp. 178–200). However, few facilities will have sufficiently well staffed personnel departments to make the measure practical.

A useful alternative has been suggested. The decision maker rates each of the applicants for a position on several dimensions, such as test score results, education, experience, apparent interest level, and the like, assigning numerical scores on each dimension to each candidate. The results can provide a systematic set of comparison data in reaching the final decision (Jauch, pp. 564–567).

Achieving Construct Validity for Hiring Nursing Home Staff

It is not enough to establish that an applicant has the technical skills needed for a job. In *Nursing Home Organization and Operation* (p. 52) Dulcy Miller suggests that when making hiring decisions, staff must realize that successful caring for frail, elderly nursing home patients is less dependent on the technical knowledge of the staff than on their compassion for others. She observes that knowing the technique of gait training for a disabled person is useless if the staff member cannot encourage the person to leave the chair.

Nursing home staff must be able to become involved with and relate successfully to sick persons, many of whom are depressed and suffering from varying degrees of disability. It is essential to discover whether an applicant is seeking the job because of a positive interest in older persons or because of an inability to get any other work. Given the complexities of meeting the requirements of federal and state laws prohibiting discrimination and the necessity to choose oftentimes from a small applicant pool, this is not an easy personnel task. However, we believe sensitivity, compassion, and caring for older persons have construct validity as hiring criteria for nursing home staff.

Miller observes that "those who are gifted in interpersonal relationships may prove to be the more satisfactory staff members, for these people can always be given additional skill training, while teaching an insensitive person to be compassionate is another matter altogether" (Miller, p. 52).

OFFERING THE JOB

Once the successful candidate is chosen, he/she should be informed by letter or interview. In either case certain information such as proposed salary, job title and level, starting date, and any other relevant information should be communicated to him/her. Normally, a period of time during which the offer may be considered is specified.

It is useful to include a personnel handbook with the offer if the applicant has not yet received one. The handbook (discussed in detail later) describes facility policy on a number of matters about which the prospective employee should be made aware as part of his/her own evaluation of the proposed position. Those not chosen for that particular position should be informed and thanked for their interest.

2.6 Training Employees

ORIENTATION

First Day on the Job

The first day on the job will leave a lasting impression (Chruden & Sherman, p. 176). It is an opportunity for the facility. The new employee nearly always brings an initial reservoir of goodwill toward the facility. The first day is normally characterized by both enthusiasm and anxiety (Meyer, pp. 14–17). A sensitively managed orientation program can help the new employee reduce anxiety and begin to build positive images of the new work environment.

Typical first day activities can include the following:

- official welcome of the new employee
- introduction to as many of the facility staff as is appropriate, particularly the employee's work group
- tour of the facility, including location of lockers for safekeeping of personal effects, eating and snack facilities, the rest rooms, parking arrangements
- instructions on use of the time clock (if hourly)
- safety rules such as infection control procedures and emergency procedures, especially those concerning fire, and staff assignments in case of fire
- explanation of patients' rights
- discussion of contents of the personnel handbook (Rogers, p. 23)

There is only one "first day on the job" for each new employee. Whether the orientation is for the director of nurses or a nurse's aide, it is equally important to the success of the organization. If the facility is organized to take notice of the new employee and attempts to meet his/her needs on the first day, this latest member of the staff will be more likely to assist the facility in meeting its needs during the following months and years (Bryan, p. 4).

Facilities of 300 beds are as capable of a personalized orientation program as those with only 30. In practice, by having a properly constituted personnel office, the larger organization may have a functional advantage over the smaller, where orientation may be left to chance and good intentions without assigned responsibility for this introduction.

Using a Checklist

Precisely because orientation is both an important and complex task, use of a checklist is valuable. Those charged with familiarizing the new staff member with the organization are thereby less likely to overlook any element of the employee's new responsibilities as they review each item on the list (Scott, S., p. 898). One researcher suggests that the use of a checklist may help reduce employee turnover by assisting each new employee to gain an initial realistic and clear set of expectations about the new position (Scott, R., pp. 360–363).

Others consider it advisable that both providers and receivers of the orientation be required to sign each activity on the checklist (Davis, p. 83; Rogers, p. 21). This maximizes the probability that the orientation will be successfully completed. When this document is placed in the employee's personnel file, the signed orientation form becomes a legal basis for establishing that the information was received. Rogers (p. 22) and Davis (p. 83) suggest that responsibility for the orientation and its documentation be vested in a single staff member, who is thus accountable for its successful completion from introduction to signed checklist.

THE PERSONNEL POLICY HANDBOOK

The personnel policy handbook, often called the employee's handbook or employee's manual, is a compilation of the facility policies that directly relate to work conditions. Whereas a job description relates to only one job, the personnel policies are general in nature and cover the entire staff.

Each facility will have its own handbook. Chains generally have sets of policies that apply to all their employees, allowing local facilities to add their own policies within the broader policy guidelines set by the chain.

The main elements most often included in such a handbook are a statement of general policies, followed by details of benefits and general information relevant to the conditions of employment. The personnel handbook can be considered the rules, or terms under which staff are hired and carry out their work.

A. Introduction or welcome to the facility

B. History or background of the facility

C. General employment policies

1. Equal opportunity employment (conforming to the Civil Rights Act).
2. Classification of employees into full time and part-time by number of hours worked per week, working hours of the facility.
3. Confidentiality of information about patients and facility matters.
4. Patients' rights statement.
5. Employee's records—confidentiality, employee access policy, usual contents: (1) application for employment; (2) preemployment checks, letters, records of phone calls; (3) credit checks; (4) performance appraisals, promotions; (5) federal and state withholding certificates; (6) correspondence; (7) disciplinary actions; (8) grievances; (9) attendance; (10) signatures for receipt of personnel policy manual, orientation activities, and in-service attendance record; (11) health records; (12) other relevant materials.
6. Reporting policies—required call-in times prior to shift if unable to come to work.
7. Progressive discipline system—generally a listing of each rule with a statement of disciplinary action, i.e., the number, if any, of oral and or written warnings before dismissal. For example, failure to follow a dress code may allow an oral warning and one or more written warnings before dismissal, whereas physical abuse of a patient could bring immediate suspension or dismissal.
8. Uniforms/appearance.
9. General conduct expected, e.g., respect, vulgarity, courtesy, attendance and punctuality, working quietly, absenteeism, visitors to employees.
10. Gifts (not permitted from patients, their family, or sponsors).
11. Eating, drinking, smoking (break policies), kitchen traffic.
12. Use of alcohol and illegal drugs.
13. Parking, telephone calls, mail, meals, lost and found.
14. Destruction of nursing home property.
15. Suggestion box, permitted uses of bulletin boards, solicitation/distribution of literature rules.

16. Probationary period, use of anniversary or other dates for personnel reviews, seniority policies.
17. Health requirements and physical examinations.
18. Employee debts, garnishment of wages.
19. Performance ratings, promotion policies and interdepartmental transfer policies.
20. Wages and salaries, time cards, pay plan, date procedures for determining payroll calculations, payrolls, deductions, overtime policy.
21. Grievance procedures.
22. Disciplinary action.
23. Hospitalization and first-aid treatment.
24. Facility's position on unions.
25. Resignaton notice and procedures.
26. On-the-job injuries.
27. In-service education requirements.

D. Benefits

1. Holidays.
2. Vacations, leave-accumulation policies.
3. Leaves of absence: sick leave, funeral leave, military leave, maternity leave, jury duty, extended leave.
4. Health benefits.
5. Retirement benefits (if any).
6. Insurance: life insurance, unemployment compensation, occupational disease insurance, workmen's compensation insurance, disability insurance.
7. Shift differential (if paid).

TRAINING

As we have noted, directing is the task of assuring that each work role is successfully communicated to the employee. Directing is the process of (1) communicating to the employees what is to be done, then (2) assisting them to perform their role successfully (Givnta, p. 19). Directing involves the communication and organizational analysis skills discussed in Part 1.

Purpose

The purpose of the orientation program is to provide an initial introduction to the new employee. The purpose of training is to communicate the organization's needs to the employees and assist them in meeting those needs. This is a continuous process, beginning formally the first day on the job, but extending for the duration of the employee's association with the facility.

In *Nursing Home Organization and Operation*, Dulcy Miller points out that employees of long-term care facilities need more than just technical skills (p. 31). According to her, they must be able to interact with and relate to sick, often depressed persons, many of whom suffer from behavioral disabilities. This is a complicated assignment, demanding a personal commitment by the employee beyond the level and quality of involvement implicit in most jobs.

Each facility has its particular philosophy of patient care, its own policies written to assist employees to achieve a high standard of care. The goal of the manager is to develop a program in which every member of the organizaton arrives at the same conclusions and makes the same decisions, given the same set of circumstances. The best way a high degree of employee conformity to facility policy goals can be achieved is through a program of continuous education, beginning the first day on the job and continuing throughout the employee's tenure.

There are several vital reasons for each facility to conduct continuous education/training programs for employees. Nursing facilities are dynamic, ever-changing organizations. As the environment of the facility is modified, so too a program of continuous education to assist the staff in accommodating to the changes is needed. Also, the individual job changes, requiring new insights. However, the most pressing reason to have a continuous training program is that with the passage of time, people forget. It is necessary to reemphasize continuously those policies that are important to the facility.

Minimum Training Program

Federal Condition of Participation 405.1121, "Governing Body and Management," mandates an ongoing facility education program. Standard H of this Condition, "Staff Development," reads as follows:

> An ongoing educational program is planned and conducted for the development and improvement of skills of all the facility's personnel, including training related to problems and needs of the aged, ill, and disabled.

> Each employee receives appropriate orientation to the facility and its policies, and to his(/her) position and duties.

> Inservice training includes at least:

> prevention and control of infections
> fire prevention and safety
> accident prevention
> confidentiality of patient information

preservation of patient dignity, including protection of his (her) privacy and personal and property rights

Records are maintained which indicate the content of, and attendance at, such staff development programs.

The Condition requires training for *all* members of the staff and that it be *ongoing*. The areas named constitute only the *minimum* required. State inspectors normally ask to review the facility records of employee training during their required periodic inspections.

In most facilities, the responsibility of assuring that training needs are met is either given to one individual or assigned to line supervisors.

Two Phases of an Employee's Training

First Phase. The primary goal of training at the beginning of an individual's employment is to bring that person's knowledge and skill up to a level satisfactory to management.

Second Phase. Once achieved, the purpose of training is to provide reinforcement, plus additional skills and knowledge for improvement of job performance and qualification for higher-level job assignments (Bryan, p. 2).

Three Steps in Establishing Training Needs

Staff members responsible for establishing the nursing facility's training program normally analyze three elements in planning for this training: (a) the organization, (b) the tasks, and (c) the person carrying out the work (Chruden, p. 181).

Organizational analysis consists of examining the facility's goals, resources, and internal and external environments to determine where training efforts need to be focused. The established policies can form the basis for such conclusions.

Task analysis involves review of job descriptions and activities essential for performing each job. The emphasis of training programs can then be placed on certain tasks that are judged to be inadequately carried out or simply in need of reenforcement because of their importance to the facility, such as fire drills and disaster preparedness.

A *person or employee skill analysis* can be made to arrive at the skills, knowledge, and attitudes required in each position. Person analysis means interpreting each position in terms of the personal attributes or behaviors necessary for performing the job acceptably.

For example, in doing an organizational analysis the administrator might conclude that an integrated team approach to patient care is a paramount goal of the facility. A review of job descriptions of team members would reveal the activities, such as patient care conferences, and the procedures used in these meetings to establish patient care plans. Person or employee skill analysis would establish employee behaviors and attitudes essential for the success of integrated team patient care. A decision may then be made as to the type and focus of any training program needed to improve delivery of integrated patient care.

Once the goal of a training program has been determined, the following four steps can be taken:

1. Formulate instructional objectives.
2. Develop instructional experiences to achieve these objectives.
3. Establish performance criteria to be met.
4. Obtain evaluations of the training effort (Chruden, p. 180).

Two Types of Training within the Facility

A wide variety of educational and training programs exists. The two major types used in nursing facilities are on-the-job and in-service training.

On-the-job training, also called instruction training, is conducted by a staff member assigned to assist the new or continuing employee to acquire the abilities needed in a position in the facility. The major advantage of on-the-job training is firsthand experience under normal working conditions for the person receiving training.

Ideally, on-the-job training permits the trainee to be an additional or extra worker for the first few days, allowing observation and progressive involvement in performing the tasks and behaviors required. A potential disadvantage to on-the-job training is the temptation for the supervisor to focus on production of work rather than teaching the new skills, especially if the trainee is part of the normal work force assigned to accomplish each day's workload.

Most training in the nursing home and other industries is on-the-job training. Many other types of training exist, however.

In-service training refers to employee education offered during the work career of the employee. Normally, in-service education consists of small seminars for groups of employees. All types of educational techniques can be employed, e.g., flip charts, films, lectures, video demonstrations, role playing, case discussions, and the like (Ruhl, p. 66).

The topics required by the Conditions of Participation, such as prevention and control of infection, fire prevention and accident prevention, lend themselves to in-service training. Prevention of infection may be held in a classroom setting with a film or discussion, whereas fire prevention may involve an actual hands-on demonstration of fire extinguishers conducted by the local fire marshal.

Programmed instruction has become a useful educational tool, either computer assisted or through use of a written manual.

Some organizations now require persons who join their staff as nurse's aides to take a training program of 1 to 3 weeks. These programs combine many of the best features of the educational approaches. At the larger level, some nursing home chains now offer training programs for personnel, especially administrators. In both of these situations the new employee is thoroughly trained and tested before being allowed to give direct services in a facility.

Other Types of Training

Numerous other types of training have been used in the nursing home field. Correspondence courses for licensure and education of nursing home administrators are permitted in certain states. Administrator-in-training programs (administrative internships) have been used by some states to give these candidates experience similar to on-the-job training. This type of training resembles apprenticeships such as medical internships and residencies in hospitals.

More formal training programs have been developed by community colleges and technical institutes for preparation of nursing home personnel such as nurse's aides and licensed practical nurses (LPNs), sometimes called licensed vocational nurses (LVNs).

EVALUATING TRAINING

Evaluation of training efforts can be difficult. While it is true that tests can be devised to measure memorization, the nursing home is seeking to assess something more complex: changes in employee behavior. To quantify behavioral changes, it is useful to state learning objectives as *behavioral objectives*.

Behavioral objectives can be measured by observing whether employees, in carrying out their duties, exhibit the behaviors sought as the objective of the training. Usually the goal is to have the employee acquire a skill or change an attitude (Wehrenberg, p. 117). Using performance-centered behavioral objectives can assist evaluation.

For example, performance-centered objectives in a nurse's aide training program might be (a) to be able to demonstrate proper procedures for turning a patient who is suffering from decubitus ulcers, and (b) to consistently greet any patients encountered in the hallways using a pleasant tone of voice.

Both of these are performance-centered objectives. Proper techniques for turning a patient who has a decubitus ulcer can be physically demonstrated by the aide in training, and the aide's demeanor toward patients encountered in the hallways can be monitored by the trainer or other staff members.

2.7 Retaining Employees

2.7.1 What the Facility Needs from the Employee

We have argued that the facility needs employees who will consistently make decisions in conformity with its policies. This is possible to the extent that each staff member can be characterized as having the following:

- full comprehension of and commitment to the facility goals, norms, values, and policies
- a high degree of interest in the job
- a genuine dedication to the well-being of the patients and the quality of care given them
- a strong positive self-image permitting the employee to see beyond his/her own needs and to be concerned, rather, with those of the patients
- skills, both technical and interpersonal, in communication and human relationships
- the capacity and willingness to make decisions in accordance with the best interest of the facility, every act contributing toward providing the highest quality of life for the patients and staff of the facility
- the ability to be self-starting, reliable, creative, and able to exercise positive appropriate leadership
- career commitment to the facility

Obviously, this is the description of an ideal employee. Few staff members will be able to embody fully all of these qualities. Practically speaking, a facility whose employees all exhibited these characteristics might be unusually difficult to manage! An entire staff of such eminently capable persons could be dysfunctional. If, however, these characteristics can be consistently encouraged and developed among the employees, the quality of life enjoyed by the residents and staff should be high.

One reason ideal employees who can exhibit all of these traits and abilities are difficult to find or train is that the employees bring their own needs into every position. Inevitably, an employee's performance is a combination of efforts to meet the needs of the facility and his/her own.

27.2 What Employees Need from the Facility

The administrator would like each employee to exhibit traits such as those listed during the hours worked at the facility, then quietly go about meeting personal needs when not at work. As indicated in Part 1, this is not what happens. The employee's personality, feelings, and behavior during the hours on the job are inevitably affected to varying degrees by personal desires and by events in life outside.

What employees require of the facility can be divided into four areas: (a) social approval, (b) self-esteem, (c) security, (d) use of power, accomplishment, service, and exercise of leadership, which are intrinsic needs.

The degree to which any one individual might seek satisfaction from employment will vary, both among the entire staff and within the same member as his/her personal situation changes over time.

SOCIAL APPROVAL

Most people rely on a network of approved and satisfying social interrelationships. Whether or not they express it openly, many of them enjoy engagement in activities sanctioned by significant others—persons to whom an individual looks for favorable regard of behavior patterns, ideas, and values. Family, members of the community, and/or one's social group are typical examples of significant others.

If the community, or significant others in the community from whom approval is sought, disapproves of the employee working at the facility, he/she will not have positive feelings about the job itself or feel that being a "good" employee is worth the effort.

SELF-ESTEEM

Adequate self-esteem is essential in order to function. Individuals need a positive self-image, that is, to feel good about themselves, what they are doing, and the world about them. Each person has need for status.

ECONOMIC SECURITY

In this case we define security as the financial benefits provided by the facility. Without sufficient income for maintenance, health insurance for eventualities, vacations for refreshment, and funds to meet future retirement expenses, an employee may remain insecure.

ADDITIONAL INTRINSIC NEEDS

Some employees expect even more of the work situation. Their intrinsic needs arise out of the essential nature of their personality. Wielding power and having authority in certain situations are intrinsic needs. Satisfaction from the process of getting things done, of achievement, is another such need, as is leadership. Giving service can be fulfilling behavior.

2.7.3 Strategies Available to the Facility to Meet Both Its Own and the Employee's Needs

Retaining satisfactorily performing employees over an extended period of time is economically desirable for the facility. The financial costs of training each employee can be high, especially if the employee participates extensively in in-service training programs offered by the facility and takes advantage of any additional on-the-job training for skills improvement.

In the nursing home setting, *employee continuity is critical for the patients themselves*, providing an important element of stability and continuity in their lives. More than in most work settings, employees in nursing homes tend to form personal relationships with the patients, often being regarded as significant friends by residents who have lost all of their family.

A contented staff, capable of contributing significantly to the quality of patient life in the facility, consists of employees who are enjoying a high level of job satisfaction and are thus enabled to provide a high level of patient care.

A FACILITY PHILOSOPHY OF HUMAN RESOURCE MANAGEMENT

What motivates employees? Every day the administrators of more than 23,000 U.S. nursing homes make decisions based on their assumptions of what motivates their staff. These conclusions reflect the administrator's beliefs about human resource management and may be consciously or unconsciously held. We will explore one general theory about employee motivation.

Theory X and Theory Y

In 1960 Douglas M. McGregor, a management theorist, published a book expounding what he called Theory X and Theory Y. McGregor wrote that the behavior of administrators is strongly influenced by their beliefs. He asserted that most business managers are Theory X types who believe that the employee naturally dislikes work, prefers to receive extensive direction from superiors, wishes to avoid taking responsibilities in the organization, has little ambition, and is motivated more by a need for security than any other factor. This approach requires that managers use fear of punishment to motivate employees, all of whom must be closely watched if work is to be accomplished.

McGregor insisted that Theory X is not valid and that managers should be guided by what he called Theory Y instead. Theory Y is based on the following assumptions (pp. 33–35):

1. Using energy to work is as natural as using energy to play or rest. The administrator can control working conditions to lead to work being a source of satisfaction, voluntarily performed, or to work being seen as a source of punishment and thereby avoided.

2. If individuals are committed to the organization's goals, they will

exercise self-direction and self-control without need for threat of punishment or of external behavior controls.

3. Rewards for achieving organizational objectives bring employee commitment; employees can achieve personal self-satisfaction in achieving organizational goals

4. The average employee, when properly motivated, will accept and also seek responsibility.

5. The preponderance of employees have the capability of exercising imagination, ingenuity, and creativity in assisting the organization to achieve its goals.

6. Most jobs underutilize the capabilities of employees.

McGregor's theory caused considerable discussion in management circles. One researcher doubted that in 1960 most managers were Theory X types. To test this, he surveyed 259 managers in 93 companies and found that managers did not completely accept either Theory X or Theory Y (Allen, pp. 1061–1067). In their opinion, reality is more complicated than either theory. Not surprisingly, a few years later this led to Theory Z.

Theory Z

Several writers proposed that, on balance, Theory Y is correct, but *what motivates employees changes over time and is dependent on changing societal values.* They argue that administrators must constantly come up with new strategies for motivating employees. In their view a straight-forward productivity-reward system is overly simplistic. Quality of life, both for the individual and for the group, while more complex and abstract, is the appropriate focus (Thierauf, Klekamp, & Geeding, pp. 108–112; White, p. 22).

MEETING THE EMPLOYEE'S NEED FOR SOCIAL APPROVAL

Individuals have a need to be part of an enterprise that is regarded by significant others as successful. Hence, approval of the nursing facility by significant others is important to nursing home employees.

In the community the word-of-mouth reputation of the facility is important. Persons and groups regarded as experts in the field (the local hospital) and other health care providers (local physicians) can be important or significant others, those whose approval is sought by the staff. Newspaper, radio, and television reports about their workplace shape employee feelings.

At the broader level, a number of regional and state organizations evaluate the facility. The fire marshal, sanitarians from the health department, various other inspectors, the regional health systems agency, and state and federal nursing home inspectors all have an impact on the facility's public image.

Quite simply, a nursing facility with a reputation for giving quality health care and maintaining a high quality of life for its residents will have little problem attracting and retaining good employees. When the operation does not meet standards established by the community, it will find recruitment a difficult task indeed.

To cite an example, in one large city a nursing home operated by the county was for 4 years attacked in the news media and threatened with decertification by state officials because its sanitation and patient care were regarded as significantly substandard. During those 4 years it was difficult to hire staff.

Nurses, janitors, physical therapists, nurse's aides, maintenance people who worked there were constantly being harangued by friends, neighbors, and workers in other health care facilities. Why were they willing to work under such conditions? After a succession of three administrators in the course of 4 years, during which the home suffered constant public attacks by both the media and individuals, an improving level of care became apparent.

Employees do care about the reputation of their organization. Community approval of their employer is important to workers, particularly in the field of health care.

MEETING THE EMPLOYEE'S NEED FOR SELF-ESTEEM

Why does one nurse's aide strive harder than another? Why does one registered nurse look for additional responsibilities at the same time that another seeks to avoid taking any? Why do wage incentives stimulate some individuals and not others? Why does a career advancement track within the facility stimulate some employees to strive to climb the ladder while others ignore the opportunities offered?

What motivates employees varies not only for the individual employee but, over time, for the same employee. Motivation is a difficult concept to define. It has been described as the factor that energizes employee behavior, directing or channeling such behavior, and sustaining it (Steers, pp. 5–6).

An individual's needs, desires, and expectations change. When one need or desire is achieved at a satisfactory level, the salience or strength of others is modified. For a nurse who has just been licensed to practice, acceptance by other nurses may be a priority until this recognition is achieved (Lorsch, p. 60). At that point other needs, such as maximizing income, may take precedence.

The complexity of motives has been described by Dunnette and Kirchner (pp. 126–129), who attempted to apply motivational psychology to the work situation. They point out the following:

1. Identifying motives is complex. Some employees will work hard to obtain more money, but why? A strongly felt need for additional money may reflect a desire for the increased status more money brings, meeting a felt need for a sense of economic security, providing a symbol of power, or simply a willingness to work harder until the car is paid off, at which point time off work may replace the desire for more money as a primary motivation.

2. Motives are always mixed. Each individual experiences a wide range of motives that strengthen and weaken as his/her circumstances change, and some needs are met while others are frustrated.

3. The same incentive—e.g., increased health insurance benefits—may generate different responses. Individuals also differ in the ease with which their needs are satisfied.

4. Some motives may recede when satisfied, e.g., hunger and thirst. Others, such as a desire for increased status or more salary, may become intensified when, for example, more status or more income is achieved.

A. H. Maslow's hierarchy-of-need concept is perhaps the most often cited human need model in the literature (see Figure 2-1).

Maslow's theory is that needs become salient, i.e., powerfully motivating, at each successively higher level mainly after the needs at each lower level are satisfactorily met. That is, until the individual has met the needs for survival and basic security (Levels 1 and 2), these will dominate until met.

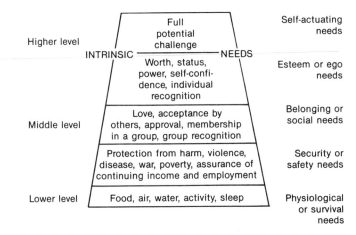

FIGURE 2-1. Maslow's hierarchy of need concept.

Once lower level needs are met to a satisfactory degree, the individual's motivation can become more dominated by social, self-esteem, and self-actuating needs (levels 3, 4, and 5). Maslow's model is widely used. In our view, it seems to be a functional and useful explanation of some of the more basic dynamics of employee motivations.

One author has pointed out that while the lower-level needs may decrease in strength when achieved, the higher-level needs, especially the need for self-actualization, tend to continue to grow stronger as they are being met (Lawler, p. 25). Examples of these types of needs or motivations are those cited above as "Additional Intrinsic Needs," such as being in authority, wielding power, accomplishing goals, and exercising leadership.

A word of caution: Each individual has a unique need pattern. In our view, what motivates an individual depends on a combination of life experiences and on his/her unique genetic makeup.

Childhood experiences such as economic deprivation may cause an employee to be anxious about financial security, no matter how much income is being earned. The social and economic class with which an employee identifies affects his/her needs. Being raised as a male or a female can influence the needs individuals will manifest on the job.

Attempts have been made to identify basic personality types. Investigators who were focusing on the causes of heart disease described two personality types. *Type A* are characterized as hard-driving, achievement-oriented people who strive to succeed to the highest level whatever the area of activity, whether in sports, job titles, or on-the-job productivity. Type A persons appear to be at increased risk of heart disease.

Type B personalities are characterized as having only moderate achievement needs, as less competitive and more satisfied with moderation, whether in sports, titles, or on-the-job productivity.

Dr. Elmer Green, the psychologist who correlated Type A and Type B behaviors with heart disease risks, commented that while Type A behavior is useful in catapulting a person to the top, "you have to be able to turn off 'A' and become 'B' if you want to live" (Green, pp. 135–142). Type A employees come to the facility with a high internalized motivation level. They are overachievers in comparison with Type B persons.

Why? What makes one individual a Type A and another a Type B personality? It appears to be some combination of genes and life experiences. The facility must provide additional external motivations for the Type B employee.

Concepts such as Maslow's hierarchy-of-need theory and others that will be discussed below are useful in predicting employee behavior. Even so, the administrator must understand that each individual has a unique need pattern.

In the following section, we discuss seven areas available to an employer seeking to retain staff through meeting needs for self-approval:

- training programs
- career paths
- performance feedback and goal setting
- recognition
- power
- respect for creative potential
- teams

Training Programs

Training programs increase employee skills and simultaneously communicate to them that those skills are valued by the management.

The programs themselves serve numerous functions. They demonstrate management's interest in the staff and provide an additional arena for exchange among employees, as well as an increased opportunity for feedback to the administration about the degree of skills and understanding of facility goals among employees. As these dynamics occur, the level of employee satisfaction can improve. With the new skills or insights, the employee experiences an increased feeling of being in tune with the goals and performance expectations of the organization.

Career Paths

Offering a career path means providing upward mobility within the organization. In a freestanding nursing home, creating career mobility is more difficult than it is within a chain that owns and operates 400 or 500 facilities.

Making career paths available within the facility communicates to the employee that the organization wants to meet his/her desires to succeed and progress in job level and income. For the nursing aide, a career path might include facility support through released time and or tuition assistance. This makes more feasible enrollment at a local technical institute to become a licensed practical nurse or a registered nurse.

The charge nurse might receive support to participate in a program to become a geriatric nurse practitioner. The kitchen worker might be assisted in attending classes that lead to qualifying as a dietetic service supervisor.

The labor market can be an influencing factor. If the home is freestanding, in a rural area with a limited number of persons in the potential pool of nurse's aides or kitchen workers, career assistance may lead to an undesirable depletion of the worker pool.

On balance, however, providing career paths that create upward mobility appears to increase worker satisfaction and improve employee retention rates. Not all of the aides will aspire to become licensed nurses, since they are not all similarly motivated. However, the availability of a career program can improve workers' attitudes. Those who choose not to participate have the satisfaction of knowing the option is available and that they may choose to exercise it if they wish. In general, the mere presence of options is important to employees.

Performance Feedback and Goal Setting

Employees receive informal feedback on their job performance on a daily basis. Formal reaction and the formal process of goal setting for an individual employee occurs under more structured circumstances. This is known as the *performance appraisal*, which normally includes establishing goals for the employee to achieve until the next scheduled performance appraisal.

Recognition

Most employees seek recognition for their work. Much of their behavior can be interpreted through *expectancy theory*, pioneered by Victor Vroom in the 1960s. Expectancy theory holds that the level of motivation to perform (make an effort at work) is a mathematical function of the expectations individuals have about future outcomes multiplied by the value the employee places on these outcomes. Vroom defines expectancy as a "momentary belief concerning the likelihood that a particular act will be followed by a particular outcome" (Vroom, p. 170).

The charge nurse who believes that working long hours and asserting her/himself on the job will lead to quick promotion to nurse supervisor is an example of an expectancy. It serves as a guideline for the charge nurse in seeking promotion to nurse supervisor. The charge nurse expects the behavior to be rewarded. Recognizing employees' expectancies can help a supervisor understand how they are motivated.

If the charge nurse's long working hours and assertiveness lead to promotion, her expectation is reinforced. According to reinforcement theory, behavior depends on reward. When rewards follow performance, performance improves. Conversely, when rewards do not follow performance, performance deteriorates. If the charge nurse had not been promoted, her performance might have deteriorated.

In *reinforcement theory* the outcome reinforces the employee's response either positively, leading to repeating the response, or negatively, leading to reduction in its use. Influencing employee behavior through reinforcement is called *operant conditioning*, literally influencing working behavior by conditioning the employee's response through rewarding the behavior.

When employees perform in a desired manner and are given praise and recognition for that behavior, the manager is engaging in what is called *behavior modification.* Behavior modification involves using operant conditioning, usually through rewards, praise, positive recognition, when an employee performs as desired by the facility.

One theorist (Rotondi, pp. 22–28) suggests the following as a pattern for modifying employee behavior to conform to facility goals:

- maintain a consistent work environment
- consciously identify the desired behaviors of employees
- decide on the rewards to be used

The performance appraisal is usually conducted on an annual basis and involves the employee and the supervisor in a discussion of a written evaluation that has been given the employee. It also sets goals for the future.

Setting work goals has a demonstrably positive effect on the motivational level and work performance of employees (Chruden & Sherman, p. 273). E.A. Locke found that individuals set work goals for themselves, whether instructed to or not. It is his contention that, given this fact, management should set goals with employees to maximize the probability that its goals will be similar to the worker's own. Within reasonable limits, employees who set or accept harder goals perform better than employees who set or accept easier ones (Locke, pp. 157–189).

Establishing work goals becomes, in effect, a contract between the supervisor and the employee. This contract serves to motivate the employee and to focus his/her efforts on the work sought by the supervisor. The goals assure that the relationship between the employee and the facility is individualized for that employee. It is an indication that the organization recognizes the presence of that employee with whom it interacts as an individual, rather than as an anonymous staff member.

- clearly communicate to the employees both the desired behaviors and the rewards
- reward desired behaviors immediately
- scale rewards to the behavioral achievement attained, i.e., vary the rewards
- minimize the use of punishments

Power—Control

Nursing facility administration needs to define policies to govern their decision making. However, this has both positive and negative aspects. The positive aspect is that the staff is given guidance and an appropriate framework within which to make decisions for the organization. The negative aspect is that deciding beforehand, through policymaking, can substantially deprive the employee of a feeling of personal involvement in decision making for the organization.

Feelings of Powerlessness

Christopher Argyris is a behavioral scientist who has observed a tendency for organizations to overlook a desire that most employees have to function in a mature, adult manner. In the literature this is referred to as the immaturity–maturity theory, which holds that most organizational designs treat employees as immature, thus frustrating their need to function as responsible adults.

Argyris believes that the typical organization tends to ignore individual potentials for competence, for taking responsibility, for constructive intentions, and for productivity. He feels that in the typical lower-level job of the nurse's aide, the laundry worker, or the housekeeper, staff members are treated as immature. This, he argues, alienates and frustrates these workers, leading them to feel justified in rejecting responsible behavior and tempting them to defy the organization by allowing the quality of their work to deteriorate.

He sees the same problems among managers who work within organizational structures that create environments hostile to trust, candor, and risk taking. In such situations, the attitudes actually encouraged are conformity and defensiveness, which tend to be expressed by producing detailed substantiation for unimportant problems and invalid information for critical issues. Argyris (p. 7) asserts that this leads to ineffective problem solving, poor decisions, and weak commitment to any decisions that are made.

Argyris is pointing to the converse of a coherent set of policies to cover all decision making in the nursing facility: little significant role in making decisions seems left to the employee. This leads to a high level of frustration among those affected.

Common reactions to frustration can be selecting an acceptable substitute goal that is attainable or engaging in behavior that is maladaptive (Chruden & Sherman, p. 275). An employee barred from making any meaningful decisions at the facility may cease trying and may concentrate energies on a leadership role in an outside voluntary organization. Or the employee relieves his/her frustration through aggressive or abusive behavior toward other employees or the patients (Chruden & Sherman, p. 276).

Combating Powerlessness: Employees As "Owners"

The solution to this problem is to make everybody an "owner." Giving all employees a sense of ownership in the facility means treating each employee as a member of the team. This can be accomplished by allowing them some control in their work and giving them information about what the facility is attempting to accomplish. Tom Peters advocates this approach in his book *A Passion for Excellence*. He calls the approach "all people as 'businesspeople'" (Peters & Austin, p. 23).

Ownership implies that all employees exercise some real portion of control in the facility. Of course, each employee does exercise some fraction of control over the workplace. It is up to the individual staff member to decide whether to give care pleasantly or in an "I don't care," "you don't deserve my respect" manner when alone with the patient.

"Businesspersons"

Tom Peters's belief is that if the organization treats every employee as a "businessperson," the employees will respond as "businesspersons" fully engaged in the facility's goal of giving quality care and committed to its success. A sense of ownership is accompanied by a feeling of control over what happens. Peters cites examples from the experimental lab and from the field.

An industrial psychologist gave the subjects in a study some difficult puzzles to work and some boring proofreading to do. While they were attempting to accomplish these tasks, the psychologist played a loud tape recording of one person speaking Spanish, two speaking Armenian, a mimeo machine in use, and a noisy typewriter.

Half of the subjects were given a button to push to stop the noise. The other half had no control over the noise. Those with buttons to push solved five times as many puzzles and had one-fourth fewer errors in proof-reading, although never once did any subject with buttons to push ever push the button. *These who perceived that they had control over their situation clearly outperformed those who felt they had little or no control.* In numerous repetitions the same results were obtained.

In the field, the same results were achieved: workers who were given buttons to push achieved superior results for the company. The Ford Motor Company plant in Edison, New Jersey, gave every worker on the assembly line a button to push that shut down the assembly line. The Ford workers shut down the assembly line 30 times the first day and an average of 10 times a day thereafter. After the first day the shutdown lasted an average of 10 seconds—just time to make this or that little adjustment, turn a bolt, or the like (Peters, pp. 20–32).

What happened at the plant? Production remained steady. Three other factors changed significantly. The number of defects dropped from 17 per car to less than 1. The number of cars requiring rework after coming off the line dropped by 97%. A backlog of union grievances plummeted. Why? Because the lineworkers felt they had some meaningful control in their jobs, they had a sense of ownership in the plant. Employees who have a sense of ownership in the facility will try to do what is best for it. The nurse's aide with this perception is also more capable of meeting his/her social needs such as self-esteem, self-acceptance, and status.

How can nurses' aides be given ownership in the facility? One director of nurses accomplished it by consulting the aides before admitting a patient to their area. When the aides told the director of nurses that the care load was too great at one particular juncture, the director of nurses refused the proposed admission.

These aides had a sense of control over their work situation. They worked harder than previously and exercised their control judiciously to make sure the quality of patient care was not compromised by over-admitting. These nurse's aides had a button to push. They never pushed it without good reason.

Why should nurse's aides be involved in running the facility? Ford Motor Company has a practice of soliciting input from all hourly workers. The assembly line workers are asked to comment on the manufacturability of parts and are members of advance design teams. Hourly workers offered 1,155 suggestions for changes in design or production for three small trucks. More than 700 of these suggestions were adopted (Peters & Austin, p. 26).

Respect for the Creative Potential of Each Employee

The "business" of every nursing facility is providing patient care. In *A Passion for Excellence*, Peters argues that there are only two ways to create and sustain superior patient care: first, by taking exceptional care of patients by providing superior services and quality of care; and second, by constantly innovating.

According to him, this is not accomplished by the genius of the administrator or by mystical strategic moves. Excellence in patient care comes from "a bedrock of listening, trust, and respect for the dignity and the creative potential of each person in the organization" (Peters & Austin, p. 20).

Quality patient care depends on the attitudes toward patients—of housekeepers, kitchen staff, laundry workers, the maintenance person fixing the lavatory, the accountant, and the secretary—as well as on the nursing staff.

Membership on a Team

We have mentioned the team concept several times and will return to it in the discussion of patient care planning in Part 5.

Industries have repeatedly rediscovered that small groups produce higher quality, more personalized service, and more innovations than do larger entities (Peters & Austin, pp. 20–32). U.S. companies, such as General Motors, Hewlett-Packard, Digital Equipment, and Emerson Electric, now limit the size of the plant they will build to between 200 and 500 employees. The Japanese organize their largest industrial plants into small teams of 10 to 40 workers.

A Natural Head Start.   The nursing home enjoys a natural advantage over these companies. The Conditions of Participation have required the small-team approach since 1973. Those who drew up the Conditions already knew what industry is beginning to realize: employees perform better when they are part of a team.

Condition of Participation 405.1124: Nursing Services, Standard D, "Patient Care Plan," mandates a care plan that is reviewed, updated, and evaluated periodically by all professional personnel involved in patient care. While not spelled out in detail, the Conditions of Participation do advocate a team approach to patient care. Team membership is a valuable tool in efforts to retain employees because it helps meet the employee's need for social involvement, communication with other employees, and meaningful personal involvement in the real work of the facility: patient care.

MEETING THE EMPLOYEE'S NEED FOR ECONOMIC SECURITY

For the purposes of this discussion, we mean by the term *security* the finance-related benefit package provided for the employees. This subject is explored later at greater length under the heading "Paying Employees."

2.8 Evaluating Employees

JOB PERFORMANCE EVALUATION: A LINE MANAGER FUNCTION

Job performance evaluation is a task assigned only to line managers. Such responsibility distinguishes staff from line management functions: staff, having no line authority in the organization, cannot be assigned line responsibility for personnel matters—hiring, evaluating, promoting, reprimanding, suspending, or firing employees.

PURPOSE OF JOB PERFORMANCE EVALUATION

The basic purpose of the job performance evaluation is to focus the energies of the employee on the level of performance that is expected of him/her (Smith, p. 45). Whereas on-the-job and in-service training are part of the directing role of the managers, job performance evaluation is a control function (King, p. 1).

The Equal Employment Opportunity Commission (EEOC) has done much to stimulate employers to keep accurate appraisal records of employees' work. Court hearings have also contributed to the desirability of carefully documenting worker performance (Chruden & Sherman, p. 230).

Three basic purposes of performance appraisals are: (a) to give employees feedback about their work performance; (b) to provide a basis (plan) for directing future employee efforts toward organizational goals; (c) to provide a basis on which managers will decide on promotions, compensation, and future job assignments (Locher & Teel, pp. 245–247).

The performance evaluation, or performance appraisal as it is often called, is a control tool. It is the process of managers assessing the degree to which an employee has performed as directed, the formulation of plans of correction, if indicated, and plans for future performance goals for that individual (Smith, p. 45; King, p. 2). The performance appraisal also strengthens the manager/employee relationship by developing a mutual understanding of expectations, goals, and measurement criteria and by allowing the employee to express his/her concerns, suggestions, and desires for the future (Smith, p. 47).

Performance evaluation occurs constantly in the facility. Every day department heads form impressions of the quality of the work accomplished in their area. Setting up a performance appraisal system is the formalizing of this process into a written evaluation periodically communicated to the employee.

Most industries use performance appraisals. A study by the Bureau of National Affairs revealed that among the industries studied, 84% had regular procedures for evaluating office personnel and 58% for evaluating line workers (Employee Performance, pp. 1–3). The majority of appraisals were given on an annual basis.

OUTLINE OF THE PERFORMANCE APPRAISAL PROCESS

The performance appraisal process operates in the following manner: First, the manager defines the functions, tasks, demands, and expectations of the job and translates them into performance criteria (Smith, p. 51; Bianco, pp. 43, 44; Baker & Morgan, p. 76). To implement this, the organization must have developed forms and procedures, including standardized methods of rating employees, to be used by supervisors in conducting appraisals.

Approximately 2 weeks before an appraisal date, the manager completes the appraisal form, sending a copy to the employee, together with notification of time and place of the evaluation. This gives the employee time to prepare for the interview.

At the interview the manager reviews the completed appraisal with the employee. Based on employee inputs during the interview, the manager may modify the appraisal if appropriate. Performance goals for the employee for the next time period are reviewed, modified if employee and manager concur, and, if possible, mutually agreed on.

At the end of the session both employee and manager sign the appraisal. Provision is normally made for any addendum the employee may wish to write or for the employee to indicate disagreement with the findings. In the event of such a difference of opinion, appeal procedures are normally available.

Most employers have policies regarding the length of time appraisals are retained in the employee's personnel file. Generally, they are kept up to 3 years and then removed and discarded by the employer.

PROBLEMS ENCOUNTERED IN THE PERFORMANCE APPRAISAL PROCESS

Whatever the importance to the facility and however rational the appraisal process may seem, resistance to its effective utilization often arises, making the program difficult to implement (Snell & Wexley, p. 117).

Typically, appraisals are given once a year at the time that the employee expects an annual raise. When a raise and the appraisal are linked, the supervisor writes an appraisal to justify his/her decision about the employee's raise or lack of it (Rodman, p. 73). This focuses the interview on rewards or absence of rewards for past performance rather than on future goals.

There are other significant reasons performance appraisal systems are difficult to implement and sustain in a facility. The managers themselves often see too little benefit to themselves for taking time to give thorough and thoughtful evaluations.

Most managers are understandably uncomfortable with the face-to-face judgmental role, frequently involving direct confrontation with the employee. Too often, these managers are not sufficiently trained in conducting employee appraisal interviews (Bianco, p. 40). Finally, the desire of the manager to be in a helping role with the employee can come into conflict with giving evenhanded appraisals (Chruden & Sherman, p. 233; Baker & Morgan, p. 74).

Because the employee may dispute and appeal the appraisal if not satisfied, the appraisal all too often appears to be a defense of the manager's written decisions and less a feedback mechanism allowing the manager and employee time to reflect on past performance and jointly to plan for the future.

Employees are naturally sensitive to appraisals inasmuch as they affect their chances for advancement, salary increases, and future recommendations at the point of a job change. Employees are concerned, therefore, that the appraising manager meet at least three of the criteria below.

Criteria for Managers

The appraiser should have adequate opportunity to observe the employee's day-to-day work and have access to any records needed to assess staff output (Smith, p. 51).

The appraiser must thoroughly understand the job requirements and be guided by clearly stated standards by which to judge the employee's efforts (Smith, p. 51).

The manager ought to judge the work from an informed viewpoint. Nurse's aides, for example, want someone trained as a nurse, who presumably understands the nature of their job, to write their appraisal.

METHODS OF RATING EMPLOYEES

Rating Scales

Rating scales are consistently used (Chruden, p. 237). They list a number of characteristics, traits, and/or requirements of the employee's position on a line or scale (Sears, p. 6). The evaluator checks off the degree to which the employee is believed to meet a trait or requirement. For example, a scale recording degree of initiative might appear thus:

Initiative
Lacks initiative   Meets requirements   Highly resourceful

Work Quality:
Needs to improve   Meets standards   Exceeds standards

Global Ratings.   Often the manager will be asked to provide a global rating for the employee. This normally is regarded as a summary score based on the components of the appraisal. Generally, each employer establishes a numeric or alphabetic scale for the facility.

For example *1* might represent the highest and *5* the lowest rating. Inevitably, the scale comes to resemble the grading system everyone has known in elementary and secondary school: whatever the symbols used, the person comes to understand that he/she is an *A*, *B*, *C*, or *D* performer—or an *F*, in which case a termination notice might be pending.

Errors Made by Managers Using Rating Scales

Three types of errors often occur when managers use rating scales.

The Halo Effect.   The halo effect occurs when a supervisor who values one particular type of job behavior, punctuality, for example, permits the presence or absence of this one trait to color several or most other trait ratings. A habitually late employee might be excellent in patient care but be rated low in most categories because the supervisor is irritated by the persistent tardiness.

The Leniency Error.   To avoid conflict, some supervisors give consistently high ratings to employees. This is known as the leniency error. The lenient supervisor's ratings are difficult to accurately compare with those of a stricter and more demanding supervisor. This has long been noticed in the school setting, where an *A* from one teacher is a rare event and represents outstanding achievement; whereas another teacher in the same subject area is known to consistently give *A*'s to over half the class.

The Error of Central Tendency. Other supervisors, on the other hand, commit the error of central tendency, consistently giving only moderate scores to employees regardless of whether their performance is poor or outstanding.

Rating by Essay

The use of essays or paragraphs describing employee progress is less frequent than rating scales. It is especially difficult to compare employees when the essay method permits supervisors simply to write whatever evaluative comments occur to them. A brief essay at the end of a rating scale can be valuable, however. Observations in essays communicate useful information about the individual that might be lost or not easily expressed through the exclusive use of rating scales.

Possible Outcomes from Appraisals

Apraisals are primarily intended to give feedback to the employee about performance to date and to provide a set of activities or goals until the next appraisal.

Some of the possible results of appraisals can be transfer, promotion, or demotion, or, in the case of a reduction in work force, they can be the basis for discharge.

Transfer. A transfer is the placement of an employee in another position that is approximately equivalent to the present position. A nurse, for example, may find that working on the heavy-care wing of a nursing facility is emotionally overburdening and may ask for a transfer to a lighter-care area, either permanently or temporarily.

Promotion. A promotion is placement of an employee at a higher level within the facility. Normally, a pay increase and additional responsibilities accompany a promotion. However, promotion of a nurse from, say, Level 1 to Level 2 may be based on either merit or seniority but may not involve new responsibilities.

There are at least two bases for promotions: merit and seniority. Seniority is concerned with length of service and tends to be automatic. The merit system relies on performance evaluations of supervisors for placement of a worker at a higher level. Under the seniority system a nurse who serves the required number of months or years at Level 1 is automatically promoted to Level 2. Under the merit system a nurse may or may not be promoted from Level 1 to Level 2, depending on evaluation decisions of the supervisor.

Demotion.   Demotion is the change of assignment of an employee to a lower level in the organization, typically with less pay, fewer responsibilities, and reduced status. Demotions, particularly if perceived as permanent, normally generate morale problems and in the nursing home setting can lead to a reduced level of caring behaviors by the demoted employee.

Demotions are often accomplished by the use of transfers. A formerly more productive employee may be transferred to another position, with pay and status remaining intact. Another alternative to demotion is promotion to a position with little responsibility or power.

Layoffs.   Layoffs are temporary dismissals and are potentially demoralizing to the remaining employees as well as to those laid off. Unambiguous layoff policies can reduce anxiety among the remaining employees. However, such policies also tie the hands of management, who might, for example, seek to retain a recent but especially valued employee.

Generally, layoffs are based on seniority but may be related entirely to merit or a combination of seniority and merit. Layoff policies are carefully scrutinized by employees for fairness and equitability in their implementation.

2.9 Paying Employees

The nursing home is labor-intensive. In most facilities wages and benefits make up more than half of the operating costs. Buttaro (pp. 3–14) estimates that 65% to 70% of nursing home expenditures are personnel costs.

Careful management of wages and benefits is one of the major sources of cost control available to the nursing home administrator.

MONEY IS LIQUID VALUE

The wages paid an employee normally determine the standard of living the employee can enjoy. Wages also affect his/her status in both the facility and the community. Wages are a statement by the facility about the relative worth of the skills of each employee.

The most liquid benefit a facility can give to its employees is the paycheck. Health insurance, sick leave, and the like, are important, but the benefit most highly valued by the employee is the dollar value of the paycheck, which provides maximum control over the product of his/her work effort.

For persons earning more than $100,000 per year, wage rates may assume less importance than other measurements of the individual's work effort. For the typical nursing home employee, however, the wage rate is salient, and even a difference of a few cents per hour can spell satisfaction or dissatisfaction with wages for an individual making comparisons with a similarly qualified co-worker.

THEORIES OF COMPENSATION

Compensation is generally considered the reward given employees in exchange for their work effort. How willing an employee may be to work hard and assist the facility toward its goals can depend on how justly the employee feels his/her wages and benefits fit his/her work effort (Belcher, pp. 13–15).

Equity Theory

According to equity theory, employees seek an exchange in which their wages and benefits are equal to their work effort, especially when compared to wages and benefits paid to similarly situated co-workers (Whitehill, p. 516). If the individual feels equitably paid, little tension may exist. If, however, he/she suspects that others with similar skills and investment of effort receive more, a tension exists that most employees will seek to resolve.

Typical worker responses to perceived inequities are to ask for a pay raise, reduce their effort, file a grievance, or, in some cases, seek employment elsewhere. Alternatively, the employee may encourage those perceived as similarly situated, but benefiting more, not to work so hard. Reactions to perceived inequities can take many forms (Ivancevich, p. 119).

WAGE POLICIES

Developing and administering compensation policies are important administrative duties. Policies should cover such areas as the following (Chruden & Sherman, p. 429):

- the rate of pay, set below, at, or above the prevailing community practice
- the discretion supervisors can exercise in differentiating an individual's pay from the set scale
- the amount of spread between pay rates for employees with seniority and pay rates for new employees
- periods between raises and the weight given to seniority and merit in determining a new pay rate

Hourly Wages or Salaries?

Most facilities distinguish between hourly employees (wage earners) and persons paid stated salaries periodically. Wage earners or hourly employees generally are required to punch in and out on a time clock and are paid only for hours worked as verified on the time card. Salaried workers, in contrast, are paid a set wage regardless of the hours worked.

HOW MUCH TO PAY: THE WAGE MIX

Determining wage rates and benefits is a complex task affected by a number of factors called the wage mix:

- the labor market
- prevailing wage rates
- cost of living increases
- ability to pay
- collective bargaining
- individual bargaining
- value of the job

The Labor Market

Once governmental requirements for minimum wage rates are met, and sometimes the influence of unions also taken into account, *supply and demand* affect the wage rates. For example, during the early decades of this century, through their organizations, physicians were able to restrict their numbers and keep them lower than the demand; this resulted in favorable influences on their incomes, which now average more than $100,000 per year. Similarly, the size of the pool of nurses available in a given area can influence the wages paid to nurses.

Prevailing Wage Rates

According to a government study, more than half of businesses surveyed indicated that the prevailing wage scale in their communities for comparable jobs was the most influential factor in determining wages actually paid.

This tends to be true for nursing facilities, which generally pay somewhat lower salaries to registered nurses and other employees than do local hospitals. One recent Massachusetts study revealed that nurse's aides earn 25% less in nursing homes than in hospitals, and RNs 23% less than RNs in hospital (Long Term Care Employee Shortage, p. 2). Other nursing facilities within the community naturally affect the wage rates that must be paid to attract the quality of staff desired, but the basic rates are heavily influenced by hospital pay scales.

Wage surveys for the community or region are taken by many organizations. They may be carried out by a single facility, or through agreements with others to share this information (Brennan, p. 25).

Cost of Living Increases

During periods of inflation, cost of living adjustments may be made in wage rates. The purpose of cost of living increases is to assist workers to maintain their purchasing power. These increases, often embodied in *escalator clauses* of labor contracts, provide for wage adjustments based on some index, usually the Consumer Price Index (CPI). The CPI is a government-defined measure of the cost of living compared to a base point, usually of a few years earlier, which is designated as 100. Any increase or decrease in the cost of living is then expressed as a percentage of the base figure of 100.

Ability to Pay

Although only 12% of industries surveyed indicated that ability to pay was the critical factor in determining wages, ability to pay may have special relevance to the nursing home industry.

For example, each state determines the reimbursement rate for Medicaid patients. If they constitute a high proportion of the patients, and if the facility is located in a state that reimburses at a low rate for Medicaid patients, the actual ability of the facility to pay prevailing wages may be affected.

If the proportion of Medicaid patients is low and that of privately paying patients is high, the institution is in a stronger position to compete with other facilities and the hospitals for highly qualified personnel.

Collective Bargaining

Where employees are unionized, nursing homes are also subject to union influences, regardless of wage rates paid.

Individual Bargaining

Individuals with especially desirable skills may be able to negotiate a higher wage than others in similar positions. When a highly qualified maintenance director or director of nurses is sought, the facility may bargain with such a person and offer him/her a premium.

WORTH OF THE JOB

How much is any single position actually worth? Inevitably, wages and benefits are a combination of market forces, prevailing wage rates, ability to pay, collective and individual bargaining, and cost of living.

The number of leading American corporate administrators who are paid over $1 million a year and the number of their perquisites (job benefits) is growing (Kessler, pp. 26–31). Star basketball and football players' annual salaries have reached $2 million a year and more. Yet the President of the United States receives only a fraction of this sum. And in the nursing home the aides generally earn a wage just above the required minimum. Why? To what extent is each of these wage levels based on the value of the job? Any of these determinations is subject to complex forces within our society.

Determining Job Worth: Factor Comparison

Points. Regardless of its difficulty, it is necessary to set wage and benefit scales within the nursing facility. In some wage-setting systems, points are assigned to each job, and wages are set accordingly. A variation of this system is to make comparisons with the key jobs.

Key Job Comparisons. In the nursing facility the wages paid to the nurses tends to become the benchmark against which the earnings of other staff members are compared and established. Nurses are the primary service providers. Their wages can be used as a yardstick for determining the comparative worth of the other jobs within the facility.

If, for example, maintenance staff who have no special training or skills are paid higher wages than the registered nurses who have met educational and licensing requirements, maintenance morale may be high and nursing morale low.

Wage Classes and Rates

To approach equity and achieve some flexibility for supervisors evaluating employees, wage classes or grades and wage rates are normally established (Brennan, p. 10). All jobs within that class are paid at the same rate or within the same rate range. A rate range is the variation permitted within a class or grade.

For example, pay for all registered nurses constitutes a pay class or pay grade. Using a rate range, registered nurses can receive differing rates of pay but still be within the rate range set for the class or pay grade established for registered nurses. Licensed practical nurses are paid at a lower rate than registered nurses. Wage rates for nurse's aides are similarly fixed.

Complications

Complications can develop when the minimum and maximum pay rates for one pay class or pay grade overlap with those for another pay class.

A licensed practical nurse who has been working for the organization for 15 years may be earning more than a registered nurse who has been on the staff for only 3 years. Similarly, a nurse's aide on the staff for 15 years who has no formal training or license may be earning more than a licensed practical nurse who has both a degree and licensure but has been with the facility for only a short time.

The extent to which the employees feel there is equity or inequity within the pay system will directly affect performance.

Government Regulations in Compensation

In addition to all of the market and other forces cited, the government participates in regulating compensation. This is discussed in Part 4 under "Regulation of Compensation."

2.10 Paying to Motivate

In *Personnel Management* Chruden observes that in recent years it has been fashionable for personnel researchers to deemphasize the importance of earnings in comparison to other job motivators. He feels the focus has been on nearly every aspect of job motivation except money (Chruden & Sherman, p. 424). However, for centuries managers have believed that people work at most jobs to earn money, and the opportunity to earn more money will motivate employees (Belcher, p. 301; Printz & Waldman, p. 84; Olian, Carroll, & Schneier, p. 78).

In our view, the conclusion that earning additional money motivates employee performance is correct. The opportunity to earn additional wages and benefits does appeal to most employees. However, when wages reach a certain level, somewhere between $50,000 and $150,000, depending on the individual and the job circumstances, more money and benefits may become less important than additional promotions with more impressive titles, larger offices, and perhaps more power. Few positions in the typical nursing home approach this happy circumstance.

WAGE MOTIVATION IN NURSING HOMES

In the typical nursing facility, more than half of the hands-on patient care is given by nurse's aides, whose wages begin at the minimum level and after years of service may rise only a few dollars above that. For these employees a raise of 25 cents per hour may be significant to help them meet their financial obligations.

Few nurses' salaries approach the point where increased income does not have an impact on their standard of living. This is also true for most other staff members. Even the facility administrator responds to promises of increased salary and benefits.

One of the reasons for this is the level of deprivation felt by these staff members when they compare themselves to other employees in the health care industry. Physicians earn, on average, well over $100,000 a year. The local hospital administrator's income will typically be twice that of the nursing home administrator. Even the local hospital nurses generally earn considerably more per hour than those in nursing homes.

Studies under combat situations in World War II established that feelings of deprivation are relative to the situation in which the individual believes himself to be acting. Nurses and other long-term care facility employees frequently compare themselves to similarly situated employees at the local hospital. When their wages are significantly lower than hospital wages for the same position, nursing home workers may feel deprived.

In our view, nursing home personnel both deserve and need more income than they normally receive. Nursing facility wage scales are limited by the necessities for economy imposed on most of them by market and governmental limitations on the daily rates the facility can charge patients. For these reasons we feel the nursing home administrator will continue to be able to use wages and benefits as incentives for obtaining the desired performance from nursing home personnel.

INCENTIVE PLANS: THE PIECEWORK APPROACH

Historically, incentive plans have focused on the differential piece rate incentive plan devised by Frederic Taylor. The more "pieces" or items the employee produced, the more money the employee made. Under the piecework approach, employees are paid by multiplying the number of units produced by the rate per unit (Printz & Waldman, p. 84).

This approach is not easily applicable to the nursing home setting. If the housekeepers are paid by the number of rooms cleaned, the emphasis will be on cleaning the rooms fast, not on cleaning the rooms well. Quality service to the residents is the "business" of the nursing home. Making beds faster, giving pills faster, assisting patients faster is not necessarily better.

DECIDING WHAT COMBINATION OF BEHAVIORS TO REWARD

The administrator must decide on the particular combination of employee behaviors to be rewarded through merit increases, bonuses, or some similar plan. For each employee group the combination of desired behaviors will be different. Most organizations finally use a trial-and-error approach to discovering the exact combination of employee behaviors to reward.

Controlling the Director of Nurses

What behaviors or combinations of behaviors should be rewarded? What nursing director behavior, for example, should be rewarded? The administrator wants the director of nurses to get the maximum reasonable productivity from nursing personnel. At the same time, the administrator seeks to offer a certain quality of patient care—a goal that requires nursing personnel to spend enough time with each patient to meet the need for social contact, as well as to attend to their strictly medical needs.

The desired behaviors must be communicated to the personnel involved and conscientiously applied by the supervisors in the performance appraisal interviews and salary decisions.

Controlling the Administrator's Behaviors

What behaviors do the corporate headquarters, the owners or the board of directors, desire of the administrator? Here again, the incentive, usually in the form of a bonus, must be designed to elicit a complex combination of behaviors in the administrator (Delaney, p. 30).

In recent years owners have discovered that cost controls under Medicare and Medicaid tend to place a financial squeeze on facility cash flow. In states offering low reimbursement rates for Medicaid patients a facility may not be able to offer the quality of care the owners seek.

They may decide to reduce the percentage of Medicaid patients in their facilities from 90% to a mix of 50% Medicaid and other patients and 50% private, paying patients. At the same time the owners may wish to keep the level of occupancy high (90%+), stay within budget, and receive no more than a minimal (2) number of deficiencies (citations for failure to meet the standards for the Conditions for Participation) from state inspectors.

Designing the Bonus

A bonus plan designed to achieve these goals might be a 25% year-end bonus offered to the administrator if all of the conditions are met by the year's end.

To further communicate corporate priorities to the administrator, reaching 50% private, paying patients might bring a 10% bonus; maintaining an average 90% occupancy, a 5% bonus; staying within budget, a 3% bonus; and keeping deficiencies at 2 or less, a 2% bonus. Thus, some bonus can be earned for achieving any of these performance goals, which, added separately, amount to a 20% bonus; when achieved simultaneously, they bring an extra 5%, for a total bonus of 25%.

ADDITIONAL TYPES OF BENEFITS

As more and more nursing homes are purchased by chains, the opportunities to offer various types of stock benefits become available as incentives designed to lead employees to become actual owners, in addition to the type of psychological ownership we advocate (McMillan & Hickok, p. 32).

A *stock option* is a right to buy a specified number of shares of stock within a specified time period, usually at a stated price. Another approach allows employees to purchase stock in the facility at a reduced purchase price, generally 10% to 15% less than market price. Any number of variations exist on employee stock purchase plans. The goal, of course, is to instill in employees a sense of ownership in the institution, leading them to behave in a facility-enhancing manner.

2.11 Controlling Benefits

Employee benefits average between 18% and 65% or more of total payroll costs. The amount in one study was 37%.

THE RISE OF BENEFITS

The rapid rise of benefits as a percentage of total payroll costs began in World War II (Carter & Shapiro, p. 562). Congress froze wages, believing that workers who remained at home and worked in the factories should not benefit more from the war effort than the soldiers fighting overseas.

American creativity at home defeated the intention of Congress. Workers began to concentrate on gaining numerous benefits, especially health insurance, in lieu of the direct wage increases proscribed by Congress. Escalation of worker benefits at a rapid rate has been in effect ever since. From 1957 to 1977 worker benefits rose from 29% to 41% of payroll costs (Employee Performance, p. 5).

Benefits as an Important Cost Factor

Employee benefits can be a significant cost factor. This can be especially true for smaller nursing homes that may have high administrative costs per employee for benefit administration, compared to larger chains, where benefit administration costs can be spread over a much larger staff.

A potential disadvantage of a large benefit package is that employees take it for granted, especially hourly employees. They may still concentrate on the dollar figure of take-home pay when thinking about their earnings in comparison to other facilities and other job opportunities.

Need to Educate Employees

To counteract this, employers must constantly remind their staffs of the value of the benefits they enjoy (Carter & Shapiro, p. 566). Aside from pamphlets and posters, probably the most beneficial educational tool is a personalized annual report to each employee showing the exact benefits currently enjoyed by them, the monetary value of those benefits, plus projections of the benefits into the future. Projecting any retirement benefits can be especially useful in convincing the employee of the advantages of remaining with the organization.

TYPES OF BENEFITS

The benefit program can be one of the most effective tools available to the employer who wishes to give staff members more of a sense of meaningful control over their economic well-being and life-style (Hoff, p. 282; Cole, p. 50). This can be partially accomplished by offering choices among available benefits. This is the "cafeteria" approach. Employees are given a total value for benefits they may receive from the facility, then allowed to select from those offered, up to a specified limit (Haslinger, p. 39).

Health Insurance. Most facilities pay for individual health insurance. Some will insure the employee's family as well. Generally, the cost is shared in such circumstances.

Life Insurance. Occasionally, free life insurance—typically a term insurance coverage—is offered. Term insurance features low premiums for high dollar coverage but has no cash, loan, or other value. An alternative is to offer coverage at reduced rates available through group insurance obtainable by the facility.

Payment for Time Not Worked. Vacation days, sick leave, an increasing number of holidays, time off for military duty, jury duty, death or grave illness in the family all have tended to be among the more valued benefits. One increasingly popular approach is to allow the employee to designate which holidays are to be taken. This has the benefit of increasing the employee's sense of control over his/her life.

Retirement Benefits. Retirement benefits are discussed in Part 4. They are attractive as a benefit but have pitfalls as a result of federal regulation of retirement plans.

Benefits Required by Law. The government mandates that facilities participate in Old Age Survivors' Insurance (OASI), pay into an unemployment compensation program, and share in worker's compensation covering injuries on the job. These are discussed in detail in Part 4.

Other Benefits

Numerous other types of benefits are offered by or under consideration by employers.

Health Programs. Health-related programs for which the employer pays all or part of the cost are becoming popular. The most frequently offered are weight reduction, smoking cessation, and exercise programs (Herzlinger, p. 70). Other benefits include counseling assistance and recreational facilities, both on and off the premises.

Flexible Time. A program allowing staff to choose the hours they will work, as long as they put in a required number of hours per day, can be perceived as a valued benefit (Rothberg, p. 32). However, in the nursing facility this may be less feasible for nursing staff committed to full care around the clock than for the accounting or housekeeping personnel. Nevertheless, allowing an employee to vary the hours of the workday, perhaps by coming in within a half-hour time span, generates a feeling of valued control over personal time (Miller, p. 2097).

Such benefits have at least two advantages: they may encourage better performance on the job, and they express the facility's concern about employees' well-being beyond their capacity to fulfill their work obligations. These programs can, however, be expensive for the employer.

2.12 Disciplining Employees

The following are some of the more common staff disciplinary problems faced by nursing facilities:

- excessive or unexcused absences or tardiness
- leaving the facility or work area without permission
- violation of rules about smoking, intoxication, narcotics, gambling, fighting, firearms
- failure to follow safety procedures
- failure to accept direction
- failure to report accidents
- failure to take patients' safety and welfare into account
- verbal, physical, or other abuse of patients
- theft, punching another employee's time card, falsifying records
- insubordinate behavior or abusive language
- failure to report their own condition of illness
- solicitation or acceptance of gratuities from patients or patients' families or sponsors
- immoral, indecent, or disorderly conduct

NEED FOR RULES AND THEIR CONSEQUENCES

Each facility should carefully state and consistently enforce policies regarding disciplinary actions. The employees must be made fully aware, before any infraction occurs, of both the facility's rules and the disciplinary action that will be its consequence (Cameron, p. 38; Hill, p. 10). Although policies and rules may have been clearly formulated, these policy statements remain meaningless unless they are continually reinforced by positive (motivating) and negative (disciplining) actions (Discenza & Smith, p. 176).

Grievance Procedures

Grievance procedures are an important safety valve for policies regarding disciplinary actions. Employees need to know that there are equitable procedures through which their reactions and views can be expressed when they feel they have been dealt with unfairly.

Progressive Discipline

For most offenses, progressive discipline—beginning with verbal warnings, followed by written warnings for any subsequent violations—makes the most sense. Progressive discipline may prevent repetition of the offending behavior after only a verbal warning, thus bringing about an early solution to the problem.

Employees who are dismissed have the right to present their case to the employment security commission, and many do. It is necessary for the employer to keep a well-documented record of having made every reasonable effort to persuade the employee to conform to facility policy before dismissal (Tobin, p. 22). Normally, administration must be able to demonstrate that disciplinary actions taken were based on rational judgments about the offending behavior, not on personal vindictiveness or excessive emotional reactions of supervisors to employee behavior (Chruden & Sherman, p. 414).

Each facility needs to define clearly its own policies governing suspension and discharge procedures. Normally, several managers, including the administrator, participate in a decision to suspend or discharge an employee.

Discharging Employees

Discharging employees, especially managers, is a painful process that generates a lot of avoidance behaviors in the facility. To avoid outright confrontation and dismissal employees often are stripped of titles and responsibilities, and raises are not given. These and similar behaviors are used by management to induce the employee to find a position elsewhere.

The process of terminating employees, especially executives, can be eased through helping that person find alternative employment. This is called disemployment, outplacement, or dehiring (Chruden & Sherman, p. 418). The managers themselves may assist the employee to find another position or hire an employment firm to do so. This is sometimes known as transferring problems.

REFERENCES TO PART TWO

Allen, L.A. (1973). M for management: Theory Y updated. *Personnel Journal*, *52*(12), pp. 1061–1067.

Argyris, C. (1972). A few words in advance. In A.J. Marrow (Ed.), *The failure of success*. New York: AMACOM.

Baker, H.K., & Morgan, P.I. (1984). Two goals in every performance appraisal. *Personnel Journal*, *63*(9), pp. 74–78.

Belcher, D.W. (1974). *Compensation administration*. Englewood Cliffs, NJ: Prentice-Hall.

Bianco, V. (1984). In praise of performance. *Personnel Journal*, *63*(6), pp. 40–50.

Brennan, E.J. (1984). Everything you need to know about salary ranges. *Personnel Journal*, *63*(3), pp. 10–16.

Brennan, E.J. (1984). Restraint of the free labor market. *Personnel Journal*, *63*(5), pp. 22–25.

Bryan, L.A. (1984). Making the manager a better trainer. *Supervisory Management*, *29*(4), pp. 2–8.

Buttaro, P.J. (1980). *Home study program in principles of administration of long term health care facilities*. Aberdeen, SD: Health Care Facility Consultants Publishers.

Cameron, D. (1984). The when, why, and how of discipline. *Personnel Journal*, *63*(7), pp. 37–39.

Carter, M.F., & Shapiro, K.P. (1983). Develop a proactive approach to employee benefits planning. *Personnel Journal*, *62*(7), pp. 562–566.

Chruden, H.J., & Sherman, A.W., Jr. (1980). *Personnel Management* (6th ed.). Cincinnati: South-Western Publishing.

Cole, A., Jr. (1983). Flexible benefits are a key to better employee relations. *Personnel Journal*, *62*(1), pp. 49–53.

Davis, W.E. (1985). *Introduction to health care Administration*. Bossier City, LA: Publicare Press.

Delaney, W.A. (1984). The misuse of bonuses. *Supervisory Management*, *29*(1), pp. 28–31.

Discenza, R., & Smith, H.L. (1985). Is employee discipline obsolete? *Personnel Administrator*, *30*(6), pp. 175–186.

Dunnette, M.D., & Kirchner, W.K. (1965). *Psychology applied to industry*. New York: Appleton-Century-Crofts.

Employee performance: Evaluation and control. (1975). Washington, DC: Bureau of National Affairs. (Personnel Policies Forum Survey No. 108).

Equal Employment Opportunity Commission, Civil Service Commission, Department of Labor, & Department of Justice (1978). Adoption by four agencies of uniform guidelines on employee selection procedures (1978). *Federal Register*, *43* (166), pp. 38290–38315.

Givnta, J. (1984). For good job training, you need a good beginning. *Supervisory Management*, *29*(6), pp. 19–21.

Gomez-Mejia, L.R., Page, R.C., & Tornow, W.W. (1985). Improving the effectiveness of performance appraisal. *Personnel Administrator*. *30*(1), pp. 74–82.

Green, E. (1977, October 17). Heart disease: New ways to reduce the risk. *Business Week, 2505*, pp. 135–142.

Haslinger, J.A. (1985). Flexible compensation: Getting a return on benefit dollars. *Personnel Administrator, 30*(6), pp. 39–46, 224.

Hershizer, B. (1984). An MBO approach to discipline. *Supervisory Management, 29*(3), pp. 2–7.

Herzlinger, R.E., & Calkins, D. (1984). How companies tackle health care costs: Part 3. *Harvard Business Review, 64*(1), pp. 70–80.

Hill, N.C. (1984). The need for positive reinforcement in corrective counseling. *Supervisory Management. 29*(12), pp. 10–14.

Hoff, R.D. (1983). The impact of cafeteria benefits on the human resource information system. *Personnel Journal, 62*(4), pp. 282–283.

Ivancevich, J.M., Szjlagyi, A., & Wallace, M. (1977). *Organizational behavior and performance*. Santa Monica, CA: Goodyear Publishing.

Jauch, L.R. (1976). Systematizing the selection decision. *Personnel Journal, 55*(11), pp. 564–567.

Jensen, J. (1981, May/June). How to hire the right person for the job. *Grantsmanship Center News*.

Kessler, F. (1985, July 22). Executive perks under fire. *Fortune, 112*(2), pp. 26–31.

King, P. (1985). Performance planning and appraisal. *Soundview Executive Book Summaries, 7*(3).

Lawler, E.E., III. (1973). *Motivation in work organizations*. Monterey, CA: Brooks/Cole.

Locher, A.H., & Teel, K.S. (1977). Performance appraisal—a survey of current practices. *Personnel Journal, 56*(5), pp. 245–247, 254–255.

Locke, E.A. (1968). Toward a theory of task motivation and incentives. *Organizational Behavior and Human Performance, 3*(2), pp. 157–189.

Long term care employee shortage taking shape nationwide. (1986). *Today's Nursing Home, 7*(10), pp. 2–3.

Lorsch, J.W., & Takagi, H. (1986). Keeping managers off the shelves. *Harvard Business Review, 64*(4), pp. 60–65.

Matheny, P.R. (1984). How to hire a winner. *Supervisory Management, 29*(5), pp. 12–15.

McGregor, D.M. (1960). *The human side of enterprise*. New York: McGraw-Hill.

McMillan, J., & Hickok, S.D. (1984). Taking stock of the options. *Personnel Journal, 63*(4), pp. 32–37.

Meehl, P.E. (1954). *Clinical vs. statistical prediction*. Minneapolis: University of Minnesota Press.

Meyer, M.C. (1977). Six stages of demotivation. *International Management, 32*(4), pp. 14–17.

Miller, D.B. (Ed.) (1982). *Long term care administrator's desk manual*. Greenvale, NY: Panel Publishers.

Now we know why they're so friendly. (1985, July 22). *Fortune, 112*(2), p. 120.

Olian, J.D., Carroll, S.J., Jr., & Schneier, C. (1985). It's time to start using your pension system to improve the bottom line. *Personnel Administrator, 30*(4), pp. 77–83, 152.

Owen, D.E. (1984). Profile analysis: Matching positions and personnel. *Supervisory Management, 29*(11), pp. 14–20.

Peters, T., & Austin, N. (1985, May 13). A passion for excellence, *Fortune, 111*(10), pp. 20–32.

Printz, R.A., & Waldman, D.A. (1985). The merit of merit pay. *Personnel Administrator, 30*(1), pp. 84–90.

Rodman, T.A. (1984). Make the praise equal the raise. *Personnel Journal*, *63*(11), pp. 73–78.

Rogers, W.W. (1980). *General administration in the nursing home* (3rd ed.). Boston: CBI Publishing.

Rothberg, D.S. (1986). Part-time professionals: The flexible work force. *Personnel Administrator*, *31*(8), pp. 29–32.

Rotondi, T., Jr. (1976). Behavior modification on the job. *Supervisory Management*, *21*(2), pp. 22–28.

Ruhl, M.J., & Atkinson, K. (1986). Interactive video training: One step beyond. *Personnel Administrator*, *31*(10), pp. 66–75.

Scott, R. (1972). Job expectancy—an important factor in labor turnover. *Personnel Journal*, *51*(5), pp. 360–363.

Scott, S. (1983). Finding the right person. *Personnel Journal*, *62*(11), pp. 894–902.

Sears, D.L. (1984). Situational performance appraisals. *Supervisory Management*, *29*(5), pp. 6–10.

Smith, K.E. (1984). Performance appraisal: A positive management tool. *College Review*, *1*(2).

Snell, S.A., & Wexley, K.N. (1985). Performance diagnosis: Identifying the causes of poor performance. *Personnel Administrator*, *30*(4), pp. 117–127.

Steers, R.M., & Porter, L.W. (1979). *Motivation and work behavior*, (2nd ed.). New York: McGraw-Hill.

Thierauf, R.J., Klekamp, & Geeding, (1977). *Management principles and practices*. New York: John Wiley and Sons.

Tobin, J.E. (1976). How arbitrators decide to reject or uphold an employee discharge. *Supervisory Management*, *21*(6), pp. 20–23.

Vroom, V.H. (1964). *Work and motivation*. New York: John Wiley and Sons.

Wehrenberg, S.B. (1983). How to decide on the best training approach. *Personnel Journal*, *62*(2), pp. 117–118.

White, E. (1984). Trust—a prerequisite for motivation. *Supervisory Management*, *29*(2), pp. 22–25.

Whitehill, A.M., Jr. (1976). Maintenance factors. *Personnel Journal*, *55*(10), pp. 516–519.

PART THREE

Budgeting and Finance

3.1 The Administrator's Role as Financial Manager

An administrator's duties encompass nearly every aspect of running the facility, from assisting in the recruitment of professional medical staff to assuring the efficient operation of the laundry department. Not surprisingly, the administrator is also finally responsible for the money coming in and going out of the facility. It is, in reality, the administrator who is the one person held accountable for the entire financial operation of the facility.

SELECTING AND EVALUATING FINANCIAL PERSONNEL

Although we will explore their individual functions in more detail later, let us say here that *the bookkeeper primarily records the daily cash transactions of the facility*, keeping track of all money going out or coming in. *The accountant uses the information compiled by the bookkeeper to generate reports on the financial standing of the facility.* The bookkeepers and accountants *record* the financial transactions, but the administrator is chief financial officer of the facility, *not* the bookkeepers and accountants.

The administrator must ensure that the bookkeeping process runs smoothly—that the bookkeeper is qualified for the job and has access to the information needed for recording all of the facility's financial transactions. Thus, the administrator must have some knowledge of bookkeeping in order to know whether this important task is carried out as it should be.

The administrator may also have to select an accountant, either as an employee or as a consultant for the facility. If the administrator manages one of a chain of nursing homes, the accountant will probably be an employee of the corporate office. The administrator should therefore have some understanding of accounting to be able to assess the accountant's performance.

More important, however, the administrator must be able to interpret the financial reports developed by the accountant. The administrator's primary role as financial manager is to use the financial information to make informed decisions about the facility. The administrator needs to know how these financial reports are prepared.

MAINTAINING ENOUGH INCOME

In addition to bookkeeping and accounting, we will also take a close look at costs. Surprisingly enough, there are many different types of costs, and we will see how looking at costs in different ways can provide the administrator with information not included in the financial reports prepared by the accountant.

As the facility's ultimate financial manager, the administrator must assure the availability of funds for conducting business: to purchase supplies and pay salaries and to meet the regular payments on any borrowed funds. Without these purchases and payments, the facility cannot operate. When money is not available to meet expenses, the facility cannot continue to operate for very long and may be obliged to close its doors.

SETTING RATES

How does the administrator guarantee that enough funds come into the facility? The administrator must know how to set rates for the services offered and how to predict the number of patients or residents who will require these services. Appropriate rates for patient care services must reflect their cost, so the administrator must be able to measure these costs.

Besides being available in sufficient amount, funds must come into the facility on a timely basis. The good financial manager understands the billing and collections procedures that keep money owed to the facility coming in regularly enough to meet financial obligations.

PLANNING AND BUDGETING

Financial management is important in planning and budgeting. To make a financial plan, or a budget, *the administrator must be able to predict both the costs of running the facility and the money it can expect to earn in the coming year(s)*. Knowledge of the facility's past financial performance and insight into the reason for earlier budget shortfalls or successes are essential for preparing a realistic and useful budget. The administrator who is not familiar with the costs and earnings of all departments in the facility cannot expect to guide the organization on a reliable path in the future.

RESPONSIBILITY TO OTHERS

Finally, by virtue of his/her position as director, the administrator is responsible for the effective operation of the nursing facility—to its patients or residents and their families, to the employees, to the owner(s) or stockholders, and to the governing body of the facility. When signs of ineffective financial management become apparent, it is to the administrator that each of these parties turns for explanation.

Because nearly every decision made will have financial implications, an understanding of financial management is incumbent on the administrator, the person ultimately responsible for the performance of the facility, even in chain-operated homes.

However good the relationship of the manager with staff or however capable he/she may be in other aspects of administration, if finances are poorly or improperly handled, the administrator is likely to be judged ineffectual by the board or the facility's owners.

3.2 Six Generally Accepted Accounting Principles

The accounting system defines the manner in which financial records should be kept, and it is used by nearly every type of organization, including nursing homes. When we speak of the financial records of an organization, we refer to the books and financial statements. Financial statements will be discussed in detail later, but here we will define the books as *a set of records that lists, in a prescribed manner, each monetary transaction (all money earned or spent) of the facility*.

Maintaining the books constitutes bookkeeping. The books are used to prepare the financial statements. *The financial statements are simply a summary of all of the transactions recorded in the books*, and they reflect the soundness of the organization's financial status.

The books and financial statements are prepared according to a series of rules known as the Generally Accepted Accounting Principles (GAAPs). These are consistent standards of accounting that allow the financial records to be understood by the various parties who have an interest in the financial position of the facility and also permit the financial statements of different homes or other organizations to be easily compared. As an introduction to the accounting system, we will discuss some of the GAAPs that affect nursing homes.

ENTITY CONCEPT

Entity is a basic concept of accounting, under which the nursing facility is regarded as a whole, entirely separate from the affairs of the owners, managers, or other employees. This means that if the owner, for instance, withdraws from or adds to the funds of the facility, this transfer must be recorded in the books to reflect the effect on its finances.

ONGOING CONCERN CONCEPT

Besides being a separate entity, the facility is regarded as an ongoing concern, meaning that it will continue to operate almost indefinitely, regardless of a change in ownership or management. Thus, the assets, those things owned by the facility, are not recorded in the books at their value as if they were going to be sold tomorrow; and all bills and other obligations are recorded in the financial records because they will ultimately be paid.

CONSISTENCY CONCEPT

Another basic rule of accounting is the consistency concept. This concept requires that the accounting reports for a facility be prepared in the same way from year to year, in order to compare accurately the reports between two or more different time periods. This does not require that the organization prepare reports in a manner that is not suitable to the needs of manangement but suggests that the method of reporting be carefully selected and that changes occur infrequently, if at all. Clearly, financial statements that are prepared in a different format every year will make comparisons difficult.

CONCEPT OF FULL DISCLOSURE

Related to consistency is the concept of full disclosure, which means that all financial information: all money spent, earned, invested, or owed by the facility, must be shown in the financial records to represent accurately the financial standing of the facility. The concept of full disclosure has important legal implications, for failure to disclose all financial information may affect the amount of taxes owed by the facility or the level of reimbursement it should receive from insurance carriers.

TIME PERIOD CONCEPT

Also known as the accounting period, the time period is the interval covered by the financial reports, usually 1 year. The accounting period should be consistent from year to year; that is, the fiscal year (the 12-month period designated for financial record keeping) should begin on the same date every year. Accounting records are frequently prepared more often than once a year, usually monthly, to provide management with current information. These shorter time periods should also remain consistent from year to year.

OBJECTIVE EVIDENCE CONCEPT

The objective evidence concept requires that the accounting records be prepared with documentable records that are kept by the facility. Every transaction should be accompanied by a documented record, that is, by a piece of paper that confirms it. These pieces of paper are the objective evidence of the transaction; they include receipts for bills that have been paid, bills (or invoices) indicating money owed by the facility, bank statements indicating interest earned periodically, or cash receipts for money received by the facility each day or designated period. These are called the *source documents* for the transactions. Objective evidence is necessary so that estimates need not be used.

Instead of estimating the cost of supplies purchased during a month, for instance, all invoices are filed in an orderly fashion and used as the objective source documents in determining the cost of supplies for the month. Estimates should be used as infrequently as possible, as this introduces an element of error and inconsistency to the accounting reports. When estimates are necessary, the process used in arriving at the estimated figure should be noted in the financial statements.

Although this is not an exhaustive explanation of the fundamental concepts of accounting, it should acquaint the reader with some of the basic accounting premises. Other important accounting concepts will be included throughout the text where they are best explained by example.

3.3 Two Approaches to Accounting: Cash Accounting and Accrual Accounting

There are two systems of accounting: cash and accrual. The difference between the two is primarily the time period in which expenses and revenues are recorded in the books. *Revenues*, the money coming into the facility, can be recorded for the period when the money from patient care is earned or when the cash payment is actually received by the facility.

Expenses, which we will define for the moment as the money spent by the facility, can also be recorded in two ways. An expense can be recorded when payment is made for items purchased. In accounting terminology, money paid out is called an *expenditure*. An expense can also be recorded when the items purchased are actually used up by the facility.

The difference in the time of recording is the difference between the two systems of accounting and results in two very different ways of preparing the financial records.

CASH ACCOUNTING APPROACH

In cash accounting, expenses are recorded when the cash is actually disbursed, and revenues are recorded when the money for patient services is received by the facility. Thus, the cash system of accounting simply records expenditures and receipts (the actual flow of cash out of and into the facility) as they occur. Organizations using the cash system of accounting therefore do not include in their accounting records "noncash" expenses such as depreciation because depreciation, the cost of wear and tear on equipment, is a cost of providing services to patients that does not involve a cash expenditure.

Cash accounting also does not recognize those expenses that are prepaid, such as insurance paid up for months or years ahead. If the premium for a 3-year insurance policy is paid in the first year that the facility is covered by the policy, an insurance expense would be recorded in the month it was paid and would be listed only as an insurance expenditure for that time period. The fact that it was a prepaid expense and would last over several accounting periods is not acknowledged. Also, money that is owed to the facility for services already provided would not be recorded as accounts receivable but would be counted as revenue only after the facility received payment.

The chief advantage of cash accounting is *simplicity*; revenues are recorded when cash is received and expenses are recorded when expenditures are made, similar to the way we balance our own checkbooks. As we shall see, recording revenues and expenses by the accrual system is not as easy.

However, cash accounting has a number of disadvantages. One is that expenses and revenues for a single time period are not attributed to that same period. For example, medical supplies might be paid for in August but actually used up over the next 4 months. The cost of providing medical services in September would not include the cost of the medical supplies, as that expense would have been recorded in August. Thus, the total cost and revenues, and therefore the real profit or loss for those months, could not be accurately measured.

As mentioned above, the cash accounting system does not recognize the very real cost of depreciation of the facility's building, or plant, major equipment, or other capital items. It also does not recognize money that is owed to creditors by the facility (known as accounts payable, a deferred expense) or money that is owed to the facility by patients for services provided (accounts receivable, a deferred revenue).

Lastly, since the only means of recording expenses and revenues is when cash changes hands, the accounting records are subject to mismanagement by those involved in the accounting process. For these reasons, the cash system is rarely used now, but it is an important concept for nursing facility administrators to understand.

ACCRUAL ACCOUNTING APPROACH

Under the accrual system of accounting, revenues are recorded when they are earned and expenses when they are incurred, regardless of the time the cash transactions take place. We can now alter our previous definition of an expense to one that is more precise. An expense will designate a cost that is used up, or "expensed."

Using the example of the medical supplies, the cost of the supplies purchased in August is expensed over the next several months. The accounting records for September would show a medical supplies expense equal to the cost of the supplies used in September, and so on. This should help the reader understand why the accounting and record-keeping procedures discussed in the next sections are so important. The accrual system requires that every expense incurred by the nursing facility be attributed to the period, usually the month, in which it is incurred and all revenues to the month in which services are rendered.

This complexity is the main disadvantage of the accrual basis of accounting, but it has numerous advantages. Most important, it allows the facility to measure the revenues earned after expenses have been paid, or losses incurred, by matching revenues and expenses for each time period. It also includes depreciation, accounts payable, accounts receivable, and prepaid expenses in the accounting records, providing a more accurate picture of the home's financial position. It is much less subject to tampering, as expenses and revenues are usually backed by several forms of objective evidence. The following discussion of accounting and record keeping will be based on accrual accounting.

3.4 The Two Main Steps in the Accounting Process: Recording Transactions and Preparing Financial Statements

RECORDING TRANSACTIONS IN JOURNALS AND THE GENERAL LEDGER

The accounting process involves two main steps: keeping the books and preparing the financial statements. *Bookkeeping is a system of recording all revenues and expenses, then matching those revenues to expenses during the same time period.* This process is necessary for the preparation of the *financial statements, which are a summary of the nursing home's financial well-being within a time period.*

The accounting process is fairly universal and will be described here in chronological order, from the chart of accounts to the preparation of the financial statements.

Chart of Accounts

The Chart of Accounts is simply a list of every account in the facility. The accounts are organized into five main groups:

assets—things owned by the facility
liabilities—things owed by the facility, or its obligations
capital—money invested in the facility, also known as the facility's net worth
revenues—earnings from operations or other sources
expenses—costs of salaries, supplies, etc., that have been used up, usually through the provision of services
fund account—for tax-exempt homes, funds for which use is restricted by the provisions of the donor

As can be seen from the sample Chart of Accounts in Table 3-1, each account has a number. The first digit indicates into which of the above categories the account falls; the second digit usually indicates a subcategory. For example, RN (registered nurse) salaries are an expense (category 5) in the nursing department and have an account number of 5251.

Note that the salary expense account number for every other department ends with *1* also. This system of classifying accounts is extremely useful, as it identifies every account of the facility and thus is a means of control; expenses, for example, are automatically applied to a specific source so that random or unauthorized expenses cannot accumulate unnoticed. The numbered system also saves time by recording a number rather than a long title on many documents. It is especially adaptable to a computerized bookkeeping system.

The Journals

Any transaction that takes place will affect some account. The journals are the first place that transactions are recorded; they are the books of original entry. Each facility will have its own system of journals, but generally there are six journals:

Cash Receipts Journal—records all cash received for services provided, sales, e.g., refreshment machines
Billings Journal—lists all bills sent for services rendered
Accounts Payable Journal (purchase journal)—records all purchases made that will be paid within the next few months
Cash Disbursements Journal—records all payments made for services and supplies used for patient care and for all other operations of the facility
Payroll Journal—summarizes all payroll checks distributed during the month
General Journal—a record of nonrepetitive entries

TABLE 3-1. Chart of Accounts, Old Well Home

ASSETS		LIABILITIES	

Current Assets   **Current Liabilities**

1101	Cash – petty	2102	Accounts Payable – supplies
1103	Cash – payroll account	2104	Notes Payable – short term
1106	Cash – operating fund	2107	Mortgage Payable – current
1112	Investments – money market fund	2109	Debts Payable – current
1114	Investments – C of D	2111	Emp. Benefits Payable
1117	Investments – depreciation fund	2113	Emp. Health Ins. Payable
1122	Accounts Receivable – Medicare	2115	Salaries Payable
1123	Accounts Receivable – Medicaid	2201	Taxes Payable – payroll
1124	Accounts Receivable – Private	2204	Taxes Payable – state
1126	Accounts Receivable – other	2205	Taxes Payable – municipal
1131	Interest Receivable	2207	Taxes Payable – federal
1163	Unexpired Liability Insurance	2221	Interest Payable

Non-Current Assets   **Non-Current Assets**

1302	Land	2303	Notes Payable – long term
1305	Land Improvements	2313	Mortgage Payable – long term
1402	Building – Main	2323	Bonds Payable
1414	Building – Welsh Hall	2401	Pensions Payable
1426	Building – garage/storage		
1430	Building Improvements	**CAPITAL**	
1502	Furniture – Main	3001	Owner's Equity
1504	Furniture – Welsh Hall	3101	Net Income (Loss)
1512	Equipment – Main		
1514	Equipment – Welsh Hall	**REVENUE**	
1516	Equipment – office	Skilled Care	
1518	Equipment – kitchen	4001	Medicare
1519	Equipment – laundry	4003	Medicaid
1521	Equipment – transportation	4005	Private
1524	Equipment – land maintenance	Intermediate Care	

Contra Assets, Accum. Depreciation

1602	Accum. Depr. – main bldg.	4103	Medicaid
1604	Accum. Depr. – Welsh Hall	4105	Private
1606	Accum. Depr. – garage/storage	4107	Other
1630	Accum. Depr. – bldg. improvements	Ancillary	
1642	Accum. Depr. – furn., main	4212	Physical Therapy
1644	Accum. Depr. – furn., Welsh	4214	Occupational Therapy
1651	Accum. Depr. – equip., main	4216	Social Services
1654	Accum. Depr. – equip., Welsh	4218	Speech Therapy – contract
1666	Accum. Depr. – office equip.	Uncompensated Care	
1668	Accum. Depr. – kitchen	4311	Contract. Discount – Medicare
1669	Accum. Depr. – laundry	4313	Contract. Discount – Medicaid
1671	Accum. Depr. – transportation	4315	Contract. Discount – Other
1674	Accum. Depr. – land maintenance	4332	Donated Care
1680	Accum. Depr. – bldg. improvements	4341	Bad Debts
		4351	Patient Refunds

TABLE 3-1. (continued)

EXPENSES

Administration

5001	Salaries – administation
5002	Salaries – clerical
5003	Consultation fees
5006	Health Insurance
5011	Payroll tax
5013	Taxes – income
5015	Taxes – property
5022	Insurance – liability
5026	Pension fund
5032	Supplies
5034	Telephone
5035	Travel
5037	Postage
5039	Licenses and Dues
5042	Repairs

Plant Operation

5101	Salaries
5106	Health Insurance
5111	Payroll tax
5122	Utility – electricity
5124	Utility – gas
5126	Utility – water
5128	Utility – sewage
5132	Supplies
5142	Repairs

Nursing

Skilled Level:

5201	Salaries – registered nurses
5202	Salaries – licensed practical
5203	Salaries – aides
5206	Health Insurance
5211	Payroll tax
5222	Pharmacy
5224	Laboratory
5232	Supplies
5237	Uniform
5242	Repairs

Intermediate Level:

5251	Salaries – registered nurses
5252	Salaries – licensed practical
5253	Salaries – aides
5256	Health Insurance
5261	Payroll tax
5272	Pharmacy
5274	Laboratory
5282	Supplies
5287	Uniform
5292	Repairs

Dietary

5301	Salary – dietician
5302	Salary – food service
5306	Health Insurance

5311	Payroll tax
5332	Supplies
5342	Repairs

Laundry

5401	Salaries
5406	Health Insurance
5411	Payroll tax
5432	Supplies
5442	Repairs
5461	Contract services

Housekeeping

5501	Salaries
5506	Health Insurance
5511	Payroll tax
5532	Supplies
5542	Repairs

Rehabilitation

Physical Therapy:

5601	Salaries
5606	Health Insurance
5611	Payroll tax
5632	Supplies
5642	Repairs

Occupational Therapy:

5661	Salaries
5666	Health Insurance
5671	Payroll tax
5682	Supplies
5692	Repairs

Social Services

5701	Salaries
5706	Health Insurance
5711	Payroll tax
5732	Supplies
5742	Repairs

Activity

5801	Salaries – beautician
5802	Salaries – crafts
5806	Health Insurance
5811	Payroll tax
5832	Supplies – beauty
5833	Supplies – crafts
5835	Transportation
5837	Special Events
5842	Repairs

Capital Expenses

5904	Interest – mortgage
5907	Interest – long term debt
5914	Debt Service – mortgage
5917	Debt Service – long term debt
5934	Depreciation – plant
5936	Depreciation – equipment

The journals are characterized by another concept of accounting: *double-entry accounting*. For each transaction, two entries are made in the appropriate journal, a debit and a credit.

A debit in accounting simply means the left side of the journal account; credit refers to the right side. When all debits and credits are totaled at the end of each month, they should be equal. Thus, for every debit entered, one or more credits are entered that equal the debit, and vice versa. Table 3-2 indicates which transactions are recorded as debits and which as credits.

TABLE 3-2. Transactions Recorded as Debits and Credits

Debit	Credit
(+) Increase in assets	(−) Decrease in assets
(+) Decrease in liability	(−) Increase in liability
(−) Decrease in capital	(+) Increase in capital
(−) Decrease in revenues	(+) Increase in revenues
(−) Increase in expenses	(+) Decrease in expenses

Journal entries are set in the shape of a *T* as in Table 3-2 and thus are often called T-accounts. Data for the journal entries are the source documents, the objective evidence referred to at the beginning of the chapter.

To illustrate the process of journalizing, we will use the example of the Billings Journal. When a bill is sent to a service recipient or client or to that person's payer, the bill represents revenues earned by the facility that it expects to receive. This account receivable is an asset because it is cash to which the facility is entitled. Thus, a bill to Mrs. Jones for $1,000 would be recorded in the debit column as an increase in assets. On the credit side, $1,000 would be recorded as an increase in revenue. This journal entry is illustrated in Figure 3-1. The source document for this entry would be a copy of the invoice sent to Mrs. Jones.

			Debits	Credits
3/02		Acc't Receivable – Jones, F.		1 0 0 0 00	
3/02		Revenue			1 0 0 0 00
3/02		Acc't Receivable – Ross, M.L.		2 0 0 00	
3/02		Revenue			2 0 0 00

FIGURE 3-1. Old Well Home billings journal.

When the billings to all service recipients for the month are entered in the journal in this manner, the sum of debits should equal the sum of credits at the end of the month. Notice that the Billings Journal is used only for the billing of a service; the service recipient's payment of the bill will be recorded in the Cash Receipts Journal. The complete transaction would be recorded as follows:

Billings Journal

	Debit _____	Credit _____
3/02	Acc/Rec $1000.00 (account receivable)	
3/02		Revenue $1000.00

Cash Receipts Journal

	Debit _____	Credit _____
4/22	Cash $1000.00	
4/22		Acc/Rec $1000.00

The credit in the Cash Receipts Journal would not be due to an increase in revenue but to a decrease in accounts receivable. Remember, under the accrual system of accounting, revenue is recognized when the services are provided, rather than when the cash is received.

Role of the General Journal. The General Journal records transactions that do not properly fit into any of the other journals. Note that the first five journals all record cash transactions; *the General Journal is used to make adjustments in the books to conform to the accrual system of accounting.*

As with medical supplies, the supplies purchased in August will be only partially consumed in that month, but the Cash Disbursements Journal would record the cash expenditure for the supplies purchased in August. Under the accrual method of accounting, only the costs of supplies used in August should be included in the August financial reports, so the total cost of providing services can be compared with the revenues earned in the same period. Therefore, an entry must be made in the General Ledger to adjust the medical supplies expenditure in the Cash Disbursements Journal to the cost of medical supplies used up in August. This is known as an *adjusting entry*.

If an expenditure of $300 for medical supplies is made in August, and the inventory records compiled at the end of August revealed that $75 remained in inventory, the adjusting entry in the General Journal would be as follows:

General Journal

	Debit _____	Credit _____
8/29	Med Supp $225.00 (an increase in expenses)	
8/29		Inventory $225.00 (decrease in asset)
8/29	Inventory $75.00 (increase in asset)	
8/29		Med Supp $75.00 (decrease in expenses)

In addition to adjustments for inventory, entries for depreciation and prepaid expenses are also recorded in the General Journal to reflect the cost of using the plant or equipment over the time period, as well as the amount of prepaid expenses used up.

Finally, the General Journal can be used to correct errors made in the other journals. The General Journal accounts are usually repeated from month to month and therefore should be standardized to the extent possible. This prevents omission of nonapparent but very real costs.

The General Ledger

At the end of each month, when all adjusting entries have been made in the journal accounts, the financial information in all journals is *posted* (written or entered in) to the General Ledger.

The General Ledger can be thought of as *a summary of all debits and credits contained in the journals for the time period*. It usually has a page for each account in the Chart of Accounts.

The purpose of the ledger is twofold. First, it keeps a continuous balance of the amount in any account for each month. It also enables a "trial balance" to be done. Before the financial statements can be prepared, the total of all debit columns in all journals must equal the total amount from all of the credit columns. By accumulating all journal entries in one book, the ledger, debits and credits can be easily added up and compared. When total debits equal total credits, the books are said to "balance," and thus a trial balance has been calculated. If total debits do not equal total credits, then there is an error in one or more of the journal entries.

Remember that under the double-entry concept of accounting, each debit recorded in a journal must be matched by a credit of an equal amount. The trial balance, therefore, indicates whether or not an error has been made in recording transactions.

With so many accounts, there is ample opportunity for error. Thus, accuracy in preparing the journal and ledger entries will save a great deal of time spent in a search for possible mistakes. The relationship between the journals and General Ledger is shown in Figure 3-2.

The General Ledger should be arranged in the order that the accounts will appear in the financial statements. Once the trial balance and profit/loss statements are prepared, the ledger is closed. This process will be discussed in the following description of the financial statements.

PREPARING THE FINANCIAL STATEMENTS: THE INCOME STATEMENT AND THE BALANCE SHEET

The financial statements are the summary of all transactions made during a particular time period and their effect on the finances of the facility. The GAAPs require that the financial statements include four reports:

1. Income statement, or profit/loss statement.
2. Balance sheet, or statement of financial position.

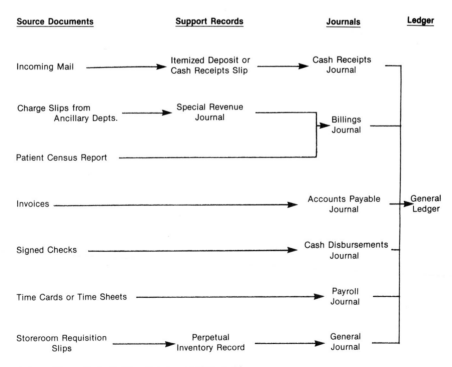

Adapted from Catholic Hospital Association, p. 14.

FIGURE 3-2. Source documents, support records, journal, ledger.

3. Statement of changes in financial position.
4. Notes to the financial statements.

The income statement and balance sheet are prepared directly from the General Ledger (Figure 3-3) and will be described below. The statement of changes in financial position and the notes to the financial statements are prepared from the income statement and balance sheet, and they will be discussed in less detail.

Profit and Loss: the Income Statement

The income statement shows whether revenues were sufficient to cover expenses, whether the facility made or lost money during the time period.

In accounting, income does not refer to the funds coming into the facility but to revenues minus expenses, or the profit or loss experienced by the facility (or income compared to expenses in not-for-profit operations). While net income indicates that the facility made money, or had some revenues in excess of expenses, a net loss indicates the facility lost money in the time period covered by the income statement. A net loss, or any negative figure on the financial statements, is usually shown in parentheses.

The income statement in Table 3-3 shows a net income of $833 for the month of July and $35,625 for the year until then. Revenues are listed first on the income statement, usually starting with the largest source of revenues. From the General Ledger, all of the revenues earned from providing room and board or other services are calculated as routine services, separated by the level of care or type of service.

When all revenues earned from providing services, or operating revenues, from the General Ledger have been computed, any deductions from revenue are subtracted from the gross operating revenues. Deductions from operating revenues might include money owed to the facility

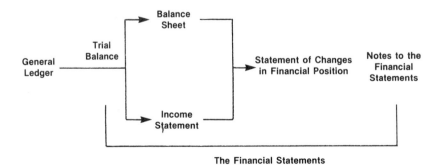

The Financial Statements

FIGURE 3-3. The financial statements.

TABLE 3-3. Old Well Home Income Statement

REVENUES	July 19X1	YEAR TO DATE
OPERATING REVENUES		
NURSING		
SKILLED	93,247	568,807
INTERMEDIATE	264,356	1,639,007
TOTAL NURSING	357,603	2,207,814
ANCILLARY		
PHYSICAL THERAPY	9,974	61,839
OCCUPATIONAL THERAPY	9,890	59,340
SOCIAL SERVICES	2,866	16,909
TOTAL ANCILLARY	22,730	138,088
GROSS OPERATING REVENUES	380,333	2,345,902
LESS DEDUCTIONS	45,640	281,508
NET OPERATING REVENUE	334,693	2,064,394
NON-OPERATING REVENUE		
MISCELLANEOUS		
MEALS	430	2,494
CONCESSION	1,358	8,691
BEAUTY SHOP	790	4,819
TOTAL MISCELLANEOUS	2,578	16,004
INTEREST	2,640	15,312
NON-OPERATING REVENUE	5,218	31,316
TOTAL REVENUES	339,911	2,095,710
EXPENSES		
OPERATING EXPENSES		
SALARIES		
NURSING		
SNF	50,452	307,757
ICF	84,741	525,394
DIETARY	15,582	93,492
ADMINISTRATION	9,551	54,441
LAUNDRY	3,409	20,454
HOUSEKEEPING	13,435	81,282
MAINTENANCE	5,287	32,145
PHYSICAL THERAPY	9,652	60,808
OCCUPATIONAL THERAPY	3,450	20,735
SOCIAL SERV	2,146	13,305
TOTAL SALARIES	197,705	1,209,812
SUPPLIES	31,393	189,928
ACTIVITY	2,065	12,390
CAPITAL EQUIPMENT	200	1,600
UTILITIES	8,764	52,584
TELEPHONE	163	1,043
INSURANCE	4,003	24,018
TAXES (REAL ESTATE)	3,313	19,878
CAPITAL COSTS		
INTEREST	27,816	166,896
MORTGAGE PAYMENT	24,029	144,174
DEPRECIATION	39,627	237,762
TOTAL CAPITAL COSTS	91,472	548,832
TOTAL EXPENSES	339,078	2,060,085
NET INCOME (LOSS)	833	35,625
INCOME TAX (@ 45%)	375	16,031
PROFIT AFTER TAX	458	19,594

that cannot be collected (known as bad debts or charity care), or they might be due to *contractual discounts*.

In the process of setting rates at which they will reimburse the facility for care, Medicare, Medicaid, or other third-party payers sometimes pay the nursing facility somewhat less than the facility's full charges. This discount from the regular price of providing care is known as a contractual discount. This discounted rate is the price at which the facility has agreed to provide care when it admits the insured patient. Contractual discounts are therefore deducted from operating revenues instead of included as an expense.

Total deductions are subtracted from the gross operating revenue to get the new operating revenue. Net operating revenues for the Old Well Home for July are $334,693. Non-operating revenues, income from sources other than direct patient care, are listed next. In July the Old Well Home earned $900 in interest from funds invested in a local bank and $4,318 from a certificate of deposit. Miscellaneous sources of revenue are also included directly from the appropriate page in the General Ledger. Miscellaneous revenues for the Old Well Home are from guests' meals, the beauty shop, or concession income.

Expenses are listed next, starting with the largest item, which is usually salaries. Nursing salaries are calculated according to skilled and intermediate levels of care, and all salaries are listed by department. The salary expense generally includes any employee benefits and payroll taxes paid by the facility.

Supplies, which are separated by department in the ledger according to the Chart of Accounts, are combined into one expense item in Old Well's income statement. We also see that a capital expense of $200 was incurred in July by the purchase of equipment.

Capital equipment is assets that will be used by the facility to provide services for more than 1 year and will not be sold in the course of operations. In addition to equipment, capital items also include such assets as the building, beds, and furniture. If we were to look at the General Ledger under the Chart of Accounts number for capital equipment expenses, we would discover that the $200 was used to purchase office equipment for the Old Well.

Further down on the income statement there is an expense called capital costs. *A capital cost is an expense related to the use of capital items.* At some earlier time the Old Well Home had borrowed money for new dining and lounge furniture and money to purchase the building, both at an annual interest rate of 13%. For the month of July the total interest expense was $27,816. Interest expenses, then, are one cost of using capital.

A mortgage payment expense of $24,029 for July is a second source of capital costs. Another cost of using capital is depreciation; the cost of wear and tear on Old Well's depreciable assets was estimated to be $39,627 for

1 month. (See section on depreciation for estimation of this expense.)

To compute the net income, or profit or loss, the total expenses are subtracted from total revenues. This gives the net income before taxes. Subtracting a percentage for income tax shows that Old Well's profit after taxes is $458. Although depreciation is a real cost of providing services, it does not represent an actual cash outflow, and depreciation may be added to the after-tax profit to give the actual cash standing of the facility.

The income statement, then, shows the operating performance of the facility for a period of time, and it is usually prepared on a monthly and annual basis.

Closing the Books

Because revenues and expenses must be measured for finite periods of time, these accounts must be brought to a sum of zero so that they can be recorded over again for a new time period. Bringing the expense and revenue accounts to zero defines "closing the books."

To close the General Ledger:

1. For all revenue and expense accounts with a credit balance, add a debit equal to the credit to bring the account to zero.
2. For all revenue and expense accounts with a debit balance, add a credit equal to the debit to bring the account to zero.

According to double-entry accounting, compensation must be made for these new debits and credits in some other account.

1. Add up all of the newly added debits.
2. Add up all of the newly added credits.
3. Subtract the debits from the credits.
4. Enter the difference in the retained earning account, as follows:
   (a) If the difference is a profit, enter it as a credit.
   (b) If the difference is a loss, enter it as a debit.

Thus, all revenue and expense accounts have been brought to zero, and the books are balanced and ready for a new time period.

Statement of Financial Condition: The Balance Sheet

Unlike the income statement, which summarized operating performance over a period of time, the balance sheet records the financial position of the nursing facility at one point in time. Whereas the income statement shows the ending balance of the revenue and expense accounts, *the balance sheet summarizes the assets, liabilities, and capital accounts of the facility*. This document is called a balance sheet because the asset accounts must balance with the liability and capital accounts. This relationship can be expressed as an equation, called the accounting equation:

$$\text{Assets} = \text{Liabilities} + \text{Capital}$$

The balance sheet for the Old Well Home for the year is shown in Table 3-4. Assets are listed on the left in order of liquidity.

Current assets refers to those possessions of the facility that will be, or theoretically can be, turned into cash within 12 months. Prepaid insurance is considered an asset because the coverage is something owned by the facility. The income statement records the proportion of the prepaid insurance that was used in the month of July ($4,003), and the balance sheet shows the amount of insurance that remains.

Non-current assets, of course, refers to those assets that will not be liquidated within the year; they usually include plant (the building), property, and equipment. These are also called *fixed assets* and are recorded at their cost at the time of purchase, rather than their current market value.

The *historic cost concept* is another basic tenet of accounting and relates to the ongoing concern concept: since capital assets will not be liquidated any time soon, their current market value is of little relevance. The value of these assets to the facility, however, must include the depreciation on plant and equipment over the years, and so this accumulated depreciation is subtracted from the historical cost of the depreciable assets. Although land usually appreciates in value over time, it does not do so simply through the operations of the facility and is therefore recorded at historic cost, with no depreciation from its value.

Depreciation, therefore, is an expense associated with the use of an asset, so depreciation is included both as an expense on the income statement and as a *contra asset* (literally, "against an asset") on the balance sheet. Note that employees are not included as an asset. This is because assets are those things owned by the facility; an organization cannot own its employees.

Liabilities are the obligations of the facility. Current liabilities are those obligations that must be met within the next 12 months, such as bills from suppliers of foodstuffs and medical or office supplies, and short-term bank loans.

On this particular date, the Old Well Home owes its suppliers $2,852. If this debt were paid tomorrow and a balance sheet made up for that day, Old Well would have no accounts payable on its balance sheet. *Notes payable* refers to loans that must be repaid within 12 months. The Old Well Home owes $33,625 to a local bank for interest on its borrowed funds, as well as a portion of a long-term debt due within the year. The non-current

TABLE 3-4. Old Well Home Balance Sheet

ASSETS	JULY 31, 19X1	JULY 31, 19X0
CURRENT ASSETS		
CASH	60,700	2,834
ACCOUNTS RECEIVABLE		
(Less Bad Debts of $9,032)	53,517	61,397
SECURITIES	225,275	10,500
INVENTORY	62,006	54,880
PREPAID INSURANCE	2,400	3,600
TOTAL CURRENT ASSETS	403,898	133,211
NON-CURRENT ASSETS		
EQUIPMENT	1,983,000	1,981,200
PLANT	5,767,004	5,767,004
Less Accumulated Depreciation	2,772,192	2,362,300
Plant and Equipment	4,977,812	5,385,904
PROPERTY	2,650,000	2,650,000
TOTAL FIXED ASSETS	7,627,812	8,035,904
TOTAL ASSETS	8,031,710	8,169,115
LIABILITIES		
CURRENT LIABILITIES		
ACCOUNTS PAYABLE	2,852	24,606
NOTES PAYABLE	33,625	355,271
BENEFITS PAYABLE	24,843	630,388
CURRENT PORTION OF		
LONG TERM DEBT:		
MORTGAGE	230,680	192,233
LONG TERM DEBT	75,000	75,000
TOTAL CURRENT LIABILITIES	367,000	1,277,498
NON-CURRENT LIABILITIES		
MORTGAGE PAYABLE	3,460,202	3,690,883
DEBTS PAYABLE	675,000	750,000
TOTAL NON-CURRENT LIABILITIES	4,135,202	4,440,883
TOTAL LIABILITIES	4,502,202	5,718,381
NET WORTH		
RETAINED EARNINGS		
YEAR TO DATE	35,625	27,507
TOTAL	370,956	335,331
OWNER'S EQUITY	3,122,927	2,087,897
TOTAL NET WORTH	3,529,508	2,450,735
TOTAL LIABILITIES AND CAPITAL	8,031,710	8,169,115

liabilities section shows which debts these are. Old Well has a payment due on its debt for new furniture, and a portion of its mortgage payment is due also.

Capital accounts, or net worth, are recorded below the liabilities. This section is also called owners' equity, shareholder's equity, fund balance, or retained earnings, depending on the origin of the funds that make up this section. It includes funds that the owners have put into the facility, whether the owners be one person, a partnership (two or more unincorporated owners), a corporation, or a charitable organization. Net worth also usually includes retained earnings, or the net income that has been put back into the facility over the years.

If the facility incurs a net loss, this amount is subtracted from the net worth. The Old Well's net worth includes the retained earnings of the year to date and the retained earnings from the facility's earlier years of operation. It also shows that the owners have invested $3,122,927 in the facility over the years. If this amount was from stockholders, it would be called shareholders' equity; if from a charitable organization, it would be a fund balance.

The most important thing to remember about the net worth is that it is not a pool of cash. The funds recorded as net worth are monies that have been put into the facility at some time; it is merely a record of these funds, not cash available for operations or investment.

Remember, the balance sheet shows the financial position of the facility for only one point in time. Its relation with the income statement is the retained earnings, which usually include the net income in the net worth.

Thus, the basic accounting equation can be expanded to

$$\text{Assets} = (\text{Liabilities} + \text{Owner's Equity}) + (\text{Revenues} - \text{Expenses})$$

Two Additional Financial Statements

Statement of Changes in Financial Position.   Also simply called the statement of changes, this financial report shows the major transactions that occurred over the period covered by two balance sheets, or the way that working capital was used during that period. *Working capital* simply refers to the current assets and current liabilities from the balance sheet. The amount of working capital available is

$$\text{Current Assets} - \text{Current Liabilities}$$

The statement of changes shows the transactions that caused the amount of working capital to change over a time period. It is therefore a very useful document for parties interested in knowing how the facility acquires and uses its funds.

Sources of funds are generally an excess of revenues over expenses of operations, interest income, and contributions to the facility (or owner's equity). Non-cash items, such as depreciation or money designated for repayment of debts, are added as a source of funds because this is still cash (a current asset) owned by the facility.

Uses of funds would include non-operating expenses such as repayment of a portion of a debt or additions to property. The uses of funds are subtracted from the sources of funds to give the change in working capital over the time period. This difference should equal the change in working capital calculated from the balance sheets at the beginning and end of the time period covered.

Notes to Financial Statements. The notes to financial statements are included to explain the accountant's interpretation or calculation of figures, or variation in the books due to a change in their organization, which may not be readily understood by those reviewing the financial statements. The financial statements are not considered complete without each of these notes.

Staff Functions in the Accounting Process

The number of staff persons in the business office and their degree of specialization will vary with the size, complexity, and ownership of the facility. In general, however, those responsible for the accounting functions will be the bookkeeper, the accountant or comptroller, and the administrator.

The bookkeeper maintains the journals and ledger and performs the trial balance. An accountant or comptroller may also check the trial balance, but his/her primary task is the preparation of the financial statements.

For all practical purposes, it is legally mandatory that a nursing facility have its books officially audited, that is, audited by a person who is a certified public accountant (CPA). It is almost impossible to do business without having the facility's books audited by a CPA, who, in effect, serves as the public's representative.

Administrators of a chain-owned facility will generally send the data from the books to a regional or corporate office, where the financial statements, as well as a variety of other schedules, will be compiled and returned.

3.5 Putting Financial Statements to Work: Working Capital, Ratio Analysis, and Vertical Analysis

The net income is an important and readily identifiable item of interest on the financial statements. What other information can be discerned from these reports? We will look at several ways the administrator can put financial statements to work. The three tools we will discuss below are (a) working capital, (b) ratio analysis, and (c) vertical analysis.

WORKING CAPITAL

Current assets minus current liabilities equals the working capital available. This can also be considered the funds available to the facility.

Suppose the administrator of the Old Well Home wants to learn if enough funds are available to purchase $60,000 worth of capital equipment for the nursing departments. Where can this information be found?

The net income for the month of July—and for the entire year—has been reinvested in the facility, as indicated by the net worth section of the balance sheet; these funds may or may not still be available. Although the net worth shows the funds that have been invested in the facility, it is *not* a pool of cash. Recall that the net worth is merely a record of the funds that have been invested in the facility over time and that most of the funds shown here are therefore not available for spending or investing.

The administrator might also check the cash accounts of the Old Well to see if the cash for purchasing the items is available. But this is not suitable either, for if the Old Well Home owes $367,000 to various creditors, as indicated by the current liabilities section of the balance sheet, any available cash may be needed to meet these obligations.

In order to get an idea of the funds available to purchase the needed equipment, the administrator must look at the amount of working capital available. The amount of current assets remaining after current liabilities have been subtracted yields the amount of money that the administrator has to work with.

The administrator finds that there is only $36,898 in working capital available to purchase equipment for the nursing departments and that the facility probably should not purchase new equipment at this time. Since current assets include relatively non-liquid accounts, such as inventory and prepaid insurance, the working capital may be calculated by excluding these accounts from the total current assets.

RATIO ANALYSIS

Another common way of analyzing financial statements is to perform a ratio analysis. Financial managers generally express the information in financial statements as a series of ratios.

There are an infinite number of ratios that may be derived from financial statements, but the discussion here will be confined to several of the more common measures of financial performance. References for Part 3 include several excellent texts that explore financial statement analysis in greater detail.

Usefulness of Ratios

Ratios are useful in several ways. First, financial ratios are no more than fractions using the numbers in the financial statement and are therefore fairly simple to calculate quickly and easily.

Ratio analysis also allows the administrator to identify trends in many measures of financial performance of the facility by comparing the same ratio for several periods. Ratio analysis of the financial statements can also be used to compare the financial performance of several facilities. It is one of the most useful tools the administrator has.

We have already mentioned that the amount of working capital available is calculated by subtracting current liabilities from current assets. A positive amount of working capital indicates that the facility is able to meet its current obligations with its current assets.

If all patient revenues were collected before or immediately after they were earned, the facility would have no need of excess working capital. But since third-party payers, such as Medicare and Medicaid, pay nursing facilities for services 1 to 6 months or more after they are rendered, the facility must maintain a certain level of working capital to meet expenses during the "lag time" before the payments are received. Even nursing homes that have exclusively privately paying patients must plan for collections of patient bills to extend over a period of weeks to months. How much working capital should the facility maintain to cover its lag time? One way to get an idea of an appropriate amount is to perform a current or acid-test ratio:

Current Ratio

$$Current\ Ratio = Current\ Assets/Current\ Liabilities$$

The Old Well Home has

$$\$403,898 - \$367,000 = \$36,898$$

in working capital. Their current ratio is

$$\$403,898/\$367,000 = 1.1$$

A current ratio greater than 1 shows that the Old Well Home is able to meet its current obligations, with a surplus of working capital. Does this mean that a current ratio of 2.5 is even better? Not necessarily; a high current ratio may show that the facility has too much money tied up in current assets and that it may make better use of some of these funds by investing them in an interest-bearing bank account.

Interpreting Ratios

Interpretation of an appropriate current ratio exemplifies a point of caution with the use of any ratio. One ratio in itself reveals very little about the performance of the facility. Ratios must be compared either over time or with the rest of the industry. A current ratio of 1.1 may be fine if the ratio for the Old Well Home in the past has been as follows:

Year 1	Year 2	Year 3	Year 4
.80	.85	.90	1.0

A ratio of 1.1 could also indicate a decline in working capital if past ratios have been much higher than 1.1. Industry comparisons are also important. If the average current ratio for the nursing facility industry, preferably in the same region, is 1.0, then the Old Well may be managing their working capital well. If, however, the industry average is 2.04, the Old Well may want to think about increasing the availability of working capital. Thus, interpretation of all ratios is relative to both past performance and industry averages. The administrator of the Old Well will find out what the appropriate current ratio is and adjust his/her own working capital to maintain that ratio.

The Quick Ratio

Another commonly used ratio is the quick ratio. The quick ratio is similar to the current ratio but is a more rigorous and representative measure of current assets, as only cash and accounts receivable, and sometimes marketable securities, are used to cover current liabilities.

$$\text{Quick Ratio} = (\text{Cash} + \text{Acc. Rec.} + \text{Mkt'ble Sec.})/\text{Current Liabilities}$$

$$(\$60,700 + \$53,519 + \$225,275)/\$367,000 = 0.93$$

The quick ratio reveals that the Old Well is not quite able to cover its current obligations with its most available assets.

Average Collection Period Ratio

The average collection period is another useful ratio, showing the average lag time of accounts receivable. Although the administrator of the nursing facility will have relatively little influence in expediting the collection of funds paid by third parties such as Medicare, Medicaid, or major private insurers, he/she should attempt to collect privately paid monies from patients as soon as possible in order to decrease working capital needs. This is therefore an important ratio.

$$\text{Average Collection Period} = 365 \times \text{Acc. Rec.}/\text{Net Operating Revenues}$$

$$365 \times \$53,517/\$334,693 = 58 \text{ days}$$

Since most insurers reimburse the nursing facility 1 to 6 months after billing, an average collection period of 58 days may be appropriate for a facility with a majority of publicly insured patients.

Accounts Payable Average Payment Period Ratio

A related ratio is the accounts payable average payment period, which shows the average number of days used to pay creditors. Too many days in the payable period may develop into a poor credit relationship with suppliers, and too few days may indicate that funds should be invested for a longer time before creditors are paid.

Average payment period = 365 × Accounts Payable/Supplies Expense

$$365 \times \$2,852/\$31,393 = 33 \text{ days}$$

Since most bills must be paid within 30 days, the Old Well Home seems to be performing well in its efforts to make timely payments to suppliers. If the average payment period were much shorter, the Old Well might consider waiting for 30 days to pay some of its creditors and investing these funds in an interest-earning account. (Banking practices are becoming much more flexible, some banks permitting regular checking accounts to draw interest on daily balances in the account.) If a discount is offered for payment within 10 days or so, as specified, early payment of accounts payable might be more cost-effective.

Net Operating Margin Ratio

The net operating margin is the proportion of revenues earned to the amount of expenses used to earn those revenues. A low operating margin may indicate that rates for services should be raised or expenses reduced.

$$\text{Net Operating Margin} = \frac{\text{Operating Revenues} - \text{Operating Expenses}}{\text{Operating Revenues}}$$

$$(\$334,693 - \$339,078)/\$334,693 = -0.013$$

The Old Well's negative operating margin shows that operating revenues do not cover operating expenses and that the administrator should consider increasing charges for services, or reducing operating costs, in order to increase the facility's operating margin. Another approach to this ratio is operating income as a percentage of revenues. This ratio is best compared with industry averages for an indication of performance.

Debt-to-Equity Ratio

The debt-to-equity ratio is a measure of the long-run liquidity of the facility, or the ability of the facility to meet its long-term debts. A small proportion of debt to equity indicates that the facility could incur more long-term debt, other things being equal, if needed; whereas a high debt-to-equity ratio probably shows that the facility may have more debt than may be advisable, all other things being equal. This ratio is of particular interest to would-be creditors.

TABLE 3-5. Old Well Home Income Statement: Vertical Analysis

	JULY 19X1	YEAR TO DATE	VERTICAL ANALYSES		
REVENUES					
OPERATING REVENUES					
NURSING					
SKILLED	93,247	568,807	26%		27%
INTERMEDIATE	264,356	1,639,007	74%		78%
TOTAL NURSING	357,603	2,207,814	100%	94%	
ANCILLARY					
PHYSICAL THERAPY	9,974	61,839	45%		3%
OCCUPATIONAL THERAPY	9,890	59,340	43%		3%
SOCIAL SERVICES	2,866	16,909	12%		1%
TOTAL ANCILLARY	22,730	138,088	100%	6%	
GROSS OPERATING REVENUES	380,333	2,345,902		100%	
LESS DEDUCTIONS	45,640	281,508	12%		13%
NET OPERATING REVENUE	334,693	2,064,394		88%	99%
NON-OPERATING REVENUE					
MISCELLANEOUS					
MEALS	430	2,494	16%		0.1%
CONCESSION	1,358	8,691	54%		0.4%
BEAUTY SHOP	790	4,819	30%		0.2%
TOTAL MISC.	2,578	16,004	100%	51%	
INTEREST	2,640	15,312		49%	1%
NON-OPERATING REVENUE	5,218	31,316		100%	1%
TOTAL REVENUES	339,911	2,095,710			100%
EXPENSES					
OPERATING EXPENSES					
SALARIES					
NURSING					
SNF	50,452	307,757	25%		
ICF	84,741	525,394	43%		
DIETARY	15,582	93,492	8%		
ADMINISTRATION	9,551	54,441	4%		
LAUNDRY	3,409	20,454	2%		
HOUSEKEEPING	13,435	81,282	7%		
MAINTENANCE	5,287	32,145	3%		
PHYS THER	9,652	60,808	5%		
OC THER	3,450	20,735	2%		
SOCIAL SERV	2,146	13,305	1%		
TOTAL SALARIES	197,705	1,209,812	100%	.59%	
SUPPLIES	31,393	189,928		9.2%	
ACTIVITY	2,065	12,390		0.6%	
CAPITAL EQUIPMENT	200	1,600		0.1%	
UTILITIES	8,764	52,584		2.6%	
TELEPHONE	163	1,043		0.1%	
INSURANCE	4,003	24,018		1.2%	
TAXES (REAL ESTATE)	3,313	19,878		1.0%	
CAPITAL COSTS					
INTEREST	27,816	166,896	30%	8.1%	
MORTGAGE PAYMENT	24,029	144,174	26%	7.0%	
DEPRECIATION	39,627	237,762	43%	11.5%	
TOTAL CAPITAL COSTS	91,472	548,832	100%		
TOTAL EXPENSES	339,078	2,060,085		100%	
NET INCOME (LOSS)	833	35,625			
INCOME TAX (@ 45%)	375	16,031			

$$\text{Debt/Equity} = \text{Long-Term Debt/Total Equity}$$

$$\$4,135,202 / \$3,529,508 = 1.17$$

Do you think this ratio shows that the Old Well may have more long-term debt than is advisable? Should Old Well consider reducing the proportion of debt? A debt-to-equity ratio of 0.5 is usually considered sound.

These are some of the more commonly used ratios. There are, of course, many other parameters of financial performance that will be of interest to the administrator, but this review should provide a substantial starting place for calculating other ratios as a matter of interest.

VERTICAL ANALYSIS

A third method of analyzing the financial statements is to perform a vertical analysis. A vertical analysis simply converts each item on the income statement, balance sheet, or other financial report to a percentage of some total item on the same document.

A vertical analysis of the Old Well's income statement, using the year-to-date values, is shown in Table 3-5. Like the ratios above, these ratios are useful when compared over time, or with other facilities. For example, an unusually high ratio of supplies to total expenses in July may indicate that supplies are being wasted or pilfered, provided there has not been a change in the type of services that would warrant a greater use of supplies. On the other hand, although their percentage for July may be higher than for any month that year, if supplies as a proportion of total expenses are consistently higher in July than any other month, then the administrator knows that this should not be a cause for concern.

The administrator can accumulate valuable information from the financial statements by performing both ratio and vertical analyses. By camparing these ratios over time and with other facilities, trends and patterns in the operation of the facility can be identified, which is perhaps one of the most important functions of financial statement analysis. Awareness of such patterns enables the administrator to pinpoint problem areas in the facility and make knowledgeable financial decisions.

3.6 Accounting Procedures that Help the Administrator Maintain Control over the Facility

Although accounting processes are similar in every institution, the procedures for managing finances will vary from facility to facility, and so will the best methods of control.

In financial management, *control* refers to the development and maintenance of systematic ways to identify problems when they occur to permit the administrator to intervene appropriately. To maintain control, the administrator and the staff normally develop policies for all office procedures. By planning them in a rational manner, staff members are able to understand the reason for the procedures and can work to facilitate them. Identification of possible financial problems as soon as they arise enables the staff to deal effectively with them through use of recognized policies.

There are several tools available to assist the administrator in controlling financial operations. Procedures should be arranged so that no single person has complete responsibility for any area of the facility's finances. A system of checks and balances can be established so that part of one person's task is completed or reviewed by another. Furthermore, each employee can be required to take vacation time so that no one has uninterrupted control of certain office tasks.

This recommendation does not imply that employees are not to be trusted but suggests that precautionary measures be in place to prevent problems. In this section we focus on some of the salient business procedures over which the administrator must exercise control.

ACCOUNTS RECEIVABLE: BILLING FOR SERVICES RENDERED BY THE FACILITY

The facility cannot receive monies for services rendered until the patient or client has been billed for them. Delays in billings have a cost: an *opportunity cost*, the opportunity that is lost to invest or use funds when cash owed to the facility is not yet in its possession. Billing that is delayed for even a few days can result in a significant opportunity cost to the facility. Billing is one of the more important functions of the business office.

Financial Review of Applicants

At the time of a resident's or patient's admission the payment source should be established. If the person is not paying for care with his/her own funds or at his/her own discretion, that person's sponsor or legal guardian must agree in writing to pay the bills. In addition, Medicare or Medicaid eligibility should be determined during the time admission is being considered. If already enrolled in either of these programs, the patient will have a card or other document indicating eligibility. Medicare will pay for skilled nursing care, provided a complicated set of conditions is met. Medicaid eligibility varies from state to state, and requirements can be checked through the office of the local fiscal intermediary (state or state-appointed agency that pays Medicaid billings).

The potential client may also qualify for welfare or other public assistance programs or may be a veteran entitled to Veterans Administration assistance. If the patient is paying privately for services, the name, address, and telephone numbers of the payer, if other than the patient, must be obtained. In short, each patient account should have a guarantor's signature to confirm an agreement for regular payment.

Because the majority of nursing facility residents enter as private payers, then convert to Medicaid when their funds are depleted, it is important for the administrator to look ahead regarding the patient's current and future ability to pay. A facility may consciously choose to admit a person, aware that his/her resources are limited and that the patient eventually may have to be subsidized by the facility itself. However, each admission ought to be processed with the greatest possible clarity about future financial obligations that the facility may face.

Patient Ledger Card

When the patient's source of payment has been confirmed, a Patient Ledger Card is made up for each resident, listing the name, room number, source of payment, and daily (or routine) service charges. The charges and the billing and collections procedures must be explained to each patient and/or sponsor.

Preparation of Invoices

Most nursing homes offer services over and above routine inpatient care. Normal additions to service include physical and occupational therapy. Some homes also offer adult day care, respite care, hospice services, and often a broad range of facility health services. In every case charge slips for each service must be collected from each service center on a daily or weekly basis, usually depending on the volume of services. Since these charges are distinct from routine room-related services, a Special Revenues Journal(s) may be created to record these charges separately.

Routine Charges

Once the ancillary charges for the billing period have been determined, they are added (in the case of residents) to the patient's routine charges. The routine charge is the charge for "room and board" services, which usually include basic nursing care, room, and meals. Some homes have developed detailed breakdowns of charges that permit patients to choose from a broader continuum of care.

Daily Census Form

The routine charge may be determined on a daily, weekly, or monthly basis and is calculated with the aid of the Daily Census Form. This is a summary of the home's occupancy that lists, for each day, admissions, discharges, and transfers by level of care (e.g., skilled, intermediate, or other), if more than one is offered in the facility. The Daily Census Form is prepared by the nursing unit(s) and is submitted to the business office each day.

Patient Census Report

A Patient Census Report is drawn up by the bookkeeper (usually for the month) by compiling the information on the Daily Census Forms (Figure 3-4). The Patient Census Report is in turn used to tabulate the total routine charge for each patient or service recipient. Routine and ancillary services are finally calculated for each patient or service recipient and entered on each patient or service recipient's Accounts Receivable Ledger card (Accounts Receivable, Invoice Supplement) (Figure 3-5) and in the Billings Journal.

To expedite the billing process, the Billings Journal should be divided

OLD WELL HOME

MONTH/YEAR	AREA
06/x1	Skilled

DAY OF MONTH

ROOM AND BED	ROOM RATE	PATIENT NAME LAST	INITIAL	PATIENT NO.	1	2	3	4	5	6	7	8	9	10	11	12	13	14	15	16	17	18	19	20	21	22	23	24	25	26	27	28	29	30	31
117	70	Jones			x	x	x	x	x	x	x	x	x	x	x	x	x	x	x	x	x	x	x	x	x	x	x	x	x	x	x	x	x	x	x
118	70	Rose			x	x	x	x	x	x	x	x	x	x	x	x	x	x	x	x	x	x	x	x											

TOTALS

	Private	Agency	Medicaid	Medicare	Other
	240.00		2100.00		
	100.00		1400.00		

TOTALS

Billings
2340.00
1500.00

FIGURE 3-4. Patient census report.

262

by payer type (private pay, Medicare, Medicaid, Veterans Administration, etc.). (The Veterans Administration, besides building new long-term-care beds of its own, is subcontracting with private nursing homes for care of the now-aging veteran population.) The billing process and services covered vary with each payer. Each bill should itemize any ancillary charges (when permitted by the payer) to expedite the processing of invoices by third-party payers.

Predetermined Contractual Discounts

We have mentioned that most third-party payers reimburse the nursing facility at a somewhat lower rate than charges that were agreed on in advance through the predetermined contractual discounts. Although the full charges may not be remitted by these payers, the precise amount of the discount is uncertain.

Medicare pays the facility on an estimated, rather than an actual, cost basis, and it is not always known if a nonroutine service needed by a patient is fully reimbursable. Normally, each state or geographical area has a designated office(s) that acts as the fiscal intermediary for both public programs and processes the home's claims (or billings) for Medicare and Medicaid reimbursement.

Billing Medicare, Medicaid, and Private Payers

The charges for all Medicaid beneficiaries are itemized, usually compiled into one composite bill covering all Medicaid patients for that month, and sent to the fiscal intermediary. For Medicare recipients a separate bill is prepared for each individual patient and sent to the Medicare fiscal intermediary. (In many states the intermediary is the same for both government programs.) For services not covered by the Medicare program, the private patient to whom they have been provided is billed separately. Bills for services provided to private patients are sent directly to the patient or to the patient's sponsor. Services must have already been rendered before third-party payers can be billed. Private payers should be billed in the same month that services are received.

Accounting for Deductions from Revenue

Besides contractual discounts, charity care and bad debts are also sources of deductions from revenue. Charity care is provided to a patient when the service is not reimbursable and cannot be paid for privately. Bad debts, on the other hand, are patient accounts that are past due but are still subject to collection.

Contractual discounts are often the largest source of deductions from revenue. Since most deductions cannot be confirmed

ADDITIONAL CURRENT ENTRIES - COMPLETE SECTION A AND B

ACCOUNTS RECEIVABLE
INVOICE SUPPLEMENT

ADJUSTMENTS TO PRIOR MONTHS - COMPLETE SECTION A AND C

S E C A	FACILITY NO.	FACILITY NAME					
		OLD WELL HOME					
PATIENT NUMBER		INVOICE NUMBER 3012-756-01	YR/MO x1/06	NUMBER /	INVOICE DATE 6/29/X1	PATIENT NAME Rose, M. L.	

STATUS CODES
1 = PRIVATE
2 = AGENCY
3 = MEDICARE
4 = VETERAN
5 = OTHER

AREA
C = CERTIFIED
S = SKILLED
I = INTERMEDIATE
R = RESIDENTIAL

P A Y M E N T S

TRAN CODE	DATE MO/DAY	OPEN ITEM	DESCRIPTION	PRIVATE	AGENCY	MEDICARE	VETERAN	OTHER	STATUS	NON-COLLECT
	/									
	/									
	/									
	/									
			TOTAL							

LEVEL
UNCLASSIFIED
SKILLED
2 - 6 INTERMEDIATE
7 = RESIDENTIAL
9 = HOLD/DOD

A C C O M M O D A

TRAN CODE	DATE MO/DAY	ROOM-BED	NO. DAYS	RATE	AREA	LEVEL	PRIVATE	AGENCY	MEDICARE	VETERAN	OTHER	STATUS	NON-COLLECT
	6/29	118	30	70.00	S	S	275.00		2100.00				
	/												
	/												
	/												
						TOTAL	275.00		2100.00				

A N C I L L

TRAN CODE	DESCRIPTION			PRIVATE	AGENCY	MEDICARE	VETERAN	OTHER	STATUS	NON-COLLECT
	PHYSICAL THERAPY					240.00				
				TOTAL		240.00				

EXPLANATION OF ADJUSTMENTS

TRAN CODE	TRAN CODE	OPEN ITEM	NO. OF DAYS	RATE	AREA LEVEL	PRIVATE	AGENCY	MEDICARE	VETERAN	OTHER	STATUS	NON-COLLECT
65												
65												
65												
65												
65												
65												
65												
65												
65												
65												
65												
65												
65												
65												
65												
65												

TOTAL

FIGURE 3-5. Ledger card.

SECTION C

265

until payment has been received, they are accounted for in the Billings Journal when known rather than estimated. The payment from public insurers will be accompanied by a Medical Assistance Remittance and Status Report. This report lists the patient's name and claim number, the service dates, the description of services rendered, the total amount billed to the program, and the allowed and non-allowed charges, with an explanation code stating why the service was not reimbursed. The T account for deductions from revenue would be:

Billings Journal

Debits _____   Credits _____

2/27   Cont. Disc. $450.00

2/27   Acc. Rec. $450.00

Resubmitting Claims

The amount of the deduction is also included on the patient's Accounts Receivable Ledger Card. If the deduction is invalid, the fiscal intermediary should be contacted for an explanation of the deduction. The claim can then be resubmitted in the next billing, accompanied by the information needed to justify the request for payment.

Medicare Cost Reconciliation Settlement

When Medicare pays a facility for providing care to patients, the amount of reimbursement is based on the cost of that care. However, instead of calculating the actual cost of providing care for each Medicare beneficiary in each facility, Medicare makes an estimate of how much the care for patients in each facility should have cost and then pays the facility periodically, based on that estimate. If this estimated amount of reimbursement received during the year is less than the cost of providing the care, Medicare will make up the difference at the end of the year by paying the facility a Medicare Cost Reconciliation settlement. (Of course, if the payments already made to the facility exceeded their allowable costs, the facility must pay back the difference.) These funds due from Medicare are recorded in the Cash Receipts Journal as follows:

Cash Receipts Journal

Debits _____   Credits _____

11/23   Due from Medicare $375.00

11/23   Cont. Disc. $375.00

Sometimes services that are not allowable by their insurer (e.g., physical therapy) will be provided to patients who cannot pay for them. These services are considered charity care and are "written off" as essentially non-billable. A special account should exist in the Chart of Accounts for this type of care, separate from other types of uncollectibles. Each facility needs policies to govern the circumstances and extent of charity care that will be given.

Free Care

The level of charity care given must be accounted for as a means of controlling the amount if a monetary or other limit is established. Charity care should also be accounted for separately in proprietary facilities, since it can be claimed as a deduction from income tax, but it is no less important to record charity care in not-for-profit homes to maintain knowledge and control over expenditures.

COLLECTING MONEY OWED TO THE FACILITY

In the nursing facility, accounts receivable are the primary, and in some cases the only, source of revenues. Delays in collecting revenues have opportunity cost. The opportunity cost of accounts receivables can be minimized if a collections policy is established and adhered to that will expedite the collection of monies owed to the facility.

Collection of nursing facility revenues is usually not the source of concern that it is in many other businesses, as routine services for private patients are usually paid for in the month that service is provided; and insurers are reliable, though sometimes slow, sources of revenues.

Bad debts may occur when the patient or the patient's sponsor fail to pay the 20% co-insurance for which he/she is responsible on bills for service paid by Medicare or when nonallowable services are provided that a private payer will not honor. Because bad debts do occur, establishment of and adherence to a collections policy is essential.

Collections Policies

An appropriate collections policy will depend on the home's past experience with its payers. For bills delinquent by 1 month, a letter is sent to the payer as a reminder that payment is past due. A telephone call to the payer should be made after an appropriate interval, approximately 2 weeks, if payment still has not been received and the payer has not otherwise contacted the facility with an explanation. The payer should then be periodically reminded of the outstanding bill. The collections policy must indicate if and under what circumstances a collections agency will be used.

Account Write-off Recommendation

Problem collections are most effectively handled with an attitude of diplomacy and firmness, and an effort should be made to accommodate the payer if there is a valid reason for delinquent payment. If a patient's account is eventually determined to be uncollectible, an Account Write-off Recommendation Form (Figure 3-6) is filled out, with one copy retained in the patient's file and another copy going to the accountant, so that the total of uncollectible accounts can be recorded in the financial statements.

Although the facility will have more control over collections from private payers, the administrator should also establish a good relationship with the fiscal intermediary or intermediaries. Properly prepared claims, as well as a pleasant and helpful attitude when dealing with the offices, may help develop a cooperative relationship with these payers.

HANDLING CASH

Cash is easily mismanaged. It is an organization's most liquid asset and can be a frequently used method of completing a transaction. It is also easily concealed.

A chain facility will usually keep only a small amount of cash on the premises, often not more than $500, as most transactions will take place in a corporate office. For those homes that do manage a large cash inflow, however, certain procedures for handling cash must be established.

Cash Handling Procedures

All cash must be handled by at least two employees, both of whom must be bonded. One person should be responsible for receiving the cash, e.g., opening the mail or taking a check in person. This should not be the same person who is responsible for making bank deposits. Checks should be stamped "For Deposit Only" in the name of the facility immediately upon receipt and a daily remittance list prepared for all cash received. One copy of this list should be retained by this employee, and another should go to the person making the bank deposits.

Cash receipt slips should then be prepared, with one copy going to the payer and another to the accountant or the accountant's file. The bookkeeper should record the cash received in the Cash Receipts Journal and also on the patient's own sheet in the Patient Accounts Receivable Ledger (Figure 3-7).

Cash should be deposited in the bank daily to prevent it from being mislaid and to earn a maximum amount of interest on available funds. At the end of each month entries in the Cash Receipts Journal are posted into the General Ledger and these figures checked against the cash receipts entries in the Patient Accounts Receivable Ledger.

Facility _____ # _____ Date _____

Patient Name _____ # _____ P__ A__ M__ VA__ Other __ Balance $_____

Admission Date _____ Discharge Date _____ Expired: Yes ☐ No ☐

Readmission Date _____ Discharge Date _____

Readmission Date _____ Discharge Date _____

Name and address of responsible party _____

_____

Home phone _____ Business phone _____

Date and amount of last payment _____

Brief History of account: (attach copy of form H-0611) _____

_____

_____

_____

Should account be assigned to a collection agency? Yes ☐ No ☐

Facility opinion by _____ Date _____

*Regional concurrence by _____ Date _____

**Corporate concurrence by _____ Date _____

If Medicare—include all intermediary correspondence.

Is coinsurance involved? Yes ☐ No ☐ If yes, please provide dates and amounts: _____

_____

_____

_____

_____ /_____
Administrator   Date

_____ /_____
Regional Controller   Date

_____ /_____
District Director/Director of Operations   Date

*For all accounts over $250.00
**For all accounts over $500.00.

FIGURE 3-6. Recommendation for write-off of uncollectible account.

ACCOUNTS PAYABLE: THE FACILITY'S BILLS

Accounts payable are monies owed to creditors for services or supplies purchased. A nursing home's creditors usually furnish foodstuffs, linens, medical supplies, pharmaceuticals, and office, housekeeping, and maintenance supplies. A file should be set up for each regular vendor or sup-

FACILITY NO. _____

DATE OF DEPOSIT 09/12/19X1

PAGE _____ or _____

FACILITY NAME Old Well Home

PATIENT'S NAME LAST NAME INITIAL	C A S H	MISCEL- LANEOUS		PRIVATE		AGENCY		MEDICARE		VETERAN		OTHER		POSTED TO INVOICE NO.
Jones, F.A.								2375	00					3012– 756–01
TOTALS FOR EA. COLUMN	Ⓐ													
	ACCOUNT	1211		1212		1213		1210		1217				

MISCELLANEOUS RECEIPTS SUMMARY		
ITEM	ACCOUNT	AMOUNT
EMPLOYEE MEALS - FOOD SALES	4820	
VENDING MACHINE INCOME	4860	
TOTAL A MUST EQUAL TOTAL B		Ⓑ

REDEPOSITED ITEMS RECEIVED FROM	AMOUNT

TOTAL OF
THIS DEPOSIT $_____
                                    ACCOUNT 1130

FIGURE 3-7. Accounts receivable receipts record.

plier, as well as a Miscellaneous Vendor file for all unusual or incidental purchases.

When a purchase order is made out and sent to the supplier, a copy of the purchase order should be placed in the appropriate file. When the order is received, all supplies should be delivered to a storeroom, with the exception of foodstuffs. A receiving slip will accompany the shipment; this should be checked against the items received and against the purchase order to make sure all items noted on the receiving slip are actually received and that all items purchased were delivered. Any back-ordered items on the receiving slip should be noted. The approved receiving slip is then placed with the purchase order in the vendor file.

Invoices from creditors are usually sent to the facility at the beginning of each month. The receiving slip and purchase order should be checked against the invoice to confirm that the unit price is the same as when the shipment was ordered and that all supplies charged in the bill were actually received.

All invoices should be approved by the administrator or designated individual and recorded in the Accounts Payable Journal by department. For example, medical supplies and pharmaceuticals may be attributed to Nursing, foodstuffs to Dietary, linens to Housekeeping, and so on. Invoices are placed in an invoice file.

At the end of the month the accounts in the Payables Journal are added, and this sum should equal the total of all invoices in the invoice file. Bills are usually payable within 30 days. Creditors should be paid on the latest possible date, unless a discount is offered for early payment, so that the funds used to pay creditors can remain in an interest-earning account as long as possible. This does not mean that accounts payable should be chronically delinquent while available funds remain in the bank; it is equally important to maintain a good credit relationship with suppliers.

At the beginning of the month the invoices in the invoice file should be used to pay all bills due in that month. Checks should be signed by two designated employees, and all payments should be recorded in the Cash Disbursements Journal at the time checks are written. Invoices should be marked "Paid" and placed in the vendor file, along with the receipt of payment statement when it is received. These source documents are retained until the end of the year for the accountant's records.

INVENTORY: CONTROLLING SUPPLIES AND EQUIPMENT

A system of inventory control is needed to measure the amount and type of supplies used by each department. We know that under accrual accounting we must be able to measure all expenses incurred in order to match them with the revenues earned in a time period. Consistent records of the cost of supplies consumed enable price and use comparisons to be made over time between departments or between services. These records are also valuable in the budgeting process.

A system of inventory control discourages waste or pilferage of supplies and provides a means of keeping supplies at optimal levels. Overstocks of supplies have an opportunity cost: the cost of monies unnecessarily tied up in inventory and a possible cost of obsolescence. Excess inventory also increases the opportunity for pilferage. On the other hand, frequent shortages of needed supplies can impinge on the quality of care and result in frustration among staff or require that costly rush orders be used to meet supply needs.

Ideally, the focal point of inventory control is a locked central storeroom (Figure 3-8). All supplies should be delivered to a central storeroom as soon as they are received. A limited number of employees should have access to central stores, usually one employee on each shift, though access to supplies must be balanced so that supplies may be obtained when needed but are not subject to unwarranted use. Smaller facilities may find a central storeroom impractical, in which case decentralized storerooms can become the responsibility of personnel in the individual departments.

Perpetual Inventory

A perpetual inventory system is recommended to maintain a precise count of inventory on hand, that is, an accurate count of supplies used and those remaining in the storeroom. At the beginning of each fiscal year, probably more often, all inventory in central stores (or the decentralized store-rooms) should be physically confirmed. This is the Beginning Inventory for the time period.

Additions to inventory are noted from the receiving slips included in each shipment of supplies. The Beginning Inventory and Inventory

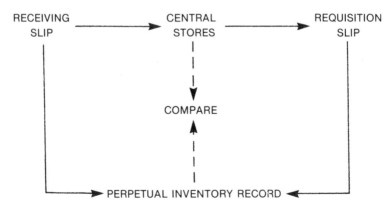

FIGURE 3-8. Perpetual inventory record.

Received by the storerooms make up the Total Available Inventory. When supplies are removed from a storeroom, a requisition slip identifying the supplies and date issued, by department, must be filled out. Supplies issued by storerooms may be taken as the supplies actually used in providing services. This, of course, does not account for those supplies remaining in each department or sublocation that have not yet been used.

For this reason, department heads should be encouraged to keep minimal levels of supplies in their departments. Requisition slips should be initialed by a department head or other designated person. Requisition slips not only provide a check on the unjustified removal of supplies from the storeroom(s) but are the objective measure of the supplies consumed during a particular period.

The receiving slips and requisition slips are the source documents for keeping the perpetual inventory record (Table 3-6). At the end of each year, or other time period, the inventory in the storerooms should be counted and compared with the ending inventory from the perpetual inventory record. If the physical count of the storerooms and the inventory record do not match, this may indicate pilferage, misuse of requisition slips, or inaccuracies in the record-keeping system.

It is advisable for the business office to maintain a list of all inventory items used by the facility, the number of items in one unit, and the current price per unit. This log acts as a reference for determining the cost of inventory used by each department and for establishing the total volume of supplies remaining in the storeroom(s).

LIFO—FIFO

To account for the effect of inflation (or deflation) on the price of inventory, the GAAP recognizes two methods of inventory costing—last in, first out (LIFO), and first in, first out (FIFO). The LIFO method

TABLE 3-6. Old Well Home Perpetual Inventory Record

ITEM #400 SYRINGES, DISPOSABLE	# UNITS	COST/UNIT	COST
JULY			
BEGINNING INVENTORY	4	$7.00	$28.00
GOODS RECEIVED	5	$7.00	$35.00
TOTAL GOODS AVAILABLE	9	$7.00	$63.00
ENDING INVENTORY	3	$7.00	$21.00
GOODS USED	6	$7.00	$42.00
AUGUST			
BEGINNING INVENTORY	3	$7.00	$21.00
GOODS RECEIVED	6	$7.00	$42.00
TOTAL GOODS AVAILABLE	9	$7.00	$63.00
ENDING INVENTORY	4	$7.00	$28.00
GOODS USED	5	$7.00	$35.00

assumes that inventory added last to stores is used first, thus making (in the case of inflation) the value of the goods remaining in inventory lower than that of the goods used to provide services. The FIFO method assumes the opposite: that the older and less expensive supplies (in the case of inflation) are used for services, and the high-priced goods remain in inventory longer. The difference in the effect of these two methods is shown in Table 3-7. Either method of inventory costing may be adopted, but the one selected should be used consistently and should be mentioned in the notes to financial statements.

PAYROLL

Payroll is another source of cash outflow. In fact, it is the largest expense in the nursing facility, accounting for 50% to 70% of total expenses. It also makes up about 85% of the home's controllable costs. *A controllable cost is a cost over which the administrator has influence.* Because it is the primary expense of the facility, accurate accounting records are essential.

The methods of recording time and earnings will probably vary by facility, but each employee should understand the payroll procedure, including the rate of pay, the pay period, date of pay, distribution of checks, and deductions from pay. Employees are usually paid on a weekly or biweekly basis. In a facility that is a part of a chain the pay period will be determined by the company.

For the individually owned facility, however, it is well for the

TABLE 3-7. Inventory

ITEM #400 SYRINGES, DISPOSABLE	# UNITS	COST/UNIT		COST				
AUGUST								
BEGINNING INVENTORY	3	$7.00		$21.00				
GOODS RECEIVED	6	$7.00		$42.00				
TOTAL GOODS AVAILABLE	9	$7.00		$63.00				
ENDING INVENTORY	4	$7.00		$28.00				
GOODS USED	5	$7.00		$35.00				
SEPTEMBER		LAST IN – FIRST OUT				FIRST IN – FIRST OUT		
BEGINNING INVENTORY	4	$7.00	$28.00		4	$7.00		$28.00
GOODS RECEIVED	5	$8.00	$40.00		5	$8.00		$40.00
TOTAL GOODS AVAILABLE	9	4 @ 7.00	$68.00		9	4 @ 7.00		68.00
		5 @ 8.00		OR		5@ 8.00		
ENDING INVENTORY	5	4 @7.00	$36.00		5	$8.00		$40.00
		1 @8.00						
GOODS USED	4	$8.00	$32.00		4	$7.00		$28.00

administrator to remember that payroll funds disbursed biweekly instead of weekly will earn a week's interest. When payroll is 50% or more of total expenses, a week of interest adds up to significant earnings in the course of a year. On the other hand, employee pay should not be withheld for unreasonable periods. The pay period, therefore, is generally determined by a reconciliation of the needs of the facility and of its employees.

Types of Pay Systems

The nursing facility will have two kinds of employees for payroll purposes: those employees who are paid an hourly rate and those who receive a salary that is less dependent on the actual hours worked (discussed in both Parts 2 and 4).

As indicated in Part 2, for hourly employees a time clock or a time sheet is used to record the time worked. If a clock is used, new time cards are made available at the beginning of each pay period. A time sheet is generally filled out by the employee's supervisor. Lunch and other breaks may be noted on these time records. At the end of the pay period the time cards or sheets are submitted to the business office.

Salaried employees generally include the personnel director, administrator, and other professional staff. They usually receive a fixed amount each pay period. Deviations from regular pay, such as a day of leave without pay or compensation for extra hours, should be approved by the administrator.

Payroll Journal

The Payroll Journal lists all paychecks disbursed in the time period, by department. At the end of the pay period the hours worked are entered in the Payroll Journal, as derived from the time cards or sheets and the salaried employees' staffing plan. Overtime (O.T.) hours are compensated at a higher rate and are listed in a column separate from the regular rate. *Gross pay* is then calculated by multiplying hours worked by the hourly rate:

$$(\text{pay rate} \times \text{reg. hrs.}) + (\text{O.T. rate} \times \text{O.T. hrs.}) = \text{gross pay}$$

Payroll Deductions

Payroll deductions must be subtracted from gross pay to arrive at the employee's net pay. They include federal, state, and sometimes municipal taxes, as well as various other deductions made by the facility.

The amount of federal, state, and local tax deducted is a percentage based on the employee's income. These percentages are supplied by the various government agencies. The Federal Insurance Contribution Act (FICA) deduction is the employee's contribution to the Social Security fund.

A certain proportion of the employee's paycheck is withheld, matched by the employer, and remitted on a quarterly basis to the Internal Revenue Service (IRS), which collects taxes for the federal government. Because this payroll tax is part of the cost of providing services, it must be attributed to the time period in which the employees were earning the wages. The cumulative amount of payroll tax is entered in the Payables Journal for each month as a credit to taxes payable and a debit to cash.

Other deductions from the employee's pay may include meals and uniform expense if these items are customarily supplied to employees by the facility. If the employee health plan requires some contribution by them, this would also be noted in the Payroll Journal as a deduction. Deductions for each employee are calculated and subtracted from gross pay to give the *net pay*. A separate column should exist for bonuses or other adjustments to net pay. At the end of each month, salary totals for each department are posted to the General Ledger. A page from a typical Payroll Journal is shown in Figure 3-9.

The employees who divide their time between two or more departments should be listed in the department where the majority of hours are spent, with a portion of their earnings and taxes allocated to the second department.

Separate Payroll Bank Account

The facility should maintain a separate bank account solely for payroll. The person preparing the payroll does not write his/her own paycheck. All paychecks should have two signatures or be approved by the administrator before being disbursed. The paycheck number and the date of issue are recorded in the Payroll Journal to identify checks that are misplaced or to stop payment on checks that are not cashed within a reasonable period of time. Checks are best distributed to each employee in person.

Preparation and maintenance of the payroll is largely a bookkeeping function, although larger homes may have a separate department devoted to this task. In recent years a number of electronic payroll services have been offered by banks and other financial service groups. A telephone call to the bank or data transmission by a telephone line–operated modem accomplishes transmission of information to the financial service, which in turn delivers the checks to the facility at an agreed-on time. The modem is an electronic device that can transmit computer data over telephone lines from the facility computer to the bank computer.

Homes that are part of a chain will have little contact with payroll functions; they usually submit the payroll records to a central office for processing. Paychecks are then sent to the facility for distribution.

TAC NO	FACILITY NAME																	PAGE	PERIOD ENDING	MAIL

PERMANENT EMPLOYEE INFO. — CURRENT PERIOD HOURS AND OTHER EARNINGS — FIXED DEDUCTIONS

		ACCT.	SHIFT 1 HOURS			SHIFT 2 HOURS			SHIFT 3 HOURS			HOL.	VAC.	SICK	OTHER HRS. CD	HOURS	OTHER EARNINGS CD	AMOUNT	CD	AMOUNT
			REG.	O/T	O/T	REG.	O/T	O/T	REG.	O/T	O/T								
NAME	EMP. NO																		
SOCIAL SECURITY	PAY RATE	SPECIAL HOURLY RAISE											accum. vacation hrs.	accum. sick hrs.					
HIRE DATE	SHIFT	SPECIAL HOURLY RATE																	
BIRTHDATE	MARI. STATUS	EXEMPS.	COMMENTS																

		ACCT.	REG.	O/T	O/T	REG.	O/T	O/T	REG.	O/T	O/T	HOL.	VAC.	SICK	CD	HOURS	CD	AMOUNT		
NAME	EMP. NO.																		
SOCIAL SECURITY	PAY RATE	SPECIAL HOURLY RATE											accum. vacation hrs.	accum. sick hrs.					
HIRE DATE	SHIFT	SPECIAL HOURLY RATE																	
BIRTHDATE	MARI. STATUS	EXEMPS.	COMMENTS																

FIGURE 3-9. Page from Payroll Journal.

PROTECTING THE RESIDENTS' ACCOUNTS

Legal Responsibilities

Nursing homes are frequently asked to safeguard the assets of their residents. The agreement to take responsibility for these assets must be confirmed through a legal contract signed by both the facility and the patient or the patient's sponsor. This contract establishes a trust relationship between the resident and the facility, and sound procedures for managing these assets must be adhered to so that the relationship is not violated. It is important to note that resident valuables and bank accounts cannot be considered assets of the facility and that fluctuations in the value of resident assets do not affect the accounts of the facility.

Use of a Safe

Resident valuables, including small amounts of cash and other personal items, should be kept in a safe in the business office. Each patient should have his/her own envelope in which these valuables are stored. When items are given to the office for safekeeping, the patient's name and the contents are entered and the date written on the envelope. The patient or sponsor should initial this information and receive a signed receipt for the items.

Separate Accounting

As a check on patient cash, a separate book should be keep to record the information, shown in Figure 3-10. When valuables are removed from the envelope, the date, contents removed, and contents remaining are noted on the envelope and in the book. A copy of a receipt signed by the patient or sponsor is kept in the envelope.

Use of Interest-Bearing Accounts

Resident funds with which the facility has been entrusted are placed in an interest-bearing checking account, separate from the accounts of the facility and all other patients. Minimal amounts of cash may be kept in the business office for the patient's daily needs. The patient or sponsor should receive a periodic summary of the resident's account, in conformity with state or other regulations.

Withdrawals of cash by the facility must be used only for the patient's needs and should be verified by the purchase receipts. Funds received by the resident, such as Social Security or other benefits, should be deposited promptly in the resident's account after the proper endorsement is obtained. A monthly record of patient accounts should be maintained by the business office, according to the monthly bank statements.

		Page _____ of _____		
		Month ending __06/30/X1__		
Facility	Old Well Home _____	# _____		

Patient Name	Beginning Balance	Deposits	Disbursements	Ending Balance
Jones, F.A.	$210.00	$90.00	$25.00	$275.00

FIGURE 3-10. Patient trust funds trial balance.

Matters such as inventory and payroll should not occupy too much of the administrator's time. However, it is important that all of these details be properly managed by the staff, and experience seems to show that when the administrator understands the fine points of financing and occasionally reviews these matters knowledgeably with staff, they tend to pay attention to details also. The result is that the administrator is thus freed to deal with broader policy while procedures such as payroll and managing patients' valuables function smoothly.

3.7 The Concept of Depreciation

We have mentioned depreciation to some extent already. Capital assets are those used to provide services during more than one time period; in the course of operations they lose value as a result of use, wear and tear, or obsolescence.

To account for this loss of value to capital assets in the accrual system of accounting, the cost of the asset is spread over the time periods that it is used. This must be done because the total cost of acquiring the asset could not properly be attributed to the month in which it was purchased, when it is actually an expense of providing services for several years to come.

IDENTIFYING DEPRECIABLE ASSETS

Assets that can be capitalized or depreciated differ from the other assets of the facility in that they are used in operations for more than one time period and will not be converted into cash within the year. Many facilities set a minimum value for depreciable assets, usually somewhere around $200. An adding machine, for example, may be used in the business office for many years, but its acquisition cost may be so low that the depreciation expense over its useful life would be negligible. The asset must be tangible and by definition must be owned by the facility. Thus, leased equipment cannot be depreciated.

All new assets meeting these criteria are considered depreciable assets. Any alterations of the present fixed asset that affect either its value or its useful life, such as renovation, are depreciable expenses. Repair of damages or regular maintenance of the asset cannot be considered part of the depreciable expense.

DETERMINING DEPRECIATION EXPENSE

There are several methods of calculating depreciation expense, but all methods are based on the historical cost of the asset, its useful life, and its salvage value. We will define these concepts first, then discuss some methods of calculating depreciation expense.

Historical Cost

The historical cost of the asset is the cost of acquiring the asset that is depreciated over several time periods. This cost should be measured carefully, as there may be hidden costs in the acquisition of a capital asset. The purchase price is included in the historic cost, but also the cost of taxes, shipping, delivery, storage, installation, assembly, interest on the money borrowed to purchase the item, and any other one-time costs associated with acquiring the asset should be included. If the asset is donated, its market value at the time it was received by the facility is used as the purchase price.

Useful Life

The useful life of the asset is the number of years the item can be expected to be used by the facility. This must be an estimation because the useful life will vary with the frequency of use and other variables. The IRS supplies useful life estimates for most assets, as do some manufacturers. Many facilities use the American Hospital Association Guide to Useful Life. The useful life may also be estimated from the home's experience with similar assets, or adjusted later if the original estimate proves inaccurate.

Salvage Value

A capital asset may have some value at the end of its useful life. This is the salvage value, and it is subtracted from the historical cost when figuring depreciation. Understandably, the salvage value is more difficult to estimate than the useful life, but when a reasonable estimate cannot be made, a certain percentage of the historical cost, usually 2% to 3% may be taken as the salvage value.

STRAIGHT-LINE DEPRECIATION

There are several methods for figuring the depreciation expense, once the historical cost, useful life, and salvage value are determined. Straight-line depreciation is a depreciation method with which the nursing facility administrator should be familiar. Here the historical cost of an asset is spread evenly over its useful life so that the depreciation expense is the same in every time period that it is in use.

Historical Cost/Useful Life = Annual Depreciation Expense

If the Old Well Home purchases new physical therapy equipment worth $20,000, with an estimated useful life of 5 years, the annual depreciation expense for the equipment would be

$20,000/5 years = $4,000 per year depreciation

After the first year the value of the physical therapy equipment on the books would be

$20,000 − $4,000 = $16,000

Hence, the $16,000 is called the book value of this asset.

Straight-line depreciation has the advantage of simplicity. It is also the basis for reimbursing depreciation expense used by most third-party payers and for these reasons is the recommended method of depreciating assets when the IRS does not prescribe useful life periods to be used with depreciable assets.

ACCELERATED DEPRECIATION

Another method of depreciation is accelerated depreciation, which attributes most of the depreciation expense to the first years of the asset's life, thus enabling the home to write it off more quickly.

Among the several types of accelerated depreciation are the sum-of-the-years digits and double declining balance. These were the most common methods of depreciation for taxpaying organizations until 1981, when Congress standardized the method of depreciation that could be used for tax purposes: the Accelerated Cost Recovery System (ACRS).

The ACRS indicates the percentage of an asset's historical cost that can be claimed as depreciation expense each year. A useful life table is supplied by the IRS; most of the nursing home's assets will be depreciated over 5 years. Since 1981, Congress has steadily lengthened the number of years over which depreciation must be calculated. The 1986 Tax Reform Act extended the time.

PURPOSES OF DEPRECIATION

We have already mentioned that depreciation must be calculated to adhere to the accrual system of accounting. To ignore the very real cost of depreciation is to underestimate the expense of providing services and to overestimate the value of the assets of the facility. For this reason, depreciation is included on the Income Statement as an operating expense and is subtracted from the historical cost of fixed assets on the balance sheet to reflect its impact on the financial position of the home.

As we have indicated, depreciation is also important for tax purposes. While any method may be used to estimate depreciation expense for the home's accounts, depreciation claimed as an operating expense and therefore a reduction in income normally is scheduled to adhere to the ACRS depreciation table. Since depreciation is a non-cash expense, it is often added to the after-tax profit to reflect actual cash flow.

Asset Replacement

Probably the most important reason for recognizing depreciation is for asset replacement. Because the asset will eventually have to be replaced, the present asset should be expensed over its useful life to accumulate the funds needed for its replacement. Chances are, however, that an asset purchased 5 years earlier will be more expensive than the original. For this reason, replacement depreciation should be based on the expected replacement cost of the asset.

Remember, however, that for tax purposes, only the actual historical cost can be used as the basis for calculating depreciation. A fund established to accumulate monies over time for the replacement would appear in the Capital or Net Worth section of the balance sheet as "Funded Depreciation."

Funded Depreciation

The importance of a funded-depreciation account should not be underestimated. For homes that do not have large cash or other liquid reserves, replacement of a capital asset without ready funds may require reliance on debt financing, a costly way of financing capital for a capital-intensive organization such as a nursing facility. The costs of debt financing can include substantial interest expense, the opportunity cost of the interest expense, and the cost of any restrictions the lender may impose on the facility's use of funds until the debt is paid.

If debt financing is not used, the facility may need to devote retained earnings or current operating funds for purchasing the asset, possibly jeopardizing its ability to meet short-term liabilities and perhaps impinging on the quality of care. Restrictions on available cash also limit the purchasing power of the facility and may require that a needed capital item be purchased on the basis of its immediate affordability, rather than its long-term benefits to the facility. In general, funded depreciation gives administration more control in the selection and purchase of capital items.

The individual chain home will probably have no need for such a fund, as this normally is managed at the corporate level. One of the strengths of corporate (investor-owned) facilities is a greater access to capital.

ENTERING DEPRECIATION INTO THE ACCOUNTING RECORDS

A portion of the depreciation expense may easily be attributed to each time period by dividing the annual depreciation expense by the number of accounting periods in the year. Since depreciation is entered in the General Journal at the end of each month, the Old Well's new physical therapy equipment depreciation expense after the first month of purchase under straight-line depreciation would be as follows:

General Journal

		Debit _____	Credit _____
1/29	Depreciation Expense	$333.33	
1/29	Reserve for Depreciation		$333.33

(Old Well could have chosen an ACRS table rate for depreciating the physical therapy equipment instead of the straight-line method, but for purposes of illustrating straight-line we have chosen not to use the ACRS table).

Categorization of Fixed Assets

The Chart of Accounts should have an account for each type of fixed asset owned by the facility. These assets can be categorized generally as

- Land and improvements
- Buildings
- Fixed equipment
- Major movable equipment
- Minor movable equipment

or in more specific categories that are more useful to the facility.

In addition, depreciation schedules should be maintained for each category of assets (Table 3-8) and for each type of depreciation if accelerated and straight-line are both used.

If two differing schedules are used to depreciate the same assets—one

TABLE 3-8. Old Well Home Depreciation Schedule

ITEM	COST	DATE PURCHASED	LIFE	METHOD DEPRECIATED	YEAR	DEPRECIATION PER YEAR ANNUAL	CUMULATIVE
PLANT: MAIN	$5,767,004.00	6/19X0	30	STRT. LINE	19X0	$192,233.47	$192,233.47
HALL WELSH					19X1	192,233.47	384,466.94
HALL & GARAGE					19X2	192,233.47	576,700.41
					19X3	192,233.47	768,933.88
					ETC.		
KITCHEN	$398,600.00	6/19X0	15	STRT. LINE	19X0	$26,573.33	$26,573.33
EQUIPMENT					19X1	26,573.33	53,146.66
					19X2	26,573.33	79,719.99
					19X3	26,573.33	106,293.32
					ETC.		

for reimbursement and one for tax purposes—there will be a difference in depreciation expense for each asset every year. Since the total amount of depreciation taken for each asset should be the same (total depreciation will equal the historical cost less salvage value), this difference between the two depreciation expenses is simply a timing difference. Depreciation in this case may be regarded as a charge that must be deferred to another time period or as revenue that is accrued if depreciation will be recognized in a later accounting period.

3.8 Using "Costs" in Managerial Decisions

In the previous section we looked at bookkeeping and control procedures that result in a current balance in each of the home's accounts. In this section we will use these records to focus on costs and their role in managerial decision making.

A focus on costs is relevant, as familiarity with the costs of the facility and cost behavior is intrinsic to the role of the administrator. As this section will illustrate, knowledge of cost behavior should give the administrator closer control over dollar flows and promote informed decision making. From the perspective of efficiency, an analysis of cost is well justified.

EFFICIENCY

Efficiency may be defined as input over output, or the amount of input used for a certain level of output. Costs, as a component of input, are generally easier to control than are revenues or other measures of output. Revenues are subject to limitation by competition from providers of similar services and government regulation through insurance and medical assistance programs. Knowledge of costs and the ability to control and reduce them permit liquidity of limited funds, making them available for other uses.

Additionally, cost-based insurers, such as Medicare, and assistance programs, such as Medicaid, require annual cost reports from providers whom they reimburse.

We have already mentioned costs in several ways. An expense was defined as that part of a cost that has been used up; thus, an expense is an incurred cost. We have also referred to opportunity cost, which is the cost of benefits foregone when funds are applied to the next best alternative.

In the last section we explained that payroll was a controllable cost, as compared to an uncontrollable cost over which the administrator has little or no influence, such as taxes, interest, or possibly required equipment. We will now introduce two new ways to look at costs and their implications for managerial decision-making.

3.8.1 Two Types of Costs: Variable and Fixed

VARIABLE COSTS

All costs can be regarded as variable, fixed, or semivariable. *Variable costs are those that vary directly and proportionately with changes in volume.* That is, if volume is increased or decreased by a certain percentage, variable costs will go up or down, respectively, by the same percentage. The cost of disposable medical supplies in the nursing department will vary directly with the number of patients served. The cost of food in the dietary department or the cost of postage for patient billing will also vary with patient volume. All three are examples of variable costs.

FIXED COSTS

Fixed costs, on the other hand, do not vary with changes in volume. The cost of the director of nursing's salary will not change with fluctuations in the number of residents. This does not mean that the director's salary cannot change at all, but it will result from an administrative decision rather than responding to patient volume. Clearly, if volume varies enough, many fixed costs will not remain the same. If patient volume increases substantially, a new administrative position in the Nursing Department may have to be created to accommodate the additional patient load. Fixed costs, then, are said to be fixed only over a relevant range of volume.

AN ADDITIONAL TYPE: SEMIVARIABLE COSTS

Semivariable costs do not fit neatly into either a variable or fixed category, as they vary disproportionately with volume. Examples of semivariable costs might be nurse's aides' salaries, which depend more on patient volume and patient service needs than does the director of nursing's salary, which does not fluctuate directly with these variables.

Utility costs that are based on ranges of usage rather than actual usage may also be considered semivariable costs. It is helpful to think of semivariable costs as having a much narrower relevant range than fixed costs. Semivariable costs are often broken down into fixed and variable components for use in calculations, and so our discussion here will be limited to fixed and variable costs for the sake of simplicity. Further analysis of semivariable costs will be left to the more advanced texts on managerial accounting to be found in the references for this section.

TOTAL VARIABLE COSTS

While total variable costs (TVC) change with volume, the variable costs per unit do not do so. If disposable syringes are $1 each, the cost per syringe per patient will be $1, whether 100 or 150 patients receive injections. Total fixed costs (TFC), however, do vary per unit with changes in volume. If the director of nursing's salary is $24,000, including benefits and payroll taxes, and he/she oversees the care of 100 patients, then the director's salary cost per patient would be $240. If the director oversees 150 patients, the cost drops to $180 per patient. Familiarity with the costs of the facility maximizes the administrator's ability to control the finances of the facility.

The behavior of variable and fixed costs is summarized in Table 3-9. As can be seen, fixed costs decrease with an increase in volume. Because the nursing facility generally has a high proportion of fixed costs, maintaining a high volume of service is of paramount concern to their administrators.

A closer study of the concept of fixed and variable costs reveals how it can be used to aid in decision making. Because all costs can be considered fixed or variable (even semivariable costs),

Total Fixed Costs + Total Variable Costs = Total Costs

TABLE 3-9. Behavior of Fixed and Variable Costs

PATIENTS	DIRECTOR OF NURSING (TFC)	FC/UNIT	DISPOSABLE MEDICAL SUPPLIES TVC	VC/UNIT
100	$24000.00	240	100	$1.00
125	$24000.00	192	125	$1.00
150	$24000.00	160	150	$1.00
	(NO CHANGE)	(CHANGE)	(CHANGE)	(NO CHANGE)

Since total variable costs are a function of the variable cost per unit and the number of units, the above equation can be expanded to

$$\frac{\text{Total Fixed Costs} + \text{Variable Costs}}{\text{Unit} \times \text{Volume Units}} = \text{Total Costs}$$

Thus, if three of these values are known, the remaining value can be calculated.

The administrator of the Old Well Home wants to find the average variable cost of medical supplies used per patient during the month. The General Ledger shows that the total costs of the nursing department of 1 month are $12,000. The administrator has determined that fixed cost accounts in that department amount to $9,000 and that medical supplies are its only variable cost. The Patient Census Report for the month shows that there have been 3,000 patient days or an average of 100 patients over 30 days. To calculate the variable cost per patient in the nursing department:

$$\frac{(\text{Total Costs} - \text{Total Fixed Costs})}{\text{Volume units}} = \frac{\text{Variable Costs}}{\text{Units}}$$

$$(\$12,000 - \$9,000)/100 \text{ patients} = \$30 \text{ per patient}$$

Thus, the variable cost of providing nursing services in this particular month was $30 per patient.

VOLUME OF SERVICE UNITS

These equations can be used to determine the volume of service units required to break even. Since total costs (TC) equal total revenues (TR) at the break-even point, TR (total revenues) can be substituted for TC (total costs) in the above equations to give the costs or volume needed to break even.

If the total costs of the physical therapy department are $6,500 per month and total fixed costs are $5,200, and the variable cost per patient visit to physical therapy is $8, how many patient visits are needed per month to break even in this department?

$$\text{Total Costs} = \text{Total Revenue}$$
$$= \$6,500 = \$5,200 + (\$8 \times \text{Volume Unit})$$

or   Volume Units = ($6,500 − $5,200)/$8
Volume Units = 162.5 visits per month

We have assumed that the physical therapists are employees of the facility and that their salaries comprise a significant portion of the fixed costs of the department. If physical therapy is provided on a contractual basis, the therapists' salaries would become a variable cost if they were paid for each visit.

Whether a facility is proprietary or not for profit, an excess of revenues over expenses is desirable in order to meet any increases in costs in the months ahead or to provide a cushion against unexpected and uncontrollable events. The above equation can be expanded to include profit also:

$$\text{Total Costs} + \text{Profit} = \text{Total Revenue}$$

or

$$\text{Total Revenue} = \text{Total Fixed Costs} + \frac{\text{Variable Costs}}{\text{Volume Units}} + \text{Profit}$$

In the last example, suppose administration has decided that physical therapy should earn a profit of 2% of total costs. How many visits must now be provided in order to earn this profit?

$$\text{Total Revenue} = \$6,500$$
$$= \$5,200 + (\$8 \times \text{Volume Unit}) + (2\% \times \$6,500)$$

or

$$\text{Volume Units} = [\$6,500 - (\$5,200 + \$130)]/\$8$$

$$\text{Volume Units} = 178.75 \text{ visits per month}$$

The example shows that 16.25 more visits (178.75 − 162.5) to physical therapy must be provided to earn a profit of 2% of total costs in this department. The administrator must ask if fixed costs will change with this increase in volume, how the additional visits might come about, and, if patient volume remains fixed, whether rates for physical therapy services should be raised instead.

3.8.2 Finding the Break-Even Point

It is often useful to illustrate the break-even concept graphically (Figure 3-11). The area under the horizontal line represents total fixed costs, which

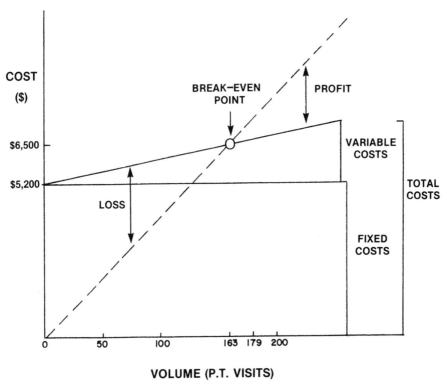

FIGURE 3-11. Old Well Home break-even graph: physical therapy.

do not vary with patient volume. A more precise representation would probably be a stair-step pattern for the fixed cost line to indicate the relevant ranges of fixed physical therapy costs.

The sloping line shows that total variable costs change with volume. The dotted line represents revenue, which meets the total cost line to indicate the break-even point.

From our calculations, we know that the physical therapy department will break even at 162.5 (or 163, rounding off) patient visits per month, but at 178.75 visits it will earn a 2% profit. The profit portion is represented by that area of the graph where the revenue line exceeds the cost line. Break-even analysis can be performed numerically or graphically. Although the former is probably more accurate, the graphic version provides a useful picture of the situation being studied.

The basic break-even equations can be adjusted to address the specific requirements of the facility in terms of volume, cost, and profit, including the effect of income tax on profit:

$$\text{Total Revenue} = \text{Total Costs} + [\text{Profit}/(1 - \text{Tax Rate})]$$

or compensation for contractual discounts by third-party payers.

At the Old Well Home, routine (room and board) fixed costs for care in the intermediate-care-facility level are $146,250, and the variable costs are $78,750 per month. The intermediate care facility has an average of 150 residents, 40% of whom are Medicaid beneficiaries. If Medicaid pays the Old Well Home $35 per day for routine care, what must the charge be to charge-based patients in order to break even?

$$\text{Total Costs} = \text{Total Fixed Costs} + \text{Total Variable Costs}$$
$$= \$146,250 + \$78,750 = \$225,000$$

$$\text{No. Medicaid patients} = 150 \times 40\% = 60 \text{ patients}$$
$$\text{No. Private patients} = 150 - 60 = 90 \text{ patients}$$

To break even, total costs must equal total revenues, so

$$\text{Total Costs} = \$225,000/\text{month}$$
$$= (\$35/\text{day} \times 60 \text{ patients} \times 30 \text{ days})$$
$$+ (?/\text{day} \times 90 \text{ patients} \times 30 \text{ days})$$
$$= \text{Total Revenue}$$

$$\text{Total Costs} = \$225,000$$
$$= (\$63,000) + (? \times 2,700)$$
$$= \text{Total Revenue}$$

$$162,000 = ? \times 2,700$$
$$? = \$60 \text{ per day}$$

Thus, the charges to private patients must be $60 per day to break even in the nursing department. Clearly, the estimate of patient volume is important in determining patient charges.

We have assumed in this discussion that fixed and variable costs are known, although in reality identification of these costs is not always clear. Depreciation, for example, may present a problem in that most capital equipment does depreciate almost directly with volume of use, but depreciation is accounted for, especially under ACRS, as a fixed cost.

Many large health care organizations rely on computer software packages to determine the fixed and variable costs, manage semivariable costs, determine the relevant ranges, and perform a variety of break-even calculations. When such aids are not available (and even when they are), the administrator should be familiar with the total costs of the facility and the operation of each department.

Break-even analysis provides useful, and indeed necessary guidelines for decision making. Although it clearly is not a definitive approach to problem solving, an understanding of the behavior of fixed and variable costs and their relation to volume and profit is an important managerial tool.

3.8.3 Additional Types of Costs: Indirect Costs and Direct Costs

Costs may also be categorized as direct and indirect. In order to discuss them, however, we must first define revenue and cost centers.

REVENUE CENTERS

Revenue centers are units of the facility, often departments, that generate revenue, usually through patient care. Revenue centers in the nursing facility will normally be nursing—providing routine care—possibly physical therapy, occupational therapy, social services, pharmacy, laboratory, and medical supplies. It may also be any other department or center earning revenue, such as a cafeteria that serves a large number of guest meals. If pharmaceuticals or medical supplies are included as part of the routine care and are not separately charged, they would not be revenue centers. In some homes all meals are not included in routine care. Extra meals in this case would provide revenue, and the dietary department would be considered a revenue center.

As homes add service areas, such as home health and hospice care, these become additional revenue centers. If the facility earns a significant amount of revenue from interest on investments, interest may also be considered a revenue center.

COST CENTERS

Cost centers are units of the facility identified with certain costs. Revenue centers are almost always cost centers because the revenue-earning departments also have costs directly associated with them. Interest as a revenue center has no costs associated with it. All other departments, such as administration, maintenance, housekeeping, and usually dietary and laundry, are cost centers, although they need not be departments. Depreciation, interest, insurance, telephone, utility, and transportation expenses may also be considered cost centers. These are all identifiable costs of the facility, and the concept of cost centers will become clearer as we proceed.

DIRECT COSTS

Direct costs are those directly attributable to a revenue center or directly providing patient care. In the nursing facility direct costs are often called resident care costs, and we will use both terms here. Direct costs of the nursing department would include all nursing salaries, payroll taxes, benefits, medical supplies, expenses associated with capital equipment used only in this department, uniforms, if they are provided, and any other costs associated directly with this department.

INDIRECT COSTS

Indirect costs are those that cannot be directly associated with a revenue-producing center yet support the functions of the resident care centers (or other care centers, such as a facility health care or an adult day-care program). Indirect costs of the nursing department would be administration, payroll, utility, housekeeping, maintenance and repair, dietary, laundry, plant depreciation, tax, and interest expenses that keep these departments running. For this reason, indirect costs are also known as support service costs.

Support Service Costs

These indirect costs must be allocated to all the revenue-producing departments that are also cost centers in order to be included in the charge for services in each revenue center and to reflect the total cost of providing that service. To find the total cost of the revenue-producing departments, then, the support costs must be spread over all revenue-producing departments in some systematic way. This process is known as cost finding, as it yields the total costs of the resident care centers (and other centers such as adult day care).

The concept of cost finding is illustrated schematically in Figure 3-12. The total costs of both the support and service, or revenue-earning centers, are shown. To find the total cost of providing patient services A and B, some portion of the support centers must be allocated to the revenue centers. Support Center No. 1 divides its support equally between service

BEFORE COST ALLOCATION:

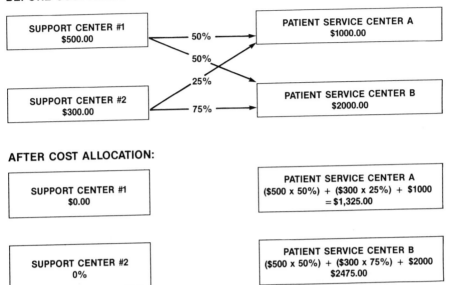

AFTER COST ALLOCATION:

FIGURE 3-12. Cost allocation between two support and two revenue centers.

centers A and B, so 50% of Support Center No. 1's costs are attributed to each Patient Service Center.

Support Center No. 2 provides more services to Patient Center B, and this is reflected in the proportion of Support Center No. 2's costs that go to Service Center B. When the costs of both support centers are allocated, the total cost of providing services A and B are known.

VALUES OF COST FINDING

Cost finding is an important managerial function for several reasons. It gives the administrator a representative picture of the entire expense of providing each service. This information is vital in deciding whether a particular service should be discontinued or supported. For example, unless all direct and indirect costs of providing a service, such as adult day care, are calculated, it is difficult to determine the cost-effectiveness of offering such a service. As we will see, cost allocation is a subjective process in that there is an almost infinite number of ways to perform cost allocation properly. Thus, the resulting costs are representative only of total costs and cannot accurately be called "actual" costs.

Cost finding is also required by Medicare, Medicaid, and most cost-related insurance organizations in order to reimburse the facility for its costs in providing care. Because of the subjectivity involved, these insurers provide worksheets and detailed guidelines for performing cost allocation.

Cost finding also facilitates the budgeting process. When budgeting is usually done on a departmental basis, an annual examination of each department's costs through the cost-finding process enables the administrator and department heads to estimate expenses with greater accuracy.

ALLOCATING INDIRECT COSTS

There are several methods for allocating indirect costs, among them the *step-down* and *reciprocal* methods. Providers who are reimbursed on a cost basis must usually use the step-down method unless another method is approved. We will discuss the step-down method in detail here and briefly explain the reciprocal method at the end of this section.

The step-down method derives its name from the shape of the completed worksheet and involves the systematic allocation of all cost centers over all other cost centers that use the "services" of the cost-center costs being allocated. Support costs are spread not only over revenue centers but also over other support cost centers.

Once a support cost is divided among the other cost centers, no more costs can be allocated to that department. Therefore, the order in which support costs are allocated affects the final cost of the revenue centers. As a rule, cost centers that are used by most of the other cost centers are allocated first.

The basis of allocation also affects the outcome of the cost-finding process. In allocating housekeeping costs to the departments that use housekeeping services, the basis for allocation might be the number of employees in the department, the square footage of the departments, or some other criteria. Likewise, administrative costs might be allocated on the basis of number of employees, total salary of employees, volume of services provided, or total revenues earned in each department. We offer these alternatives as examples only; clearly, the basis for allocation can vary widely.

Third-party reimbursers will indicate the basis for allocation that should be used for homes with insured patients, but in any case it should remain consistent to enable comparison of the resulting costs in different time periods.

The Step-Down Process

Cost allocation is best illustrated through a step-by-step example of the step-down process. The one provided in Tables 3-10 and 3-11 is necessarily

TABLE 3-10. Old Well Home Step-down Worksheets: Preliminary Worksheet

Cost Centers	Capital (sq. ft.)	Plant (sq. ft.)	Admin. (1) (- FTE)-(1)	Main. (1) (sq. ft.)	Laundry (lbs. dry)	Housekeep (sq. ft.)	Dietary (meals)	Soc. Serv. (visits)	P.T. (visits)	O.T. (visits)	SNF	ICF	TOTAL
Support & Revenue Centers													
Administration	3.0%	3.0%											
Maintenance(2)	1.5%	1.5%	0.5%										
Laundry	9.0%	9.0%	3.0%	9.4%									
Housekeeping	8.0%	8.0%	7.4%	8.4%	5.0%								
Dietary	10.%	10.%	7.3%	10.5%	15.0%	12.8%							
Social Services	0.5%	0.5%	0.1%	0.5%		0.6%							
Physical Therapy	7.0%	7.0%	2.5%	7.3%	2.5%	8.9%							
Occupational Therapy	2.0%	2.0%	0.4%	2.1%	2.5%	2.6%							
Nursing, Skilled	15.0%	15.0%	30.0%	15.7%	30.0%	19.1%	25.0%				97.0%		
Nursing, Intermediate	44.0%	44.0%	48.8%	46.0%	45.0%	56.1%	75.0%				3.0%		
TOTAL	100.0%	100.0%	100.0%	99.8%	100.0%	100.0%	100.0%	100.0%	100.0%	100.0%	100.0%	100.0%	

1. -FTE = Full Time Equivalent Employees
2. Total Maintenance costs include all utility costs.

297

TABLE 3-11. Old Well Home Step-down Cost Allocation

Cost Centers (Total Costs)	Capital 116580	Plant 109550	Admin. 328338	Main. (1) 76826	Laundry 73583	Housekeep 189476	Dietary 434797	Soc. Serv. 29851	P.T. 128457	O.T. 56953	SNF 797352	ICF 1269366	TOTAL 4611129
Support & Revenue Centers													
Administration	33,497.40	3,286.50	365,121.90										
Maintenance	16,748.70	1,643.25	1,825.61	97,043.56									
Laundry	100,492.20	9,859.50	10,953.66	9,126.95	204,015.30								
Housekeeping	89,326.40	8,764.00	27,109.02	8,112.84	10,200.77	332,899.03							
Dietary	111,658.00	10,955.00	26,653.90	10,141.05	30,602.30	42,444.63	232,454.87						
Social Services	5,582.90	547.75	365.12	507.05	0.00	2,122.23		38,976.06					
Physical Therapy	78,160.60	7,668.50	9,128.05	7,098.74	5,100.38	29,711.24			265,324.50				
Occupational Therapy	22,331.60	2,191.00	1,460.49	2,028.21	5,100.38	8,488.93				98,553.61			
Nursing, Skilled	167,487.00	16,432.50	109,536.57	15,211.58	61,204.59	63,666.59	58,113.72				125,0334.75		
Nursing, Intermediate	491,295.20	48,202.00	178,179.49	44,620.63	91,806.89	186,755.35	174,341.15				38,670.15	2,523,237.86	
TOTAL	1,116,580.00	109,550.00	365,121.90	96,847.05	204,015.30	333,190.31	232,454.87	38,976.06	265,324.50	98,553.61	1,289,004.90	2,523,237.86	4,215,096.92 (1)

(1) Differences due to rounding

simplified; cost allocations for most health care organizations are usually performed by computer because of the volume and complexities involved in larger, more departmentalized, or multiprogram facilities.

1. Identify the revenue centers of the facility. Nursing services should be divided by levels of care because they will have different direct and indirect costs. The revenue centers in the Old Well Home are the skilled nursing facility (SNF), the intermediate-care facility (ICF), physical therapy (P.T.), occupational therapy (O.T.) and social services (Soc. Serv.).

2. Identify the direct costs of the revenue centers, and add them up to arrive at the total direct costs for each revenue-earning department. The total direct costs for the Old Well's revenue centers are shown below the department heading in Table 3-11.

3. Identify all indirect, or support, costs and cost centers. For the Old Well, support cost centers are dietary, housekeeping, laundry, maintenance, administration, plant, and capital costs. Telephone, taxes, insurance, and legal fees have been included in administration. Utilities such as gas, electricity, and water are included under plant, though they could have been grouped under administration or some other cost center.

Capital costs represent all depreciation and interest expenses. Depreciation could have alternatively been subsumed under each department with capital equipment and the cost of plant depreciation alone allocated over all cost centers. These are some of the alternatives that exist for identifying cost centers.

4. Analyze the functions of each cost center and decide whether and in what way each cost center provides support services to the other cost centers. It is through these service relationships that the order of the allocation is decided. Because capital costs, plant, and maintenance are used by all other cost centers, these costs are allocated first. Capital costs are applied to maintenance but not vice versa, so maintenance will follow capital costs on the step-down worksheet. However, the order of allocation is not always that clear-cut.

Maintenance provides services to administration in the repair and upkeep of office machinery and the like, but administration also provides services to maintenance through, for example, the processing of maintenance employees' payroll. These reciprocal relationships are accommodated by the reciprocal method of allocation, but other arrangements must be made in the step-down method.

Because revenue centers do not provide services to the support centers, they should be listed last to "accumulate" the costs of the support centers. Sometimes revenue centers provide services for other revenue centers. The service relationship between revenue centers determines their order. Insurers will usually indicate the order of allocation, but whatever order is used, it should remain consistent from year to year.

5. Select the basis of allocation for all support costs. This may also be decided for the facility by third-party payers, but it should represent the criteria that determine the extent of services provided by departments and the ease in measuring the criteria. For example, using number of employees or square footage of a department is probably more representative of required housekeeping services, easier to measure, and more consistent than number of wastebaskets or average salary of the employees in the cost center. The basis of allocation used for the various cost centers in the Old Well is indicated under the cost center heading.

6. Prepare a preliminary worksheet for reference when performing the step-down allocation. This worksheet indicates the percentage of costs from each cost center that will be allocated to all other cost centers.

For the Old Well, administration is allocated on the basis of the number of employees in each cost center. No administration costs are allocated to capital, plant, or administration, but housekeeping has 7.4% of the Old Well's employees. So 7.4% of total administration costs are allocated to this cost center. Laundry has 3% of total employees, so 3% of administration costs go there. In this way the preliminary worksheet is constructed. Note that when indirect costs are allocated, 100% of that cost center's costs must be allocated; thus, the percentages should add up to 100% (or 1) along the bottom of the worksheet.

7. Using the preliminary worksheet, prepare the step-down worksheet, listing all revenue centers last, and allocate the total costs of each cost center to the subsequent cost centers on the step-down worksheet.

When the first cost center is spread over all of the appropriate departments, add to the portion from the first cost center just allocated the total cost of the next cost center, and spread this new total cost for the second cost center over the following appropriate cost centers.

Let us review the Old Well's step-down worksheet. When all capital and plant costs have been spread over all of the departments, with some amount of capital, interest, or utilities expense, the next cost center, administration, now reflects a higher total cost because a portion of capital and plant costs have been allocated to this department. This new total cost of $365,121.90 is spread over all departments that use administrative services, and so on. In this way, all indirect costs are included in the costs of other cost centers.

8. When all indirect costs are allocated to the revenue centers, the revenue centers will have new total costs, the sum of all indirect allocated costs, and their own total direct costs.

Occasionally, revenue center costs may need to be allocated to other revenue centers. Nurse's aides who normally work in the intermediate-care level may regularly work several hours a week in the skilled-care department, or special supplies from the skilled-care department may periodically be needed for intermediate-care residents. In this case, some percentage of the new intermediate-care facility cost should be added to the new skilled-nursing facility cost. Thus, the total cost of providing resident care is included in the new costs of the revenue centers.

At the Old Well, 3% of skilled-nursing-level costs have been allocated to the intermediate-care level because of its apparent uses of the services of the skilled-level facility on a regular basis.

Other Methods of Cost Finding

Two other approaches to cost finding are the reciprocal and cost-apportionment methods. The reciprocal is similar to the step-down method, except that it recognizes reciprocal services provided between cost centers, such as administration and maintenance. Because of the calculations involved and the extent of these services in most organizations, reciprocal allocation is performed by computer.

RATE SETTING

One of the primary uses of the cost-finding process is to develop a basis for setting rates for the services provided by the revenue centers. Once the costs of the revenue centers are known, *the average cost per unit of service can be calculated by dividing the total cost of the revenue center by the expected service volume.*

The unit of service must first be determined. In the physical therapy department a visit might be defined in terms of the time spent with the therapist, one continuous session of therapy, or all therapy received in 1 day. Social service visits also usually require definition. Again, most third-party payers will provide a definition of a service unit for the services they reimburse.

The average cost per unit of service offers a basis for rate setting, since rates should approximate the cost of providing the service. But other factors, such as demand for services, competitive rates, expected inflation rates, and contractual discounts and frequency of uncollectibles must be considered in setting appropriate rates.

3.9 Budgets and Budgeting

Most of us know what a budget is. Although we may not have had a hand in the preparation of financial statements, we probably have drawn up budgets for our own finances or even contributed to the budgeting process in an organization. In this section we will first discuss preparation of the budget, its uses and benefits, and then the budgeting process itself.

CONSIDERATIONS IN BUDGETING

The budgeting process in the nursing facility is a period of planning. The physical budget is more than a record of anticipated expenses for the next fiscal year. It represents a careful examination of internal and external changes that management believes will affect the operations of the facility and the strategy to deal with these changes for some time to come. Thus, the budget is a reflection of the administrator's short- and long-term goals for the facility. Many health care organizations also prepare less detailed budgets for the 2, 3, or 5 years following the next fiscal year as a guide for the organization's long-term goals and objectives.

Health care organizations characteristically have a number of objectives. While developing strategies to reduce expenses during the budget process in an effort to maintain a certain net income, it is easy to forget the objective of providing a high quality of care to service recipients. As a reflection of the home's priorities, this objective must remain intact throughout the budgeting process.

The budget is a tool to be used by the administrator and staff throughout the year, rather than a document that, once completed, is filed away and remains only in the memory of the budget participants. The budget is not a static document with fixed expenditure and revenue levels but one that should be altered as internal and external conditions change. It provides a meaningful comparison between actual and projected expenditures and revenues. Adjustments between budget items can be made any time after the budget is completed.

The budget, then, is not to be regarded simply as one of the many financial records prepared by the business office in the course of the year but as a product of the home's direction, objectives, and priorities that can be used as a managerial tool throughout the year.

3.9.1. Two Methods of Budget Preparation

Budgeting can be done in any number of ways, and each individual nursing facility or chain will develop its own particular style. In general, two methods of budget preparation are used: the *top-down* and the *participatory* method.

TOP-DOWN APPROACH TO BUDGETING

With the top-down approach, the administrator alone prepares the annual budget with little or no guidance from department heads. This method is most suitable for smaller homes with few departments, where the administrator is familiar with all of the costs of the facility. Top-down is also often the approach used by chains, in which case the local administrator is given a "suggested" budget with the corporation's goals already built into it. The top-down method is quick but has the disadvantages of possibly stifling innovation or of imposing an unpopular or unrealistic budget on department heads or chain facility administrators.

THE PARTICIPATORY APPROACH

The participatory method of budgeting requires input from staff members on several levels of the organization. The administrator provides guidelines for the preparation of departmental budgets, prepared by the department heads and other key personnel. These budgets are then reviewed by the administrator, adjusted as necessary, and combined into one organizational budget.

Participatory budgeting is more appropriate for larger homes. Although it is time-consuming, participatory budgeting furnishes an opportunity for communication between the administrator and department heads, and results in input into the budget from those who are most knowledgeable about the daily operation of the individual departments.

Participatory budgeting will be used to describe the budgeting process in this section, as it is considerably more involved than the top-down approach. However, the process described is equally applicable to the latter.

We have already indicated one purpose of budgeting: to plan for the next fiscal year and the several years beyond in terms of expenses, revenues, goals, and objectives.

Additionally, budgeting can promote communication between the administrator and staff, especially participatory budgeting. The budget allows the administrator to communicate expected changes to staff in the facility, as well as the administrator's long-term goals for the facility. It also reveals the administrator's own expectations of the staff in operating their departments. The budgeting process allows department heads to express their needs and concerns in carrying out their functions.

Participatory budgeting augments the role each participant plays in the operations of the facility. Department heads and others become more aware not only of the costs of their areas and the resources available to the facility but also of the needs of the other departments. Budgeting also brings greater recognition of their own roles to the participating staff, and although the budget process is often time-consuming and frustrating, the staff is rewarded by the knowledge that their expertise and experience are valued.

Finally, the budget communicates information about the facility to external parties who have an interest in its status, such as the board of directors or stockholders, third-party payers, planning agencies, rate review commissions, and unions. The administrator must often be able to justify proposed expenses and revenues to these parties.

3.9.2 Five Steps in the Budgeting Process

There are any number of ways to prepare the budget, whether by the administrator alone or with the input of key personnel. The optimal method will depend on, among other considerations, the size of the facility, whether it is free standing or a unit in a small or large chain, and the administrator's time constraints.

In designing the budgeting process the administrator first decides what information is desired and how detailed it must be and then maps out the logistics of the activity. The administrator determines who the participants will be. In the case of top-down budgeting the administrator and perhaps other administrative personnel, such as the bookkeeper, comptroller, or business manager, will be involved. Participatory budgeting usually includes the administrator, the accountant or comptroller, bookkeeper, personnel director, and department heads and their assistants. The budget timetable must also be defined. At least 2 to 5 months before the beginning of the next fiscal year should be allowed for the entire process.

STEP 1: ASSESSING THE ENVIRONMENT

The initial step in the budgeting process is the assessment of the external and internal environments. The budget cannot be prepared in a vacuum. The political, economic, and social environments outside the nursing facility walls are obviously not static. Although the administrator does not have control over these aspects of the external environment, ignorance of the trends affecting the nursing facility industry, and failure to anticipate their effects on the operations of the facility, leaves the administrator less able to deal effectively with changes. Such trends may occur as one or more of the following:

- increased or decreased competition
- altered reimbursement policies
- amended licensing laws
- revised quality review regulations
- swings in the economy
- inflation, deflation, or stagnation
- reduction in the potential service population
- changes in disease patterns among patients

Some, if not most, of these fluctuations in the external environment may affect the plans and operations of the facility.

STEP TWO: PROGRAMMING

After the external environments and their effects on the facility have been evaluated, the home's objectives for the coming year are determined. This process is sometimes known as programming; in effect it results in a program for the facility to follow. Through programming the administrator can alter internal operations over which he/she has control to respond to the external influences on the facility.

How might an administrator use programming to cope with external events? In periods of rising inflation the cost of living goes up. This usually results in a demand for higher wages. If the administrator is aware of this trend, an objective might be to index the salaries, that is, raise them by a certain percentage to approximate the increased costs of living by a certain time during the following year. An increase in salary expense can then be included in the budget, thereby preventing a situation in which funds are not set aside for this purpose. Such an oversight could result in recruiting problems, high staff turnover, or a strain on operating funds when a salary increase is finally provided.

Other considerations for programming are changes in (a) service volume, (b) services offered, (c) payer mix, (d) personnel needs, and (e) capital needs. The cumulative effect of expected external and internal events should determine the objectives of the facility for the next year, which in turn form the basis of assumptions made in the budgeting process.

The completed budgeting process should result in four types of budgets: the operating budget, the cash budget, the capital budget, and the pro forma financial statements.

STEP 3: DEVELOPING THE OPERATING BUDGET

The operating budget has two parts: the *expense budget* and the *revenue budget*.

The Expense Budget

The expense budget, the type with which we are most familiar, lists the anticipated expenses of the facility for the coming year and is prepared largely by the department heads. The budget timetable should indicate when the final departmental expense budgets are due.

It is important that those preparing any portion of the budget be well aware of the type of information needed. The heads of all service units should indicate the expected patient service volume, while support departments (such as dietary) should be able to estimate the number of meals that will be served. Budgeting offers an opportunity for communication between departments. After all, dietary must learn the expected patient volume in the different nursing-care levels to be able to calculate the number of meals that will be served.

Additionally, department heads should review staff positions and note any recommended changes in the staffing pattern. In larger homes recommendations for salary changes may be the responsibility of the personnel director and may be based on competitive salaries in the community or union agreements if employees are so organized. Table 3-12 shows a salary recommendation form for budgeted changes in administrative salaries at the Old Well Home.

Department heads should also check equipment in their departments for repair or replacement needs. Included in this assessment would be estimates of the costs of repair or replacement, supported by professional estimates, manufacturer pamphlets, and the like. If equipment needs are extensive, it may be worthwhile for department heads to develop a plant and equipment budget for their departments, which will facilitate preparation of the capital budget. A departmental plant and equipment budget for the Old Well's nursing department is shown in Table 3-13.

The cost of supplies and other expenses are often a significant portion of departmental costs. Any change in the volume of supplies needed and the cost per unit should be noted on the budget (Table 3-14). Catch-all or miscellaneous categories should be kept to a minimum, as there can be little control over unidentified costs.

Anticipated expenses should be broken down by months or another customary accounting period used in the facility. Monthly expense budgets also facilitate preparation of the cash budget.

Determining Expenses. In determining expenses several strategies can be used. One tactic is to increase all of the current year's expenses by a certain percentage. Although this method is quick, it defeats the purpose of budgeting and the effort involved in environmental assessment and programming.

It is more productive for the department head to identify monthly and yearly trends in costs and utilization to help predict expenses. For example, occupancy of the skilled-care unit might be consistently below average during the winter holidays but regularly above average in late January and February. Identification of such trends is useful in budgeting for monthly costs and volume levels. It is also often helpful to identify the source of variances in the current year's budget and allow for them in the preparation of the new budget.

In setting up the expense budget a checklist can be used to make sure all expense items in departments are included. A good source for this checklist is the Chart of Accounts, which should list all expense accounts by department.

All budget participants ought to know how and by whom the final budget levels are decided. Finally, the organizational expense budget is separated by months, and the individual department budgets retained for comparison of actual with budgeted performance in each department throughout the year. The Old Well's completed expense budget is shown in Table 3-15.

TABLE 3.12. Old Well Home Department: Administration

DEPARTMENT: ADMINISTRATION
SUPERVISOR: M.J. BORDERS
DATE: 10/24/X1

NAME	POSITION	HRS/WEEK	FULL TIME/ PART TIME	DATE OF EMPLOYMENT	CURRENT RATE	PROJECTED CHANGE %	PROJECTED CHANGE $	ANNUAL WAGE
BORDERS, M.J.	ADMINISTRATOR	40	FT	12/24/XO	$16.50	5%	$17.33	36,036.00
GOODWIN, J.A.	ASST. ADMIN.	40	FT	5/9/X8	$10.64	5%	$11.17	23,237.76
BIGGS, M.T.	BOOKKEEPER	40	FT	3/28/X8	$7.00	5%	$7.35	15,288.00
WANCHECK, W.W.	SECRETARY	40	FT	5/16/X7	$6.00	3%	$6.18	12,854.40
LUX, C.C.	ACCOUNTANT	30	PT	6/12/X1	$8.00	3%	$8.24	17,139.20
TOTAL		190						104,555.36

TABLE 3-13. Old Well Home Nursing Department: Equipment Needs

DEPARTMENT: NURSING (INTERMEDIATE LEVEL)
SUPERVISOR: S.E. ADAMS
DATE: 10/15/X1

EQUIPMENT NEEDED	REASON FOR REQUEST	ESTIMATED COST
TWO (2) CHAIR SCALES	To weigh non-ambulatory patients	2 @ $3,577 = $7,154
FIVE (5) COLLAPSIBLE WALKERS	Old walkers in disrepair, collapsible easier for patients to use.	5 @ $550 = $2,750
TOTAL		$9,904

TABLE 3-14. Old Well Home Administration Department Change Request

DEPARTMENT: ADMINISTRATION
SUPERVISOR: M.J. BORDERS
DATE: 10/22/X1

EXPENSE	ACTUAL COST 19X1-X2	BUDGETED 19X2-X3	% CHANGE	REASON FOR CHANGE
Health Insurance	5,780	6,274	8.5%	Increase in insurance rates
Payroll Tax	7,388	7,319	−0.9%	
Supplies	11,580	12,940	11.7%	Increase in cost of supplies
Liability Insurance	26,330	26,330	0.0%	
Property Insurance	21,700	21,700	0.0%	
Income Tax	15,750	18,000	14.3%	Expected increase in net income
Property Tax	38,960	39,750	2.0%	
Telephone	2,230	1,950	−12.6%	Attempt to reduce telephone usage
Travel	3,450	3,600	4.3%	Continuing Education — May
Postage	43,550	46,340	6.4%	Increase postal rates
Licenses, Dues	1,325	1,240	−5.4%	
Repairs	1,500	1,545	3.0%	
TOTAL	179,543	186,988	4.1%	

The Revenue Budget

The second section of the operating budget is the revenue budget, which projects the monthly income for the next fiscal year. The revenue budget need not be prepared on a departmental basis; fewer departments are involved in determining revenues than in determining expenses, and non-operating revenues are generally under the control of the administrator. Also, service revenues are based on the prices charged for services, which are determined by administrative decision. Hence, the revenue budget is usually prepared at the administrative level.

TABLE 3-15. Old Well Home 19X2–19X3 Summary Expense Budget

ACCOUNT	PROJECTED (ANNUAL)	SALARIES	DEPARTMENTAL
ADMINISTRATION			
SALARIES	104,560		
HEALTH INSURANCE	6,274		
PAYROLL TAX	7,319	118,153	
SUPPLIES	12,940		
INSURANCE:			
LIABILITY	26,330		
PROPERTY DAMAGE	21,700		
TAXES:			
INCOME (@45%)	18,000		
PROPERTY (@1.5%)	39,750		
TELEPHONE	1,950		
TRAVEL	3,600		
POSTAGE	46,340		
LICENSES & DUES	1,240		
REPAIRS	1,545		
TOTAL ADMINISTRATION			291,548
PLANT OPERATION			
SALARIES	57,890		
HEALTH INSURANCE	3,473		
PAYROLL TAXES	4,052	65,416	
UTILITIES	109,550		
SUPPLIES	8,670		
REPAIRS	2,740		
TOTAL PLANT			186,376
NURSING			
SNF: SALARIES	552,340		
HEALTH INSURANCE	33,140		
PAYROLL TAXES	38,664	624,144	
SUPPLIES	89,468		
PHARMACY	57,670		
LABORATORY	23,070		
REPAIRS	2,700		
UNIFORM	300		
TOTAL SNF	797,352		
ICF:			
SALARIES	927,740		
HEALTH INSURANCE	55,664		
PAYROLL TAXES	64,942	1,048,346	
SUPPLIES	150,600		
PHARMACY	51,540		
LABORATORY	12,680		
REPAIRS	5,400		
UNIFORM	800		
TOTAL ICF	1,269,366		
TOTAL NURSING			2,066,7˙
DIETARY			
SALARIES	170,590		
HEALTH INSURANCE	10,235		
PAYROLL TAX	1,1941	192,767	
SUPPLIES	234,530		
REPAIRS	7,500		
TOTAL DIETARY			434,797
LAUNDRY			
SALARIES	37,330		
HEALTH INSURANCE	2,240		
PAYROLL TAX	2,613	42,183	
SUPPLIES	7,450		

TABLE 3-15. (continued)

ACCOUNT	PROJECTED (ANNUAL)	SALARIES	DEPARTMENTAL
REPAIRS	3,500		
CONTRACT SERVICES	20,450		
TOTAL LAUNDRY			73,583
HOUSEKEEPING			
SALARIES	157,430		
HEALTH INSURANCE	9,446		
PAYROLL TAX	11,020	177,896	
SUPPLIES	10,380		
REPAIRS	1,200		
TOTAL HOUSEKEEPING			189,476
PHYSICAL THERAPY			
SALARIES	105,670		
HEALTH INSURANCE	6,340		
PAYROLL TAX	7,397	119,407	
SUPPLIES	7,550		
REPAIRS	1,500		
TOTAL PHYSICAL THERAPY			128,457
OCCUPATIONAL THERAPY			
SALARIES	42,560		
HEALTH INSURANCE	2,554		
PAYROLL TAX	2,979	48,093	
SUPPLIES	7,260		
REPAIRS	1,600		
TOTAL OCCUP THERAPY			56,953
SOCIAL SERVICES			
SALARIES	24,240		
HEALTH INSURANCE	1,454		
PAYROLL TAX	1,697	27,391	
SUPPLIES	2,460		
TOTAL SOCIAL SERVICES			29,851
ACTIVITY			
BEAUTY SHOP:			
SALARIES	7,680		
PAYROLL TAX	538	8,218	
SUPPLIES	2,340		
TOTAL BEAUTY SHOP	10,558		
CRAFTS:			
SALARIES	12,750		
PAYROLL TAX	893	13,643	
SUPPLIES	5,320		
TOTAL CRAFTS	18,963		
TRANSPORTATION	3,870		
SPECIAL EVENTS	3,400		
TOTAL ACTIVITY			36,790
CAPITAL COSTS			
INTEREST:			
MORTGAGE	276,816		
LONG TERM DEBT	56,972		
TOTAL INTEREST	333,788		
DEBT SERVICE:			
MORTGAGE PAYABLE	288,350		
DEBTS PAYABLE	18,927		
TOTAL DEBT SERVICE	307,277		
DEPRECIATION:			
PLANT	192,230		
EQUIPMENT	283,285		
TOTAL DEPRECIATION	475,515		
TOTAL CAPITAL COSTS			1,116,580
TOTAL SALARY		2,367,503	
TOTAL EXPENSES			4,611,129

The nursing facility, as we recall from the Income Statement, has two sources of income: operating or patient service revenues and non-operating revenues. Both of them must be considered in the revenue budget.

Operating Revenue Estimates. To estimate operating revenues, all revenue centers are listed, with the number of patients appearing by type of payer. Total patient service revenues are calculated by multiplying the expected service volume in each revenue center by the charge per unit of service. As we discussed in the section on cost finding, rates for services may be determined in several ways. For publicly insured patients, the allowable rate per unit of service may be somewhat less than charges; the reimbursable rate should be used in projecting revenues for these patients.

For privately paying patients, charges can be based on the cost plus profit for providing the service, using the results of the cost-finding process and break-even analysis. Rates may also be based on competitive charges for similar services in the community or on the price that the market will bear.

Non-Operating Revenues. Non-operating revenues, such as interest income, borrowed funds, and charitable donations, are dependent on any number of factors but are relatively predictable on a monthly basis. These revenues are added to the monthly operating revenues to arrive at the total expected revenues. The revenue budget for the Old Well is shown in Table 3-16.

Total revenues can then be compared with total budgeted expenses. If revenues seem inadequate to meet expenses, the administrator can check the validity of the predicted service volume. If service levels seem reasonable, the administrator can seek to increase patient service volume, reduce budgeted expenses, or raise rates.

Using the Operating Budget: Variance Analysis

As a managerial tool, the operating budget is used throughout the fiscal year to measure performance by a technique called *variance analysis*. Variance analysis is simply a comparison of actual versus budgeted monetary and volume values at the end of each month.

Actual expenses that deviate significantly from the budgeted amounts can be investigated to identify the source of the variance. Such variances may be anything from an inadvertent miscalculation of costs or patient volume to serious mismanagement by a particular department. Once the source of variances is known, the budget can be adjusted accordingly or the cause of the variance can be eliminated. Budget variance analysis provides the administrator with an important means of control over the finances of the facility.

TABLE 3-16. Old Well Home 19X2–X3 Summary Revenue Budget

PATIENT REVENUE ROUTINE CARE: CARE LEVEL: BY PAYER	CENSUS (Pt days/year)	200 BEDS 95% OCCUPANCY CHARGE/DAY PER PT.	CONTRACT DISCOUNT (avg.)	ANNUAL REVENUE
SNF (50 BEDS)				
Medicare	10,403	$70.00	10%	655,358
Medicaid	2,601	$70.00	12%	160,199
Private	4,334	$70.00	0%	303,406
SUBTOTAL	17,338			1,118,962
ICF (150 BEDS)				
Medicaid	26,006	$66.00	15%	1,458,951
Private	24,446	$66.00	0%	1,613,428
Other	1,560	$66.00	3%	99,895
SUBTOTAL	52,013			3,172,274
TOTAL REV.	69,350			4,291,236

ANCILLARY CARE: SERVICE BY PAYER	ANNUAL VISITS	CHARGE PER VISIT	CONTRACT DISCOUNT	ANNUAL REVENUE
PHYSICAL THERAPY				
Medicare	6,045	$22.00	10%	119,691
Medicaid	1,257	$22.00	12%	24,336
Private	2,430	$22.00	0%	53,460
SUBTOTAL	9,732			197,487
OCCUPATIONAL THERAPY				
Private	5,640	$18.00	0%	101,520
SOCIAL SERVICES				
Private	1,008	$16.00	0%	16,128
TOTAL ANC.	16,380			315,135
TOTAL PT. CARE				4,606,370

OTHER REVENUE

INTEREST: SOURCES	RATE	AVG. BALANCE	ANNUAL EARNINGS
Account, National Bank	8.50%	$6500.00	7,053
Certificate of Deposit Account Maturing:			
10/15/XX	11.50%	$2500.00	2,788
2/15/XX	12.25%	$4000.00	4,490
TOTAL INTEREST INCOME			14,330

MISC INCOME: SOURCES	ANNUAL VOLUME	AVG. CHARGE/UNI	ANNUAL REVENUE
Guest Meals	1,370	$3.45	4,727
Concession			13,995
Beauty Shop	1,560	$5.00	7,800
TOTAL MISC. INCOME	2,930		26,552
TOTAL OTHER INCOME			40,852
TOTAL REVENUE			4,647,222

STEP 4: THE CASH BUDGET

The next step in the budgeting process is preparation of the cash budget. As its name implies, it is prepared on the cash basis of accounting, although it is based on the revenues and expenses from the operating budget. Note that the operating budget is prepared on the accrual basis of accounting: projected revenues are based on the income earned in the time period, not on the amount of cash received for services during the month.

The cash budget estimates the cash inflows and outflows for the next 12 months, enabling the administrator to identify months with cash shortages and overages. This information can be used to defer nonurgent expenditures to a month with high cash inflows or retain overages in 1 month to cover anticipated cash shortages in the next. The cash budget is an invaluable tool; indeed, many health care administrators rely on the cash budget for daily operations and sometimes prepare weekly or even daily cash budgets a month in advance.

Determining Cash Inflows and Outflows

To develop the cash budget, cash inflows and outflows must be determined. Because the facility has less control over cash inflows, especially those received from third-party payers, projecting them is somewhat involved. First, all payer sources must be identified. These will usually be private payers, Medicare, and Medicaid. Then the lag time between the billing of services and receipt of payment is determined. Most private payers do so within 30 days of billing, but time lags for Medicare and Medicaid may be anywhere from 20 to 90 days or more, depending on the state and the fiscal intermediaries involved. This can be used to measure the percentage of revenues that will be received from each payer in each month.

In Part I of Table 3-17 no payment will be received by the Old Well Home in February for services provided to Medicare patients in January. In March, 40% of January's Medicare revenues will be received, and in April, 60%. Time lags for all payers can be confirmed from the Accounts Receivable Ledger dates.

Next, the proportion of all patient revenues received from each payer is calculated. At the Old Well, Medicare is responsible for 15% of total patient revenues, Medicaid for 40%, and private payers for 42%. We now know the percentage of patient revenues by payer and the percentage of funds that is usually received from each payer in a particular month. Multiplying these two percentages together in Part II of Table 3-17, we can learn the percentage of total revenues received from each payer in each month. For example, in March the Old Well will receive 40% × 15% = 6% of the total revenues earned in January from Medicare. Based on the

TABLE 3-17. Old Well Home Projection of Monthly Cash Inflows, 19X2−X3

I

SOURCE OF REVENUES (Less Uncollectibles)	% OF TOTAL REVENUES	% REVENUES RECEIVED IN MONTHS AFTER BILLING: MONTH 1	MONTH 2	MONTH 3	MONTH 4	TOTAL
MEDICAID	40%	0%	40%	50%	10%	100%
MEDICARE	15%	0%	0%	40%	60%	100%
PRIVATE	42%	60%	35%	5%		100%
OTHER	3%	20%	75%	5%		100%

II

SOURCE	MONTH 1	MONTH 2	MONTH 3	MONTH 4
MEDICAID	0%	16%	20%	4%
MEDICARE	0%	0%	6%	9%
PRIVATE	25%	15%	2%	0%
OTHER	1%	2%	0%	0%
% TOTAL REVENUE RECEIVED BY MONTH	26%	33%	28%	13%

III – CASH INFLOWS

MONTH OF BILLING:	PROJECTED REVENUES:	MONTH REVENUES RECEIVED (+ ACCTS. RECV.) JAN. 394019	FEB. 437200	MARCH 384670	APRIL 376220	MAY 372450	CASH INFLOW PER MONTH, JAN–MAY
JANUARY	263,544	101,656.90					365,200.90
FEBRUARY	119,784	129,829.26	112,797.60				362,410.86
MARCH	30,078	111,310.37	144,057.04	99,244.86			384,690.63
APRIL		51,222.47	123,509.00	126,748.77	97,064.76		398,545.00
MAY			56,836.00	108,669.28	123,964.49	96,092.10	385,561.87
JUNE			50,007.10	106,282.15	122,722.28	279,011.53
				48,908.60	105,217.13	154,125.73
					48,418.50	
TOTAL		**394,019**	**437,200**	**384,670**	**376,220**	**372,450**	**2,329,546.50**

monthly revenues in the revenue budget, these proportions can be used to determine the cash receipts for each month.

When cash inflows from patient services are known, monthly cash receipts from non-operating sources are computed to give total cash receipts for each month (Part III of Table 3-17).

Cash outflows are somewhat easier to estimate, as most cash disbursements, such as salaries and supplies, are made at prespecified intervals. Using the expense budget and the home's experience with suppliers and other creditors, the amount of cash disbursements can be determined for each month. Monthly cash inflows are compared with monthly cash outflows and the difference noted as part of the cash budget (Table 3-18).

As with the operating budget, the cash budget is updated as conditions or needs change throughout the year, whatever the reason. The cash budget can be a useful planning tool.

TABLE 3-18. Old Well Home Cash Flow Budget, FY 19X2–X3

	JAN.	FEB.	MARCH	APRIL	MAY	JUNE	JULY	AVG. NET INCOME JAN.–JULY
BEGINNING CASH BALANCE	4,760	-15,079	2,432	2,667	11,387	13,039	20,879	
CASH RECEIPTS:								
PATIENT CARE	365,201	362,411	384,691	398,545	385,562	374,800	368,790	
OTHER	3,460	3,570	3,115	2,875	3,870	3,650	3,420	
TOTAL CASH AVAILABLE	373,421	350,902	390,238	404,087	400,819	391,489	393,089	
CASH DISBURSEMENTS:								
SALARIES %	197,240	197,240	197,240	197,850	197,850	197,850	197,850	
SUPPLIES	32,350	28,300	30,500	22,650	31,600	32,360	32,420	
UTILITIES	9,560	9,340	9,121	8,230	7,860	7,740	7,860	
INSURANCE	35,849						35,849	
TAXES				18,000			39,750	
CONTRACT SERVICES	5,670		15,410	3,470				
OTHER	107,830	113,590	135,300	142,500	150,470	132,660	87,450	
TOTAL DISBURSEMENTS	388,499	348,470	387,571	392,700	387,780	370,610	401,179	
ENDING CASH BALANCE	-15,079	2 432	2,667	11,387	13,039	20,879	-8,091	27,235

STEP 5: THE CAPITAL BUDGET

The capital budget is simply a summarization of all anticipated capital expenditures in the budget year. Although many capital purchases and projects may be needed, all might not be readily affordable in the course of a single year. The capital budget is the result of the decision on the capital projects that will be undertaken, and, most important, how they will be financed.

Pro Forma Financial Statements

The budget process concludes with the development of the pro forma financial statements. We have discussed the preparation of the financial statements; the pro forma statements are preliminary financial statements based on budgeted amounts. The pro forma income statement, for instance, is derived from the operating budget and shows the net income (or loss) expected under the budgeted expenses and revenues.

The budgeting process can be costly in terms of time for the administrator and all other budget participants. However, it involves a thorough investigation of the home's finances through such tools as cost finding, break-even analysis, rate setting, programming, and cash flow analysis. Through this process, budgeting familiarizes the administrator with the costs of running the facility and maximizes his/her ability to manage its finances successfully.

REFERENCES TO PART THREE

Catholic Hospital Association. (1977). *Guide to accounting principles, practices, and systems*. St. Louis, MO: The Catholic Hospital Association.

Neumann, B.R., Suver, J.D., & Zelman, W.N. (1984). *Financial management: Concepts and applications for health service providers*. Baltimore, MD: National Health Publishers.

Rhoads, J.L. (1981). *Basic accounting and budgeting for long term care facilities*. Boston: CBI Publishing.

Suver, J.D. (1982). Financial management techniques for the long term care administrator. In D.B. Miller (Ed.), *Long term care administrator's desk manual*. (pp. 3001–3128). Greenvale, NY: Panel Publishers.

Suver, J.D., & Neumann, B.R. (1981). *Management accounting for health care organizations*. Oak Brook, IL: Healthcare Financial Management Association.

PART FOUR

Laws and Regulatory Codes

A nursing home operation is subject to numerous regulations. Some of them guide the administrator in daily management of the facility, whereas others, such as health planning, are referred to only occasionally. We have attempted to provide a logical order to the sequence in which the many laws and regulations are presented in Part 4. Section 4.1 is a reproduction of the law that originally established nursing home administration as a profession. Although it was enacted much later (1970) than many of the laws that are presented in sections 4.2 through 4.8, we consider this to be an appropriate starting point.

Sections 4.2 through 4.5 first discuss laws governing the actual physical shape of the building (4.2), then laws governing the type of program to be presented in the building (4.3), and finally laws that regulate relationships between the administrator and the employees in the facility (4.4 and 4.5).

Sections 4.6 and 4.7 are examinations of health planning regulations concerning planned expansion and of voluntary standards available to the facility.

The following are reproduced word for word *with author's commentary noted separately in parentheses*: Federal Regulations Establishing State Boards for Education and Licensure of Nursing Home Administrators; Conditions of Participation for Skilled Nursing Facilities. All emphasis is the author's.

We do not quote directly the Specifications for Making Buildings and Facilities Accessible to and Usable by Physically Handicapped People. We do not attempt to reproduce literally the specifications for adapting buildings to the handicapped because there are innumerable exceptions noted in the specifications that would make the learning task over-whelming. However, we do present all of the points in these specifications. We have spared the reader only the exceptions and some of the further specifications and alternative ways of meeting these requirements.

In every case, nevertheless, original copies of each of these documents will be indispensable for actual management of the facility.

4.1 A Law Establishing and Regulating Nursing Home Administration as a Profession

NURSING HOME ADMINISTRATION

In February 1970 the federal government published rules and regulations requiring that states receiving Medicaid Title XIX assistance monies establish state programs to license nursing home administrators: Federal Regulations Establishing State Boards for Education and Licensure of Nursing Home Administrators. Licensing; Training and Instruction Programs. Title 45—Public Welfare; Chapter 11—Social and Rehabilitation Service, Department of Health, Education and Welfare (currently called Health Care Financing Administration, Department of Health and Human Services) (*Federal Register*, 35:41, pp. 3968–3970).

The effect was to establish a national regulation program: 49 of the 50 states had Medicaid programs, and all 50 states moved immediately to establish the licensing boards (or equivalents).

Part 252.40 of the regulations, below, defines then describes the responsibilities assigned in these federal regulations to the state nursing home administrator licensing boards. Part 252.44 deals with the subject areas in which nursing home administrators are to be trained. These are the two parts covered in this text.

252.40. State Programs for Licensing Administrators of Nursing Homes

(a) Purpose. This section delineates the procedures to be followed by States for compliance with the requirement for participating in a title XIX program to establish programs for the licensure of nursing home administrators.

(b) Definitions. When used in this section:

1. "**Nursing Home**" means any institution or facility defined as such for licensing purposes under State law, or if State law does not employ the term nursing home, the equivalent term or terms as determined by the Secretary (of Health and Human Services).
2. "**Nursing home administrator**" means any individual who is charged with the general administration of a nursing home, whether or not such individual has an ownership interest in such home, and whether or not his (/her) functions and duties are shared with one or more other individuals.
3. "**Board**" means a duly appointed State board duly representative of the professions and institutions concerned with the care of chronically ill and infirm aged patients, established for the purpose of carrying out a State program for the licensure of administrators of nursing homes.
4. "**Agency**" unless otherwise indicated, means the agency of the State responsible for licensing individual practitioners under the healing arts licensing act of the State.
5. "**License**" means a certificate or other written evidence issued by a State agency or board to indicate that the bearer has been certified by that body to meet all the standards required of a licensed nursing home administrator under this section.
6. "**Provisional License**" [Persons who were already active nursing home administrators at the time these regulations came into effect were given a provisional license and required to complete a 100 hour course (similar to the one outlined below) before July, 1972.]

(c) State Plan Requirements (establishment of state licensing boards; definition of duties and powers of state licensing boards)

Effective July 1, 1970, a State plan for medical assistance under title XIX of the Social Security Act must include a State program for the licensure of administrators of nursing homes, which:

1. Provides that no nursing home within the state may operate except under the supervision of an administrator licensed in the manner provided in this section.

(Note that the above paragraph requires *all* nursing homes in the state to operate under an administrator licensed by this board, *not only those that have Medicaid patients.*

In this indirect manner, federal regulation writers are able to effectively introduce sweeping rules for all nursing homes in the state, regardless of whether these homes participate in Medicaid.)

2. (State Board must) provide for licensing of nursing home administrators by the single agency of the State responsible for licensing individual practitioners under the healing arts act of the State, or in the absence of such an act or agency, a State licensing board representative of the professions and institutions concerned with the care of chronically ill and infirm aged patients and established to carry out the purposes of Section 1908 of the Social Security Act.

(Functions and Duties of the Board)

1. Develop, impose and enforce standards which must be met by individuals in order to receive a license as a nursing home administrator, which standards shall be designed to insure that nursing home administrators will be individuals who are of good character and are otherwise suitable, and who by training OR experience in the field of institutional administration, are qualified to serve as nursing home administrators.

2. Develop and apply appropriate techniques including examinations and investigations, for determining whether an individual meets such standards.

3. Issue licenses to individuals determined, after the application of such techniques, to meet such standards, and *revoke or suspend licenses previously issued by the agency or board* in any case where the individual holding such license is determined substantially to have failed to conform to the requirements of such standards.

4. Establish and carry out procedures designed to insure that individuals licensed as nursing home administrators will, during any period that they serve as such, comply with the requirements of such standards.

5. *Receive, investigate, and take appropriate action with respect to any charge or complaint filed with the agency or board to the effect that any individual licensed as a nursing home administrator has failed to comply with the requirements of such standards and*

6. Conduct a continuing study and investigation of nursing homes and administators of nursing homes within the State with a view to the improvement of the standards imposed for the licensing of such administrators and of procedures and methods for the enforcement of such standards with respect to administrators of homes which have been licensed as such.

(Power to license and regulate nursing home administrators resides in the states, not in the federal government. *States license* and monitor the performance of members of the medical professions. Hence, *the federal government does not and cannot delegate* responsibilities discussed above because these powers to license and regulate belong to the states in the first place.

The effect of these federal rules and regulations, however, is the same as if the federal government actually had the power to require and regulate the licensing of nursing home administrators. This confusing situation arises when two governmental bodies behave as if both had original jurisdicton. Although the federal government does not have original jurisdiction, it does control the purse strings and as a consequence does make rules.

Because the states have original jurisdiction in the licensing and monitoring of nursing home administrators, state licensing boards may be given *any powers* the state legislature or executive branch may delegate to them. Although state licensing boards for nursing home administrators may be obliged to meet federal requirements, these boards do not receive their authority from these regulations and are not limited in scope by them.)

(e) Federal Financial Participation

Federal financial participation is *not* available to defray the costs incurred by the licensing board in establishing and maintaining standards for the licensing of nursing home administrators.

252.44. Grants to States for Training and Instruction Programs for Waivered Nursing Home Administrators

(This section provided money to states to train persons who were already nursing home administrators when these educational requirements were put into effect in 1970. Although never directly stated in the title of this section, a core of knowledge consisting of the following nine areas is established by this section as recommendations to the state boards.)

Development of Program of Training and Instruction

To provide a basis for future licensure reciprocity between states, and to provide that the content of examinations and programs of training and instruction contain sufficient amounts of appropriate information relating to the proper and efficient administration of nursing homes, the following detailed guideline categorization of nine basic areas of the core of knowledge which it is deemed an administrator should possess are set forth as recommendations for appropriate use by State agencies and boards.

1. Applicable standards of environmental health and safety:
   (i)   Hygiene and sanitation

  (ii) Communicable diseases
  (iii) Management of isolation
  (iv) The total environment (noise, color, orientation, stimulation, temperature, lighting, air circulation)
  (v) Elements of accident prevention
  (vi) Special architectural needs of nursing home patients
  (vii) Drug handling and control
  (viii) Safety factors in oxygen use
2. Local health and safety regulations: guidelines vary according to local provisions.
3. General administration:
  (i) Institutional administration
  (ii) Planning, organizing, directing, controlling, staffing, coordinating, and budgeting
  (iii) Human relations:
     (a) Management/employee interrelationships
     (b) Employee/employee interrelationships
     (c) Employee/patient interrelationships
     (d) Employee/family interrelationships
  (iv) Training of personnel:
     (a) Training of employees to become sensitive to patient needs
     (b) Ongoing in-service training/education
4. Psychology of patient care:
  (i) Anxiety
  (ii) Depression
  (iii) Drugs, alcohol and their effect
  (iv) Motivation
  (v) Separation reaction
5. Principles of medical care:
  (i) Anatomy and physiology
  (ii) Psychology
  (iii) Disease recognition
  (iv) Disease process
  (v) Nutrition
  (vi) Aging processes
  (vii) Medical terminology
  (viii) Materia Medica (drug reactions)
  (ix) Medical Social Service
  (x) Utilization review
  (xi) Professional and medical ethics
6. Personal and social care:
  (i) Resident and patient care planning
  (ii) Activity programming:
     (a) Patient participation
     (b) Recreation

    (iii) Environmental adjustment: Interrelationships between patient and:
        (a) Patient
        (b) Staff (staff sensitivity to patient needs as a therapeutic function)
        (c) Family and friends
        (d) Administrator
        (e) Management (self-government/patient council)
    (iv) Rehabilitation and restorative activities:
        (a) Training in activities of daily living
        (b) Techniques of group therapy
    (v) Interdisciplinary interpretation of patient care to:
        (a) The patient
        (b) The staff
        (c) The family

7. Therapeutic and supportive care and services in long-term care:
    (i) Individual care planning as it embraces all therapeutic care and supportive services
    (ii) Meaningful observations of patient behavior as related to total patient care
    (iii) Interdisciplinary evaluation and revision of patient care plans and procedures
    (iv) Unique aspects and requirements of geriatric patient care
    (v) Professional staff interrelationships with patient's physician
    (vi) Professional ethics and conduct
    (vii) Rehabilitative and remotivational role of individual therapeutic and supportive services
    (viii) Psychological, social, and religious needs, in addition to physical needs of patient
    (ix) Needs for dental service

8. Departmental organization and management:
    (i) Criteria for coordinating establishment of departmental and unit objectives
    (ii) Reporting and accountability of individual departments to administration
    (iii) Criteria for departmental evaluation (nursing, food service, therapeutic services, maintenance, housekeeping)
    (iv) Techniques of providing adequate professional therapeutic, supportive and administrative services
    (v) The following departments may be used in relating matters of organization and management:
        (a) Nursing
        (b) Housekeeping
        (c) Dietary

    (d) Laundry
    (e) Pharmaceutical services
    (f) Social service
    (g) Business office
    (h) Recreation
    (i) Medical records
    (j) Admitting
    (k) Physical therapy
    (l) Occupational therapy
    (m) Medical and dental services
    (n) Laboratories
    (o) X-ray
    (p) Maintenance
 9. Community interrelationships
    (i)   Community medical care, rehabilitative, and social services resources
    (ii) Other community resources;
          (a) Religious institutions
          (b) Schools
          (c) Service agencies
          (d) Governmental agencies
    (iii) Third party payment organizations
    (iv) (Health Systems Agencies)
    (v)   Volunteers and auxiliaries
{F R Doc 70-2276; Filed, Feb. 27, 1970, 8:45 a.m.}

4.2 Fire Safety: The Life Safety Code®*

The National Fire Protection Association is a private, nonprofit organization with headquarters in Quincy, Massachusetts. It is not a government agency, nor does it write federal regulations. However, because the federal regulations for licensing nursing homes require adherence to the Life Safety Code, these fire safety standards have, in effect, the force of law for nursing homes.

The National Fire Protection Association has more than 150 committees, one of which is the Committee on Safety to Life, which establishes and revises these standards. The committee has met since 1913 and currently has 11 standing subcommittees (Lathrop, p. xiii).

The Code has evolved over the years, benefiting from the hindsight gained from the experience of fire after tragic fire. This Code represents the collected wisdom on fire prevention and fire containment.

The regulations published in the *Federal Register* in 1974 required that skilled nursing facilities "meet such provisions of the Life Safety Code® of the National Fire Protection Association as are applicable to nursing homes" (405.1134 A). These regulations have been revised regularly, with new editions in 1967, 1970, 1973, 1976, 1981, and 1985. The regulations described in the following sections are from the 1985 Life Safety Code® edition.

The actual wording of the Life Safety Code® is not used in the following pages. The major concepts and a number of the essential features of the Code presented below are *summaries* of the Code presented for study

* Reprinted with permission from NFPA 101, Life Safety Code®, Copyright ©, 1985, National Fire Protection Association, Quincy, MA 02269. This reprinted material is not the complete and official position of the NFPA on the referenced subject which is represented only by the standard in its entirety.

purposes. The Code itself is not quoted. Under no circumstances, then, should the reader treat this material as a substitute for obtaining and using the actual Code.

The *Life Safety Code*® *Handbook* by James K. Lathrop, which offers highly useful interpretations of the Life Safety Code, and copies of the Code itself may be ordered from the National Fire Protection, Inc., Batterymarch Park, Quincy, MA 02269.

HEALTH CARE OCCUPANCIES (SECTION 31-4 OF THE FIRE SAFETY CODE)

31–4.1 Attendants, Evacuation Plan, Fire Exit Drills

All nursing homes and hospitals must have a plan for the protection of all persons on their premises and for their evacuation from the building in case of fire. Written copies of this plan must be available to all supervisory personnel.

All employees must be periodically trained and informed of their duties in implementing the plan. In addition, copies of the plan must be available at all times for the telephone operator or at the central security office.

All beds must be easily movable, should evacuation be necessary. Emphasis should be placed on moving patients who are in the room of fire origin and others who are directly exposed to the fire and on maintaining in their rooms the patients who are not immediately threatened during the fire (Lathrop, p. 756).

Fire exit drills must include actual transmission of a fire alarm signal along with a simulation of fire conditions. Residents, however, need not be physically moved outside the building during a fire drill.

Quarterly drills on all shifts are required. All personnel, including administrative staff, maintenance personnel, and interns must be trained, as well as the nurses on duty each shift. A minimum of 12 drills must be held each year. Use of a coded alarm is permitted on drills conducted between 9:00 p.m. and 6:00 a.m.

All employees must be instructed in life safety procedures and use of devices.

31–4.2 Procedure in Case of Fire

Prompt and effective actions must be undertaken by personnel. Required actions include

- removing any occupants directly involved
- transmitting the appropriate fire alarm to warn others in the building

- isolating the fire area by closing doors
- performing evacuation duties as prescribed in the facility's fire safety plan

Each facility must have a written fire safety plan that includes the following:

- using alarms
- transmitting alarms to the fire department
- responding to alarms
- isolating the fire
- evacuating the area
- preparations for evacuation of the building
- putting out the fire

All personnel must be trained in using fire alarms and responding to fire alarms. Particular attention should be placed on training in the use of a code phrase under the following circumstances: (a) when the person who discovers the fire must go to the aid of an endangered patient and (b) when the building's alarm system fails to function properly. A staff member who hears the code phrase announced shall first activate the nearest fire alarm station, then immediately perform his/her duties prescribed under the facility fire safety plan.

Evacuation plans should stress closing doors of as many patient rooms as possible in order to shut out smoke spreading from a fire, and, if possible, to confine the fire in a room.... In studies of fires in health care institutions in which the staff closed doors, the fire spread was readily confined and the life loss was either nil or small. In many recent serious loss-of-life fires in health care facilities, staff either did not close doors or else reopened them. The fire spread was sizable, and the life loss was high. (Lathrop, p. 758)

Two important concepts contained above:

- More persons die of smoke inhalation than of direct burning by flames; hence, smoke is often the most dangerous element threatening patient safety.
- Fire needs oxygen to spread. Keeping doors closed denies oxygen to fires, thus possibly containing them close to the point of origin.

31–4.3 Maintenance of Exits

Appropriate servicing to assure functionality of doors for evacuation must be maintained. Where exits are ordinarily locked, adequate staff to assist occupants to safety must be on duty at all times.

31–4.4 Smoking

Smoking regulations must be written, enforced, and include at least the following:

1. No smoking allowed in rooms, wards, or areas where flammable liquids, combustible gases, or oxygen are used or stored, or any other location determined to be hazardous. No Smoking signs must be posted in all such areas.
2. Patients judged "not responsible" may be permitted to smoke *only* under the direct observation of a staff member.
3. In areas where smoking is permitted, noncombustible ashtrays must be provided.
4. Smoking areas must be furnished with metal containers with self-closing covers into which ashtrays are to be emptied.

Smoking in bed or discarding smoking materials into ordinary waste containers not designed for receiving them lead the list of causes of fires in health care occupancies.

The most rigid discipline with regard to prohibition of smoking may not be nearly as effective in reducing incipient fires from surreptitious smoking as the open recognition of smoking and the providing of suitable facilities for smoking. (Lathrop, p. 759)

31–4.5 Bedding, Furnishings, and Decorations

Draperies. Draperies, curtains (both at windows and around cubicles), and any similar decorations or furnishings must meet flame-resistance standards set by Standard Method of Fire Tests for Flame Resistant Textiles and Films (NFPA 701).

Furnishings and Decorations. Decorations or furnishings of an explosive nature are prohibited. Only flame-retardant decorations may be used in health care occupancies. Decorations must pass both the large- and small-scale tests of NFPA 701, Standard Methods of Fire Tests for Flame Resistant Textiles and Films. Exception: combustible decorations of such limited quantities that a hazard of fire development or spread is not present, such as photographs and paintings.

Waste containers, such as wastebaskets, must be of noncombustible or approved materials.

The purpose here is to try to contain any fire that may start in a waste container. A combustible container or container that collapses during fire exposure will help spread the fire. If the trash container is adjacent to a bed, there is a high probability that the bed linens will ignite regardless of whether or not the container is approved. This fire spread scenario is very common in health care facilities. (Lathrop, p. 759)

NEW HEALTH CARE OCCUPANCIES

Different standards sometimes apply to residential–custodial care facilities (i.e., buildings used for lodging or boarding four or more persons who are incapable of self-preservation because of age or physical limitation).

Only those sections that pertain to skilled and intermediate nursing facilities are cited, and not all of the requirements are included in all details. Numerous exceptions are cited in the full document to which the reader should refer when planning a new building.

GENERAL REQUIREMENTS (SECTION 12-1)

New nursing facilities and hospitals must either meet the standards given here or demonstrate equivalent safety. Alternative designs are allowable if they are deemed to provide equivalent safety.

12-1.1 Objective. The goal is to provide fire safety through containing the fire to the room of its origin, thereby reducing the need to evacuate the building.

Total Concept. Design, construction, and operation of nursing facilities should aim at minimizing the need for evacuating occupants from the building. Because the adequacy of evacuation to protect occupants cannot be guaranteed, further protection should be provided by:

- Appropriate building design, construction, and use of compartments (separation into fire areas)
- Plans for discovering and putting out fires
- Fire prevention plans, adequate training of the staff on how to isolate the fire and move occupants to safety

The basic approach here is to "defend in place."

Any new buildings (additions) conforming to these standards must be separated from any nonconforming structure by a fire barrier with a minimum rating of 2-hour fire resistance.

Communicating openings (e.g., hallways) in dividing fire barriers must be only in corridors and protected by approved self-closing fire doors; otherwise the doors must normally be kept closed.

If a nursing home is located in a building with another classification (e.g., a business or a doctor's office), the two occupancies must be separated from each other by construction having a fire resistance of 2 hr.

12-1.6 Minimum Construction Requirements. Stories are counted from the primary discharge story to the highest habitable floor. At least 50% of the primary level must be level with or above ground (see Figure

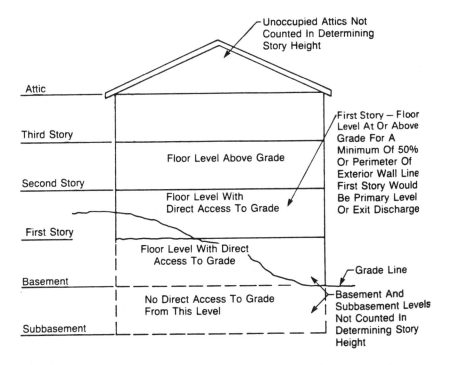

FIGURE 4-1. Building section view illustrating grade line and story designations.

1985 National Fire Protection Association, Inc. Reproduced with permission of the National Fire Protection Association, Inc.

4-1). When a building is one story high, the following types of construction are permitted:

Type I-443, I-332, II-222 (i.e., fire resistive and protected noncombustible)
Type II-111 (protected noncombustible)
Type II-000 (unprotected noncombustible, if automatic sprinkler)
Type III-211 (unprotected noncombustible, if automatic sprinkler)
Type IV-2HH (heavy timber, if automatic sprinkler)
Type V-111 (protected wood frame, if automatic sprinkler)

Facilities two or more stories high may be of Type I-443, Type I-332, or II-222, i.e., fire resistive and protected noncombustible.

Multistory buildings must be of noncombustible materials with a minimum 2-hr fire-resistive rating. An exception is allowed for buildings completely protected by automatic sprinklers. Type II-111 buildings can be a maximum of three stories where a complete system of electrically supervised automatic sprinklers is provided.

In Type I and Type II buildings, all of the interior walls must be noncombustible or of limited-combustible materials. Noncombustible describes a material that in the form it is used and under the conditions anticipated will not aid combustion or add appreciable heat to an ambient (spreading) fire.

Openings in walls that must meet fire- or smoke-resistance requirements must be protected using suitable appliances such as metal plates, masonry fill, or other products approved for the purpose in order to keep fire or smoke from penetrating the partition.

12-1.7 Occupant Loads. Occupant load calculations for determining exit requirements must be calculated by projecting at least one person per 120 sq. ft of floor area in sleeping areas and at least one person per 240 sq ft in inpatient health care treatment areas, and/or the actual expected count of persons.

MEANS OF EGRESS REQUIREMENTS (SECTION 12-2)

Doors opening to the outside must have panic hardware that releases when pressure is applied from the direction of exit travel.

12-2.2.2 Interior Stairs

New Stairs. Excepting handrails projecting no more than 3½ in., a minimum clearance of 44 in. is required. Riser height *maximum* is 7 in.; riser height *minimum* is 4 in. Tread depth must be a minimum of 11 in. At least 6 ft 8 in. of headroom must be provided. Height between landings can be no more than 12 ft.

Slip-resistant treads with no projections that could trip occupants are required.

Handrails. Handrails are required on each side of new stairs and ramps, and must continue the full length of the stairway. Handrails must be not less than 30 in. or higher than 34 in. above the tread.

Handrails must have a clearance of at least 1½ in. from the wall, be capable of withstanding a load of 200 lb, and be continuously graspable. Handrails that are not continuous between flights shoud be extended horizontally a minimum of 12 inches.

12-2.2.3 Smokeproof Towers

According to Lathrop,

> A smokeproof tower is a stair enclosure designed to limit the penetration of heat, smoke, and fire gases from a fire in any part of a building.

This smoke control system should limit the entrance of products of combustion into the tower to a level where, during a period of 2 hours, the atmosphere of the [stair enclosure] will not include a quantity of air emanating from the fire area that is more than 1 percent of the volume of the air in the stairwell. (p. 69)

Each set of stairs must have doorways complying with standards relating to the other doorways in the facility. Doors must open in the direction of exit travel and have approved windows or be fire doors of a self-closing type.

12-2.2.4 Horizontal Exits

A horizontal exit is a protected way of moving from one area to another in the same building or in an adjoining building on approximately the same level. Single doors are permitted as a horizontal exit if they open in only one direction and are 44 in. wide or more.

Nursing and hospital facility horizontal exists must be 8 ft (or wider) corridors. The openings to these corridors must be protected by two swinging doors, each at least 44 inches wide, opening in opposite directions. An appropriate vision panel must be placed in each door.

On each side of the horizontal exit there must be a total of at least 30 sq ft of floor space per patient when the square footage of corridors, treatment rooms, patient rooms, lounge, dining, or other low-use areas is calculated (6 ft per occupant on each side of a horizontal exit on stories not housing patients).

12-2.2.5 Class A Ramps

Ramps are of special interest to nursing facilities inasmuch as they impose less restriction on movement by residents/patients than do stairs.

One can consider ramps and steps simply as prosthetic devices for assisting the human organism in climbing from floor to floor.... When one must consider the energy cost of both horizontal and vertical movement, one finds that a ramp with a gradient of less than about 8 degrees is more economical than any stairway that is likely to be encountered in normal activity. (Lathrop, p. 84)

Lathrop quotes from the National Bureau of Standards study: "For certain occupancies, such as schools and institutions (e.g., nursing facilities) ramps are believed to be more satisfactory and their use in these buildings is recommended" (Lathrop, p. 84).

The National Safety Council has suggested the following guideline:

Grade	Preference
20–50 degrees	Stairway
7–20 degrees	Stairway and landings
Under 7 degrees	Ramps

(National Safety Council Safe Practices, Pamphlet No. 2, National Safety Council, 425 N. Michigan Avenue, Chicago, IL, 61034)

When ramps are used as exits, they must be wide enough to accommodate 30 persons per exit (22 persons per stair exit unit is required). Exception: If a facility has an approved automatic sprinkler system, the capacity can be increased to 45 persons per ramp (horizontal exit) and to 35 persons per stair exit.

Ramps are of two classes, A and B. Nursing homes must use Class A ramps in all instances except where the height of the ramp is 1 ft or less (Class B). Exit capacity for a Class A 44-in.-wide ramp is normally one ramp per 100 persons. Nursing homes are required to have one ramp per 30 persons using ramps and one exit per 22 persons using stairs.

Minimum width: Class A, 44 in.; Class B, 30 in.
Maximum slope: Class A, 1 in 10; Class B, 1 in 8.
Maximum height between landings: Class A, no limit; Class B, 12 ft.

When used as an exit, a ramp must be separated from other parts of the facility by a 1-hr fire-resistance rating for facilities three stories or less and by a 2-hr fire-resistance rating if four or more stories high. Openings must be protected with self-closing fire doors and used solely for exit purpose, e.g., no storage.

Ramp slope must not vary between landings. Landings must be level. Any change in direction of travel must be accomplished at a landing. Ramps must have slip-resistant surfaces.

5-2.6.2 Outside Ramps. Outside ramps must meet the same specifications as those inside and be protected with *a grill at least 4 ft high in buildings over three stories high.*

Ramps may be used from doors 2 or 3 ft above or below grade. Balconies or landings should be level with the building floor.

Several additional detailed requirements exist.

12-2.2 Exit Passageways. All floors and fire sections must be equipped with at least one exit, consisting of a door leading directly outside the building, an interior or exterior stair, a smokeproof tower, and a ramp or an exit passageway.

No fire area can be served solely by horizontal exits. A horizontal exit provides a protected means of passage from one part of a building to another part of a building, but does not provide exit to the outside (Lathrop, p. 35).

12-2.4 Number of Exits. Each floor or fire section of a facility must have at least two exits that are located remotely from each other. A door to the outside or to an outside stair, smokeproof tower, ramp, or interior stair must be provided in each fire section.

Means of egress must be provided for every 30 persons in the case of horizontal travel, and for every 22 persons when the means of egress is stairs. All aisles, corridors, and ramps used as exit accesses must be at least 8 ft wide and free of obstructions. The minimum width of doors in the means of egress from sleeping rooms shall be 44 in.

12-2.5 Arrangement of Means of Egress. Each patient sleeping room must have a door leading directly to a corridor used as an exit access. Each corridor must have at least two exits consisting solely of corridors or lobbies. No aisle, corridor or passageway may have a dead end in excess of 30 ft.

12-2.6 Measurement of Travel Distance to Exits. *Travel distance* must be a maximum of 100 ft between any room door used as an exit access and the exit itself and no more than 150 ft between any point in a room and the exit. Exception: when automatically sprinklered, the travel distance in each case may be increased by 50 ft.

No point in a sleeping room or suite may be more than 50 ft from an exit access door.

12-2.7 Discharge from Exits. Every required exit ramp or stair must lead directly outside at grade or be an enclosed passage meeting all fire-resistance regulations at grade.

12-2.8 Illumination of Means of Egress

The means of egress must be illuminated, and the illumination must be continuous. The floors of means of egress must be illuminated at all points to values of not less than 1 footcandle measured at the floor.

Exit illumination must assure that the failure of any one lighting fixture will not result in darkness in that area. This means the arrangement of lights, circuitry, auxiliary power, and so on, must assure continuity of lighting under all circumstances. Duplicate light bulbs, overlapping light patterns, and overlapping dual electrical circuits can accomplish this.

5-8.2 Sources of Illumination. Egress illumination must be from a dependable source, such as the local electric utility. Battery or portable lamps are not permitted as the primary means of illuminating an exit.

Batteries may be used for auxiliary power provided they will be automatically kept charged and will burn adequately for 1½ hr when used.

12-2.9 Emergency Lighting

Emergency lighting must be provided. If you must switch to a different type of power to maintain continuous lighting, no appreciable interruption may occur.

When an electric generator with its own source of power is used, the changeover must be accomplished within 10 sec. That is, when an auxiliary electricity generator is used, it must be capable of coming on line, i.e., restoring power, within 10 sec after any electrical interruption; 1 foot-candle of illumination must be provided for 1½ hr in the event of failure of normal lighting Automobile batteries are not permitted because they discharge easily and have a short life.

Provision must be made for emergency lighting that is automatically available, not requiring manual intervention for continuous operation, whenever normal power to the facility is interrupted.

For example, two separate lighting systems with independent wiring could be used. One system would be wired to the public utility, the other to the emergency electricity generator, which normally runs on gasoline or diesel fuel. The batteries must be automatically recharged whenever they have been used.

Buildings equipped with or relying on the use of life-support systems for patient care are normally required to meet higher NFPA 76A standards than those for facilities with life-support equipment for emergency purposes only.

Some states demand that skilled-nursing facilities meet the NFPA 76A standard to provide adequate emergency lighting for the building. As a matter of practicality, most skilled-nursing facilities would want to meet the NFPA 76A requirement so that (a) they can provide adequate lighting during the inevitable power outages that occur due to lightning, trees falling across power lines during storms, normal equipment failure over time, and so on; and (b) by conforming to NFPA 76A during construction the management can have the option of installing and using life-support equipment at a later date without expensive building modifications.

Health facilities that house life-support systems have special requirements. Lathrop comments: "NFPA 76A Standard for Essential Electrical Systems for Health Care Facilities (Boston, 1977) requires emergency power supplies be arranged and protected so as to minimize the possibility of a single incident affecting both normal and emergency power supplies simultaneously."

Circuits are to be run separately. Emergency and normal circuits are "joined" at the transfer switch. Damage to the transfer switch would interrupt normal and emergency power supplies simultaneously.

The transfer switch is therefore a critical item and should be separated from any potential source of fire, including the emergency generator and attendant fuel supply.

To assure that emergency generators remain in readiness, they must be inspected weekly and run at least 30 min per month under load.

Emergency power requirements seem to fall between the cracks in both of the conditions of participation (see 405.1134 B, as well as NFPA 12-2.8 and NFPA Section 5-8, both of which address the emergency power issue). What is required is lighting in all means of egress and electrical power to maintain fire detection, alarm, and extinguishing systems and, where present, life-support systems.

Neither set of regulations addresses itself to providing lighting at the nurses' stations or any other areas necessary to maintain continuing functioning of the facility at a minimum level of care in the event of power failures.

Typically, state codes make up for this omission by requiring emergency power systems that at least cover nursing stations and other vital functional areas, if not also requiring lighting for patient rooms as well.

It would seem that, simply as a matter of practicality, the provision of enough lighting to facilitate normal or near-normal functioning of the facility is cost-effective for each new facility, although not required in the Conditions of Participation or the NFPA Code.

5-10 Exit Marking

Access to exits must either be clear or be marked by easily seen signs. Signs must be spaced so that the nearest sign is never more than 100 ft from the exit access.

Every exit sign must be of a size, distinctive color, and design to make it readily visible and in clear contrast to decorations, interior finish, or other signs.

5-10.2 Size of Signs. Letters on exit signs must be at least 6 in. tall and ¾ in. wide.

Signs must be lighted and visible in the normal and emergency lighting modes. (Additional requirements are outlined in the Code giving amount of light intensity required, and so forth.)

The path of travel to exits must be clearly marked with arrow exit signs, and doors that are not exits or the way to an exit must be marked Not an Exit.

12-2.11 Special Features

Normally, locks are not permitted on patient room doors. However, key locks restricting access from the hallway to the room are permitted so long as egress from the room is not inhibited.

Doors to the outside of the building may be locked from the inside. However, doors inside the building on access corridors must not require a key to operate.

When doors are locked, e.g., in a ward of patients who tend to wander, remotely controlled releasing or master keys in the immediate possession of readily available staff must be provided.

Exit doors and smoke-barrier doors ideally should be kept shut at all times. Functionally, however, nurses, aides, and other staff must pass up and down these halls hundreds of times a day. Recognizing this, provision is made for these doors to be held open by automatic-release devices.

Doors in such areas as mechanical equipment rooms, smoke-barrier areas, or hazardous areas may be held open only by devices that release automatically when a fire alarm is activated. Such doors should be closable by (a) the manual alarm system, (b) the smoke detection system, and (c) any automatic fire extinguishment system.

PROTECTION (SECTION 12-3)

12-3.1 Protection of Vertical Openings

To maintain floor-to-floor separation of multistory facilities, 2-hr fire-resistive enclosures are required around vertical openings, which must be of fire-resistive construction, and 1-hr fire-resistive enclosures in all other buildings.

Doors protecting openings in stairway enclosures must be self-closing after anyone walks through them and normally should be kept closed. *The automatic door-closing devices permitted in the hallways are not permitted for stairway doors.* Stairway doors should be marked: Fire Exit—Keep Door Closed.

12-3.2 Protection from Hazards

Lathrop notes: "Hazardous areas are spaces with contents which, because of their basic nature [as in the case of flammable liquids] or because of the quantity of combustible materials involved, represent a significantly higher hazard than would otherwise be typical of health care facilities" (p. 372).

Hazardous areas must be protected by fire barriers with a fire resistance rating of 1 hr or a complete automatic extinguishment system. Hazardous areas include mechanical equipment rooms, the laundry, kitchens, repair shops, handicraft shops, employee locker areas, and gift shops.

The following must have both 1-hr fire resistance and a complete extinguishment system: soiled linen rooms, paint shops, trash collection rooms, and rooms or spaces, including repair shops, used for the storage of combustible supplies and equipment in quantities deemed hazardous by the authority having jurisdiction.

Cooking Facilities

Numerous regulations govern cooking facilities. NFPA 96, Standards for the Installation of Equipment for the Removal of Smoke and Grease-Laden Vapors from Commercial Cooking Equipment apply. A major focus is the requirement for a regularly serviced, fixed, automatic fire-extinguishing system for cook stoves in nursing home kitchens.

12-3.3 Interior Finish

The interior walls must meet Class A interior finish standards. Exception: in patient rooms of four or fewer persons Class A or Class B finishes may be used.

Class A interior finish—flame spread, 0–25; smoke development, 0–450—includes any material classified at 25 or less on the flame-spread test scale and 450 or less on the smoke test scale. Any element thereof when so tested shall not continue to propagate fire.

Class B interior finish—flame spread, 26–75; smoke development, 0–450—includes any material classified at more than 25 but not more than 75 on the flame-spread test scale and 450 or less on the smoke test scale.

12-3.4 Detection, Alarm, and Communication Systems

This is an extensive section with numerous provisions and exceptions. The following are some of the more important requirements.

Each building must have a manually operated fire alarm system that is electrically monitored. This means that when any component part of the fire alarm system malfunctions, a continuous "trouble indication" alert is sent electronically to a continuously attended location.

The fire alarm system must be arranged to notify all building occupants when any alarm station is activated. The local fire department (or its equivalent) must be automatically notified whenever any fire alarm station is activated. Codes for identifying fire zones are permitted.

Emergency Control. Activating any fire alarm station must automatically activate all appropriate devices, e.g., the sprinkler system, alarms, door releases.

New nursing homes must have automatically operated smoke-detection systems. Smoke detectors must be located no farther apart than 30 ft and not more than 15 ft from any wall.

The automatic smoke detection and fire detection systems must both be connected electrically. An exception is made when patient sleeping rooms have their own independently operated smoke detection systems.

> Lathrop makes the following useful observations: manual pull stations should be located along the natural routes of egress and located so as to adequately cover all portions of the building.
>
> Manual pull stations should always be located so that anyone qualified to send an alarm may summon aid without having to leave the zone of his or her ordinary activities or pass out of the sight and hearing of people immediately exposed to or in direct view of a fire.
>
> The operation of a manual fire alarm station should automatically summon attendants who can assist in removing physically helpless occupants. (p. 375)

12-3.5 Extinguishment Requirements

New health care facilities must have an automatic sprinkler system (some exceptions are allowed for one-story buildings). Whenever the main sprinkler system valve closes (permits water to begin flowing), an alarm signal at a continuously staffed station must sound.

Each facility must provide portable fire extinguishers in accordance with Standard for the Installation of Portable Fire Extinguisher, NFPA 10, and these extinguishers must meet all local codes.

Hand fire extinguishers are required on every floor and in every hazardous area. The travel distance to any extinguisher may be no more than 75 ft to a Class A extinguisher, 50 ft to a Class B or C extinguisher. Short persons must be able to reach fire extinguishers.

Every extinguisher must be in operating condition at all times. Fire extinguishers must be *checked quarterly* by the local fire department. Fire extinguishers must be *serviced annually* by a qualified examiner who must show the date that the inspection and servicing was accomplished on an attached tag.

12-3.6 Construction of Corridor Walls

Every corridor must have partitions separating them from other areas. These partitions must be continuous from the floor underneath the area to that of the floor above. Any openings, e.g., for pipes, must have a 1-hr fire-resistance rating. (Numerous exceptions are added.)

Corridor doors may have wired and fixed glass up to 1,296 sq in. in area, provided they are mounted in a steel or other suitable frame. Doors that protect corridor openings must be substantial, e.g., 1¾ in. thick and of solid wood or constructed to resist a fire for 20 min or more. (Several exceptions exist.)

12-3.7 Subdivision of Building Spaces

Smoke barriers are required as follows: (a) two or more compartments (smoke barriers) are required in any story housing more than 50 occupants or used by any inpatients for sleeping, and (b) smoke compartments must be limited to a maximum of 150 ft in length. A fire-resistance rating of at least 1 hr is required for smoke barriers (see Figure 4-2).

At least 30 sq ft per patient of usable building space must be provided on each side of a smoke barrier. When no patients are housed on a floor, at least 6 sq ft of usable space must be provided on each side of a smoke barrier.

Smoke barrier doors must be 1¾-in.-thick solid bonded core wood or construction that will resist fire for at least 20 min.

12-3.8 Special Features

Each patient's room must have a window or door to the outside to permit access to fresh air and/or to vent the fire to the outside. Sills must be no higher than 36 in. from the floor. If windows require tools or keys to be opened, these tools or keys must be readily accessible to the staff.

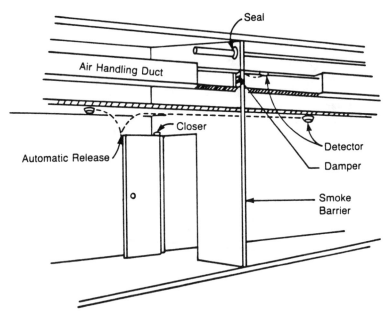

FIGURE 4-2. Typical penetrations of a smoke barrier.

Use of portable space heaters is not permitted. Lathrop comments: "A major concern of the Code is to prevent the ignition of clothing, bedclothes, furniture, and other furnishings by a heating device. Therefore, 12.5.2.2 prohibits portable heating devices in areas used by patients" (p. 387).

EXISTING FACILITIES

Requirements for existing facilities do not vary significantly from those for new ones. The degree of overlap may be about 95%.

Each time the requirements are revised, subtle improvements are introduced and numerous small changes made. For example, new minimum stair-tread depth is 11 in. in the 1985 Code, whereas existing minimum stair-tread depth was less in previous years.

The previous edition required Fire Exit—Keep Door Closed signs on both sides of an exit. The new code instructs that the sign be placed only on the side from which egress is made. This is to prevent confusing this sign with an exit sign, leading a person in a mistaken direction.

CONCLUDING OBSERVATIONS

The administrator who is planning new construction must meet state and local codes as well as the Life Safety Code® requirements cited here.

Sometimes conflicts will arise among codes and jurisdictions. The administrator should meet at least the Life Safety Code® requirements or obtain an exception from appropriate officials if deviating from Life Safety Code standards in order to comply with local codes.

Many areas have been left uncovered. There are, for example, additional sections in the Life Safety Code® on utilities, heating, ventilation, air conditioning, elevators, rubbish chutes, incinerators, laundry chutes, and so on that have not been discussed.

The reader is urged not to attempt to use this introduction for construction purposes or as a reference manual. We strongly advise the purchase of the latest *Life Safety Code® Handbook*. The third edition, based on the 1985 edition of the Life Safety Code®, edited by James K. Lathrop, is available.

The *Life Safety Code® Handbook* is an essential tool for administrators (for ordering information see p. 329). It is the administrator's job to understand the Code and its basic requirements in order to assure that his/her facility is in basic conformity with regulations and to work intelligently with engineers, architects, and state building code officials in planning any nursing facility construction project.

4.3 American National Standard Specifications for Making Buildings and Facilities Accessible to and Usable by Physically Handicapped People

In 1959 the President's Committee on Employment of the Handicapped invited the American National Standards Institute (ANSI) to join forces in calling a conference to set up standards that would lead to improvement in meeting the needs of handicapped persons in American buildings and construction (ANSI, foreword).

The resulting standards were approved in 1961, reapproved in 1971, then revised extensively after a 2-year study sponsored by the U.S. Department of Housing and Urban Development (1974–1976). The current version was approved in 1980 (ANSI, foreword).

Unlike the federal Conditions of Participation, which we quoted verbatim, only a summary of the salient aspects of these standards is offered here. While not especially lengthy, these standards contain many more specifications in inches and other types of measurements than we include. The published standards manual provides many helpful illustrations incorporated in the written descriptions.

1980 STANDARDS

Following is a summary of the essential points for introductory information and study purposes. Do not use this is a representation of the standards in full detail. A well-illustrated 68-page manual is available from American National Standards Institute, 1430 Broadway, New York, NY 10018.

The standards may be seen in overview as listed below:

4.1   Accessible Elements and Spaces
4.2   Space Allowances and Reach Ranges
4.3   Accessible Route
4.4   Protruding Objects
4.5   Ground and Floor Surfaces
4.6   Parking and Passenger Loading Zones
4.7   Curb Ramps
4.8   Ramps
4.9   Stairs
4.10 Elevators
4.11 Platform Lifts
4.12 Windows
4.13 Doors
4.14 Entrances
4.15 Drinking Fountains and Water Coolers
4.16 Water Closets
4.17 Toilet Stalls
4.18 Urinals
4.19 Lavatories and Mirrors
4.20 Bathtubs
4.21 Shower Stalls
4.22 Toilet Rooms
4.23 Bathrooms, Bathing Facilities, and Shower Rooms
4.24 Sinks
4.25 Storage
4.26 Size and Spacing of Grab Bars and Handrails
4.27 Controls and Operating Mechanisms
4.28 Alarms
4.29 Tactile Warnings
4.30 Signage
4.31 Telephones
4.32 Seating, Tables, and Work Surfaces
4.33 Assembly Areas
4.34 Dwelling Units

The purpose of these standards is

to make buildings and facilities accessible to and usable by people with such physical disabilities as the inability to walk, difficulty walking, reliance on walking aids, sight and hearing disabilities, incoordination, reaching and manipulation disabilities, lack of stamina, difficulty interpreting and reacting to sensory information, and extremes of physical size. Accessibility and usability allow a disabled person to get to, enter and use a building or facility. (ANSI, p. 9)

These standards also apply to new construction, remodeling, alteration, and rehabilitation of existing facilities.

4.1 Accessible Elements and Spaces

The first specification is that sites, exterior facilities, accessible buildings, and accessible housing must meet the standards established in paragraphs 4.2 through 4.34 and summarized below.

4.2 Space Allowances and Reach Ranges

Wheelchair passage width: Minimum passage for a single wheelchair shall be 36 in. continuously and 32 in. at any point, e.g., a door opening. See Figure 4-3.

Width for wheelchair passing: Minimum width for two wheelchairs to pass is 60 in.

Wheelchair turning space: (to make a 180-degree turn) minimum clear space of 60-in. diameter or a T-shaped space.

Clear floor or (outdoors) ground space for wheelchairs: For a single stationary wheelchair and occupant, 30 in. by 48 in. is required (knee space under some objects may be included).

Relationship of maneuvering clearances to wheelchair spaces: One unobstructed side of the wheelchair space must adjoin or overlap an accessible route. If in an alcove, additional space must be allowed.

High forward reach: When a wheelchair occupant can reach forward only, the maximum height of the reach forward shall be 48 in. If the reach forward is over something like a desk (which must be located 20 to 25 in. above the floor), the maximum height of the forward reach shall be 44 in. See Figure 4-4.

Side reach: When reaching sideways, objects must be located between 9 in. and 54 in. above the floor. If reaching sideways over an object, e.g., a desk or shelf, the depth of the side reach must be no more than 24 in.

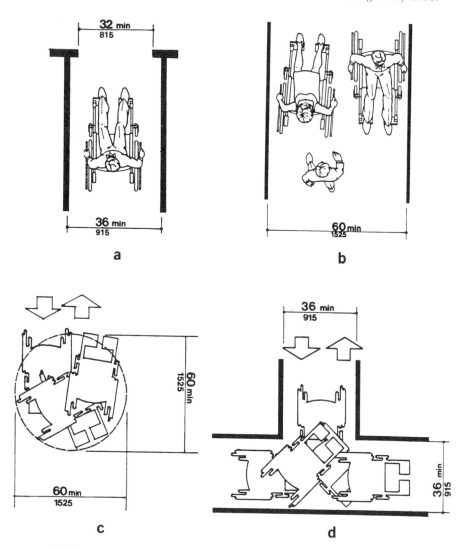

FIGURE 4-3 Wheelchair turning space: **(a)** minimum clear width for single wheelchair; **(b)** minimum clear width for two wheelchairs; **(c)** 60-in (1525-mm)-diameter space; **(d)** T-shaped space for 180° turns.

4.3 Accessible Route

All walks, halls, corridors, aisles, and other spaces that are part of an accessible route must comply.

Location: At least one accessible route shall be provided from public transportation stops, accessible parking and passenger loading zones, and

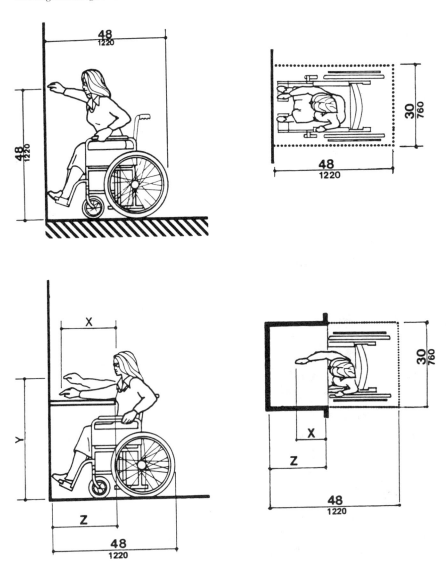

FIGURE 4-4. Forward reach. *Top*: High forward reach limit. *Bottom*: x shall be ≤ 25 in (625 mm); z shall be ≥ x. When x < 20 in (510 mm), then y shall be 48 in (1220 mm) maximum. When x is 20 to 25 in (510 to 635 mm), then y shall be 44 in (1120 mm) maximum.

public streets or sidewalks to the accessible building entrance(s) they serve. At least one accessible route shall connect accessible buildings, facilities, elements, and spaces that are on the same site, including all accessible dwelling units and all accessible spaces within those units on the site.

Width: The minimum clear width of an accessible route shall be 36 in. (except 32 in. at doors). If a wheelchair must turn around an obstruction, the minimum clear width is a 42-in.-wide route (each side of obstruction) and a 48-in.-deep turn space beyond the obstruction, e.g., a door.

Passing Space: If the accessible route is less than 60 in. wide, passing spaces at least 60 in. by 60 in. must be located not more than every 200 feet. (A T-intersection of two corridors, or walks, etc., is accepted as a passing space).

Head room: at least 80 in.

Surface texture: stable, firm, relatively non-slip under all weather conditions.

Slope: must be less than 1:20 (cross slopes, e.g., one pedestrian path crossing another pedestrian path, must be less than 1:50). (A 1:20 slope means 1 in. of drop is allowed over a distance of 20 in.).

Changes in level: up to ¼ in. permissible; between ¼ and ½ in. beveled edge is required with a slope no greater than 1:2; changes in level over ½ in. must meet ramp requirements. Stairs are not allowed.

Doors: see page 356.

Egress: A reasonable number (but at least one) of all accessible routes shall serve as emergency exits or connect to an accessible place of refuge.

Protruding Objects

Object located between 27 and 80 in. above the floor must protrude no more than 4 in. into any hall or passageway or walk. Objects with their leading edge 27 in. high or less may protrude any amount from the wall. Freestanding objects mounted on posts or pylons may overhang 12 in. when mounted between 27 in. and 80 in. above the floor, e.g., a telephone booth. In no case may protruding objects reduce the clear width of an accessible route or maneuvering space. See Figure 4-5.

Head room: At least 80 in. is required.

Ground and Floor Surfaces

General: must be stable, firm, and relatively non-slip under all weather conditions.

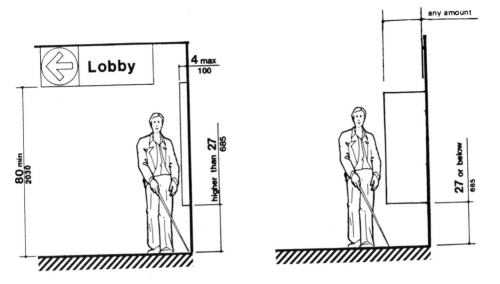

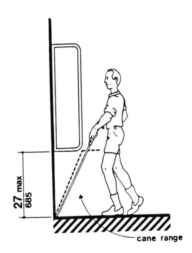

FIGURE 4-5. Protruding objects. *Top*: walking parallel to a wall. *Bottom*: walking perpendicular to a wall.

This material is reproduced with permission from American National Standard Specifications for Making Buildings and Facilities Accessible to and Usable by Handicapped People, ANSI A117.1-1980, copyright by the American National Standards Institute. Copies of this standard may be purchased from the American National Standards Institute at 1430 Broadway, New York, NY 10018.

Changes in level: up to ¼ in., no edge required; beveled edge required if between ¼ and ½ in.; ramp treatment required if over ½ in.

Carpet: must be securely attached, firm or no pad, with maximum pile height of ½ in., level cut, and trim along exposed edge that conforms to changes in level (see paragraph above).

Gratings: maximum width of openings: ½ in. If in walkways, the ½-in. openings must be perpendicular to dominant direction of travel.

4.6 Parking and Passenger Loading Zones

Parking zones: if provided, must be of a reasonable number, with shortest possible access route to an accessible entrance. Spaces shall be at least 96 in. wide with minimum of 60-in.-wide access aisle (two spaces may share one access aisle).

Signage: shall be standard handicapped symbol placed so that it remains visible when a vehicle is parked in the space.

Passenger loading zones: must have access aisle at least 48 in. by 20 ft adjacent and parallel to the vehicle pull-up space.

4.7 Curb Ramps

Location: wherever an accessible route crosses a curb. See Figure 4-6.

Slope: 1:12 (exceptions allowed for existing construction but never greater than 1:8).

Width: 36 in.

Sides: if located where pedestrians walk across it, must have flared sides with slope no greater than 1:10.

Tactile warnings: required (see "Tactile Warnings" below), especially at uncurbed intersections.

4.8 Ramps

Ramp: is any part of an accessible route with a slope greater than 1:20.

Slope and rise: Least possible slope is to be used. Maximum slope: 1:12 with a clear width of 36 in. and a maximum rise of 30 in.

Landings: level landings required at bottom and top of each run, as wide as widest ramp run leading to it and at least 60 clear in. in length. If changing directions, a 60-in.-by-60-in. landing size is required.

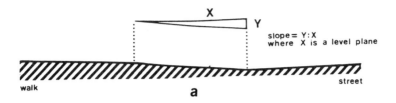

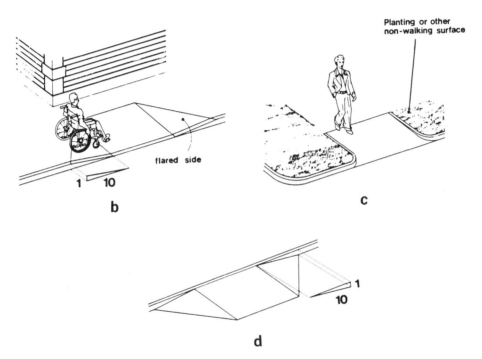

FIGURE 4-6. Built-up curb ramp. (**a**) measurement of curb ramps slopes; (**b**) flared sides; (**c**) returned curb; (**d**) sides of curb ramps.

Handrails: required if rise is 6 in. or more and length of ramp is 72 in. or more. Must be on both sides and continuous on inside rail when switchbacks occur. If not continuous, e.g., ramp connects to flat section, handrails must extend 12 in. beyond the top and bottom of the ramp and be parallel to the flat surface. Clear space between handrail and any wall must be 1½ in.

Cross slope: maximum of 1:50.

Edge protection: if dropoff, minimum of 2-in.-high curb or appropriate wall, railing, or projecting surface.

4.9 Stairs

Treads and risers: On any given flight of stairs, riser heights and tread widths must be uniform. Treads must be no less than 11 in. apart, measured from riser to riser. Nosings (projections) must project no more than 1½ in. See Figure 4-7.

Handrails: required. See "Ramps" above. Also, at the bottom, the handrail shall continue to slope for the distance of one tread past the bottom riser, then extend parallel to the floor or ground surface for 12 in. Gripping surfaces must be uninterrupted by posts or other construction elements. See Figure 4-8.

Tactile warnings: required (see "Tactile Warnings").

Outdoor conditions: Water must not be able to accumulate on walking surfaces.

4.10 Elevators

Numerous detailed requirements are set forth in addition to those for compliance with the American National Standard Safety Code for Elevators, Dumbwaiters, Escalators, and Moving Walks (ANSI A17.1-1978 and A17.1a-1979).

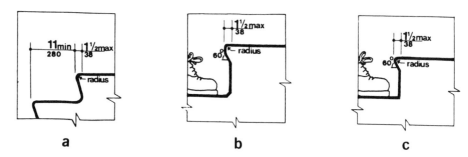

a   **b**   **c**

FIGURE 4-7. Usable tread width and examples of acceptable noisings. (**a**) flush riser; (**b**) angled nosing; (**c**) rounded nosing.

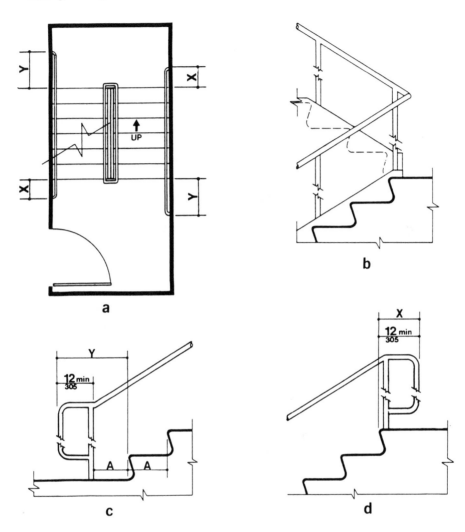

FIGURE 4-8. Stair handrails. (**a**) plan; (**b**) elevation of center handrail; (**c**) extension at bottom of run; (**d**) extension at top of run.

Platform Lifts

Platform lifts are permitted if no other possibility exists. They must conform to "Space Allowances and Reach Ranges" above (clear floor or ground space for wheelchairs).

4.12 Windows

If intended for operation by occupants, at least one window is required per accessible space. Maximum of 5 lb of pressure exerted by occupant to operate window is allowed.

4.13 Doors

Revolving doors, turnstiles: may not be the only means of passage at an accessible entrance or along an accessible route.

Clear width: must be a minimum of 32 in. at opening.

Extra maneuvering clearances at nonautomatic doors: required.

Doors in series: must have at least 48 in. between them. Doors must swing in the same direction or away from the space between them.

Thresholds: maximum of ½-in. rise (¾ in. for exterior sliding doors); must be beveled with a slope no greater than 1:2.

Hardware: must be easy to grasp with one hand, not requiring tight grasping or pinching to operate. Lever-operated mechanisms, push-type mechanisms and U-shaped handles are acceptable. Sliding glass doors must have usable hardware on both sides.

Door opening force: Fire doors: per local ordinances; others: maximum for pulling or pushing a door open: exterior hinged, 8.5 lb; interior hinged, 5 lb; sliding or folding, 5 lb.

Automatic doors and power-assisted doors: should be slow-opening and low-powered: not opening back to back faster than 3 s nor with a force of more than 15 lb.

Entrances

A reasonable number shall be provided in conformity with Paragraph 4.3, "Accessible Route," above.

Drinking Fountains and Water Coolers

Spouts: shall be no higher than 36 in., located at the front of the fountain, flowing parallel with the front of the unit and at least 4 in. high (to allow for a cup or glass to be inserted under the stream of water). See Figure 4-9.

Controls: operable with one hand, easily grasped, maximum of 5 lb of pressure to operate.

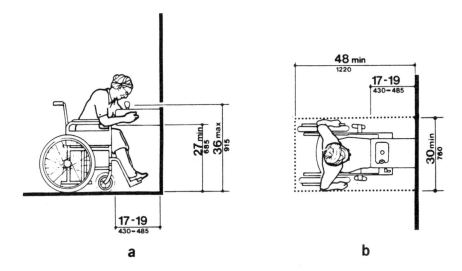

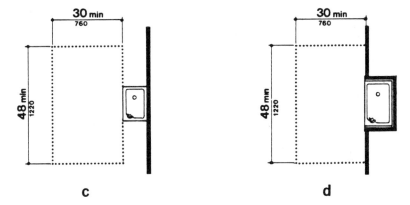

FIGURE 4-9. Drinking fountains and water coolers. (**a**) spout height and knee clearance; (**b**) clear floor space; (**c**) free-standing fountain or cooler; (**d**) built-in fountain or cooler.

Clearances: Wall- and post-mounted cantilevered units must have clear knee space 27 in. from floor to bottom of fountain, be 30 in. wide and 17 to 19 in. deep, plus clear floor space in front 30 in. by 48 in. to allow a person in a wheelchair access to the fountain while facing forward. Freestanding or built-in units with no space under them must have a clear floor space in front of at least 30 in. by 48 in.

4.16 Water Closets

Toilets not in stalls: must meet clear floor space requirements and may have either right-handed or left-handed approach.

Height: 17 to 19 in. measured to the top of the toilet seat.

Grab bars: must be provided on side wall(s) and back wall (33 to 36 in. high).

Flush controls: hand operable with 5 lb or less pressure, easily grasped, maximum of 44 in. high if wall-mounted.

Toilet paper dispensers: to be located within reach, maximum of 19 in. high on side wall.

4.17 Toilet Stalls

Toilet stalls must meet numerous dimension requirements. They may be of a specified standard or alternative size, must include grab bars, and (if less than 60 in. deep) must provide for 9 in. of toe clearance under the front and one of the side partitions.

4.18 Urinals

Urinals may be wall-hung or stall type with elongated rim a maximum of 17 in. above the floor; clear floor space of 30 in. by 48 in. is required; hand-operated flush lever (5 lb maximum force required to operate) not more than 44 in. above the floor.

4.19 Lavatories and Mirrors

Lavatories (see Figure 4-10): shall be mounted with at least 29 in. clearance between floor and bottom of apron, with at least 8 in. of knee depth clearance and 6 in. of toe depth clearance under the drain pipes, plus a 30-in.-by-48-in. clear floor space.

Hot water and drain pipes under lavatory shall be wrapped and any sharp or abrasive surfaces protected.

Faucets may not require more than 5 lb pressure to operate.

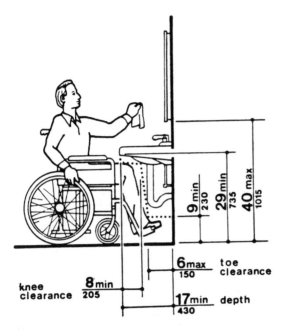

FIGURE 4-10. Lavatory clearances.

This material is reproduced with permission from American National Standard Specifications for Making Buildings and Facilities Accessible to and Usable by Physically Handicapped People, ANSI A117.1-1980, copyright 1980 by the American National Standards Institute. Copies of this standard may be purchased from the American National Standards Institute at 1430 Broadway, New York, NY 10018.

Mirrors: shall be mounted with the bottom edge no higher than 40 in. above the floor.

4.20 Bathtubs

Bathtubs must meet floor space requirements depending on arrangement of bathroom fixtures. They must have the following:

an in-tub seat or a seat at the head of the tub.
grab bars and controls (5 lb pressure or less to operate) located on near
  side of tub enclosure
a shower spray unit with a hose at least 60 in. long usable as a hand-held
  shower or fixed shower spray.

4.21 Shower Stalls

Shower stalls must meet size requirements; have grab bars, controls, and shower hand-held sprayer unit as required for tubs; and provide a seat.

4.22 Toilet Rooms

Doors, clear floor space, water closet, urinals, lavatory, and mirrors must be located and sized according to requirements already reviewed for each of these.

4.23 Bathrooms, Bathing Facilities, and Shower Rooms

They must meet requirements as outlined above for doors, toilets, urinals, tubs, and so on. In addition, any medicine cabinet provided must be located so as to have a usable shelf no higher than 44 in. above the floor.

4.24 Sinks

Height: counter or rim to be no higher than 34 in. from the floor.

Knee clearance: clearance at least 27 in. high, 30 in. wide, and 19 in. deep shall be provided underneath sinks.

Water depth: maximum of 6½ in. deep.

Clear floor space: at least 30 in. by 48 in. in front of sink, extending a maximum of 19 in. under the sink.

Exposed pipes, abrasive, sharp surfaces: must be covered.

Faucets: no more than 5 lb of pressure to operate.

4.25 Storage

Clear floor space: at least 30 in. by 48 in., allowing frontal or parallel approach by wheelchair. See Figure 4-11.

Height: 48 in. high maximum for frontal reach, between 9 and 54 in. high for side reach.

Clothes rods: maximum of 54 in. high.

4.26 Size and Spacing of Grab Bars and Handrails

Diameter or width: shall be 1¼ to 1½ in. or provide equivalent gripping surface. See Figure 4-12.

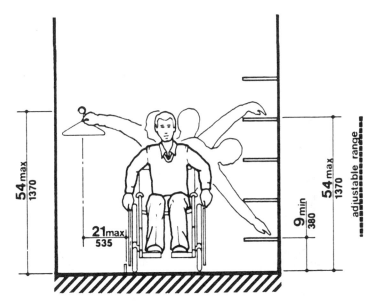

FIGURE 4-11. Storage shelves and closets.

This material is reproduced with permission from American National Standard Specifications for Making Buildings and Facilities Accessible to and Usable by Physically Handicapped People, ANSI A117.1-1980, copyright 1980 by the American National Standards Institute. Copies of this standard may be purchased from the American National Standards Institute at 1430 Broadway, New York, NY 10018.

Space between handrail and wall: must be 1½ in.

Bending and sheer stress point: must be 250 lb or greater.

Grab bars: must not rotate within their fittings.

Edges: must have a minimum radius of ⅛ in. (i.e., no sharp edges allowed).

4.27 Controls and Operating Mechanisms

Electrical and other communications switch receptacles: must be located at least 15 in. above the floor.

Clear floor space: must allow a forward or parallel approach by a person in a wheelchair.

Operation: must be operable by one hand and must not require tight grasping, pinching, or twisting of the wrist, with a maximum force of 5 lb.

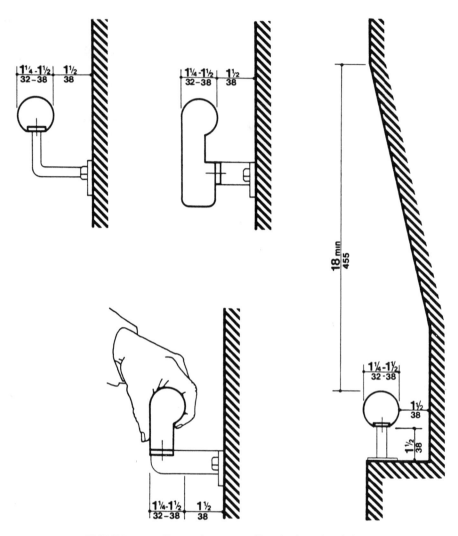

FIGURE 4-12. Size and spacing of handrails and grab bars.

This material is reproduced with permission from American National Standard Specifications for Making Buildings and Facilities Accessible to and Usable by Physically Handicapped People, ANSI A117.1-1980, copyright 1980 by the American National Standards Institute. Copies of this standard may be purchased from the American National Standards Institute at 1430 Broadway, New York, NY 10018.

4.28 Alarms

Audible emergency alarms: must produce sound that exceeds prevailing equivalent sound level in the room or space by 15 dB or exceeds the maximum sound level with a duration of 30 by 5 dB, whichever is louder. Sound levels from this equipment must not exceed 120 dB.

Visual alarms: shall be electrically powered, internally illuminated emergency exit signs, flashing as a visual alarm in conjunction with audible emergency alarms. Flashing frequency shall be less than 5 Hz and connected to the audio emergency alarm system.

Sleeping accommodations: shall have a visual alarm connected to the building emergency alarm system or a 110-V receptacle into which such an alarm could be connected.

4.29 Tactile Warnings

On walking surfaces: shall consist of exposed aggregate concrete, rubber, or plastic cushioned surfaces, raised strips, or grooves and must contrast with the surrounding surface. Grooves may be used indoors only.

Tactile warnings on doors to hazardous areas: (e.g., to warn blind persons of boiler room, loading platform, or other hazardous areas) shall have hardware with a roughened texture.

Tactile warnings at stairs: all stairs (except those in enclosed stair towers or set to the side of the path of travel) shall have a tactile warning at the top of stair runs.

Tactile warnings (36 in. in length) shall be placed at hazardous vehicular areas and at reflecting pools.

Standardization: tactile warnings shall be standardized (consistent) within a building.

4.30 Signage

Character width-to-height proportions: are specified.

Color contrast: either light characters on a dark background or dark characters on a light background.

Raised or indented characters: are specified as to size and font type.

4.31 Telephones

Clear floor or ground space: 30 in. by 48 in. required.

Mounting height: the highest operating part must be 48 in. for frontal approach, 54 in. for side approach, 54 in. for corner approach.

Enclosures: Side reach overhang shall be no greater than 19 in. deep and at least 27 in. high. Full-height enclosures (i.e., regularly shaped booths) shall be 30 in. wide (minimum).

Equipment for hearing impaired persons: Telephones shall be equipped with a receiver that generates a magnetic field around the receiver cap, and equipped with a volume control. *Controls:* pushbutton type (where available).

Telephone books: must be accessible to persons in wheelchairs.

Cord length: at least 29 in.

4.32 Seating, Tables, and Work Surfaces

Seating: at least 30 in. by 48 in. of clear floor space.

Knee clearances: at least 27 in. high, 30 in. wide, and 19 in. deep.

Height of work surfaces: from 28 to 34 in. from the floor or ground.

4.33 Assembly Areas

Minimum number: at least two wheelchair locations and two listening systems.

Size of wheelchair locations: Each wheelchair location must consist of space for *two* wheelchairs and be 48 in. by 66 in. for rear or forward access and be 60 in. by 66 in. for side access, thus accommodating two persons in wheelchairs.

Placement of wheelchair locations: must be dispersed throughout the seating areas with lines of sight comparable to all viewing areas and be located on an accessible route that also serves as a means of egress in case of emergency.

Surfaces: shall be level and comply with Paragraph 4.5, "Ground and Floor Surfaces," above.

Access to performing areas: (e.g., stage, dressing rooms, or wherever performers are) shall be provided by an accessible route.

Placement of listening systems: If the listening system provided serves individual fixed seats, then such seats must be located within a 50-ft viewing distance of the stage and have a full view of the stage.

4.34 Dwelling Units

This is a new section of the standards, not described here. It specifies standards for all aspects of living units and would be of special interest to continuing-care retirement communities and others who offer individual rooms and apartments as well as skilled and/or intermediate nursing care.

An appendix offers additional information and details on such matters as wheelchair turn spaces, telephones, and other aspects of adapting environments to physically handicapped persons.

4.4 Organization and Operation of the Nursing Facility

CONDITIONS OF PARTICIPATION FOR SKILLED NURSING FACILITIES

The requirements set by the federal government for nursing homes to obtain reimbursement through Medicaid (Title 19 of the Social Security Act) or Medicare (Title 18 of the Social Security Act) for services to patients are reproduced on the following pages.

All of the Conditions of Participation are quoted directly, giving the original wording. Where the material has been summarized in a few places, it appears in brackets [...]. Author's own observations or clarifications, appear in parentheses (...). The "Historical Note" is the author's commentory.

Readers will want to familiarize themselves with all of the material, but certain points are of special interest. They appear in boldface.

HISTORICAL NOTE

As we have noted, the two pieces of legislation most directly affecting the nursing home industry were passed by Congress in 1965 and 1966 (Smith, pp. 7–8; Williams & Torrens, p. 170; Kart, p. 292; Wilson, p. 36).

The Original Legislation

Medicare was passed in 1965 as an amendment to the Social Security Act (originally passed in 1935). Medicare provided health insurance to older Americans (Rogers, pp. 56–58). The next year (1966) Congress passed additional health legislation that has profoundly shaped the nursing home industry: Medicaid. Medicaid provides medical assistance to medically indigent persons (those who cannot afford to pay for health care they need) and was passed by Congress as Title 19 of the Social Security Act of 1935 (Hogstel, p. 76; Freymann, pp. 30–32).

After an extended implementation period and several additional amendments to the Social Security Act, the Social Security Administration prepared an extensive set of rules, or minimum conditions, which it considered any nursing facility receiving federal funds should meet (Smith, pp. 8, 10; Miller, 1982, p. 7042; Rosenfeld, Gaylord, & Allen, p. 57; Freymann, p. 32).

Proposed rules were published in the *Federal Register* on July 12, 1973. So many comments were received that the Secretary (head of the Department of Health, Education and Welfare, of which the Social Security Administration was an agency) extended the usual 30-day period for public comment to 60 days, ending September 13, 1973. The Department of Health Education and Welfare (DHEW) changed its name to Department of Health and Human Services (DHHS) in 1981. Officials made several changes in response to public comments and on January 17, 1974, published these final rules, which are still in effect (*Federal Register*, 39(12), Part 3, pp. 2238–2249).

Importance to Nursing Home Industry

These rules are of overriding importance to the nursing home industry because, directly or indirectly, most nursing homes must comply with them. Homes that expect to be reimbursed for services to Medicare or Medicaid patients must meet these conditions for participation (Boling, pp. 198–199; Miller & Barry, p. 32; Freymann, p. 31).

Nursing homes are licensed by the states (Wilson, p. 41). However, most states have relied very heavily on these federal Conditions of Participation in writing their own standards for licensing nursing homes (Smith, p. 10). The net effect is that nearly every nursing home, directly or indirectly, is obligated to comply with the federal standards (Miller & Barry, pp. 22–25; Wilson, p. 41).

These new rules did bring some clarity to the industry. Nomenclature (what to call something) for the various levels of nursing care facilities had been a source of confusion at the federal level (and still is at the state level).

The Conditions of Participation given below are the first introduction of the term *skilled nursing facility* (SNF), the previous federal term having been *extended care facility* (ECF). These Conditions of Participation established the current designations of skilled nursing facility (SNF) and intermediate-care facility (ICF).

Conditions of Participation for intermediate-care facilities are different. There are fewer requirements for charge nurses, nurse staffing, and physician services and none for a medical director (Vladeck, p. 151; Wilson, p. 39). Intermediate-care facilities are for persons who do not need 24-hr-a-day nursing care but must live in a protective environment so that their health needs are constructively supervised in an institutional setting to prevent deterioration and disability.

A second contribution to clarity made by these regulations is their application to both Medicare and Medicaid patients, ending a period of confusion when separate federal guidelines had been set for these two groups.

PROPOSED CHANGES IN THE CONDITIONS OF PARTICIPATION: AN OVERVIEW

In the intervening years, consumers, providers, and government officials have sought to make changes. President Carter appointed a 2-year commission that proposed recommendations seen as favoring consumer interests. Comprehensive changes were proposed.

Before the Carter administration could obtain Congressional action on its proposed changes, Ronald Reagan was elected. President Reagan froze the Carter commission's proposals. In their place, in the "interest of reducing the amount of federal regulations," the President urged that inspection requirements be reduced and simultaneously cut back on the amount of federal monies available to the states for inspecting nursing homes. These measures, viewed as favoring provider interests, were hotly opposed by consumer groups.

1981 Moratorium

In 1981 Congress enacted a moratorium on implementing proposed changes to nursing home regulations, then extended that moratorium to 1982. Finally, the National Academy of Science's Institute of Medicine was authorized to begin a 22-month study of these regulations in November 1983.

This panel, composed of 20 persons, was charged with reviewing such areas as survey and certification procedures, the Conditions of Participation, enforcement mechanisms, and the federal and state roles in enforcement.

States, using federal money, conduct the on-site inspections of nursing home facilities to determine whether a facility meets the federal Conditions of Participation.

The Conditions of Participation were born in controversy. Since they came into effect on February 19, 1974, they have stirred up further dissension among providers, consumers, and the government officials who wrote them.

Not many months after the Conditions were published, the DHEW commissioned "Operation Common Sense," involving a group of federal regulation writers who committed themselves "to revise and recodify [these] regulations to produce clear, readable, and helpful documents" (HCFA, p. 7042). In the process of making the regulations more easily understood, these federal employees attempted to introduce "needed" policy changes at the same time (HCFA, p. 7042).

By 1976 a drive, called the "Long-Term Care Facility Improvement Campaign" (LTCFIC), was on within the DHEW. It began by issuing a monograph supporting the idea of a comprehensive patient-assessment mechanism.

Out of this grew a 3-year project called the Patient Care Evaluation Project (PACE). PACE staff tested two versions (PACE I and PACE II). Criticisms were that the instrument brought "burdensome paperwork," that it put "too much emphasis on the medical model" (for the nursing home), and that "evidence was lacking that PACE produced either cost effectiveness or benefit" (HCFA, p. 7043). However, the federal government was preparing to move.

In response to rumblings received from its regional offices, state agencies, and the general public, Health Care Financing Administration (HCFA), the federal agency that administers Medicare and Medicaid, published a general notice in the June 8, 1978 *Federal Register* that it planned to revise these Conditions of Participation. It invited public comment.

The response by 1,200 organizations, individuals, and providers was impressive. Hearings were held in California, Georgia, the District of Columbia, Maryland, and Illinois. In addition, 620 comments were received. "Most commenters," HCFA reports, "urged us to find ways to ease the burdens of regulation" (HCFA, p. 7044). In the summer of 1980 HCFA published what it assumed to be the new Conditions of Participation to replace the long-criticized 1974 Conditions.

HCFA officials ran into heavy seas. President Carter, in whose administration all of these changes had been proposed, lost to President Reagan, who rejected the proposed revisions, using the Tax Equity and Fiscal Responsibility Act of 1981 as his vehicle.

In the paragraphs below we summarize the changes proposed in the 1980 Conditions of Participation that were never adopted. Understanding the proposed changes will give the reader some insight into the mood of the country from 1975 to 1981.

CHANGES PROPOSED BY HCFA: 1980

Proposed change. Elevated patients' rights to a Condition of Participation. Purpose: to "strengthen enforcement capabilities" (HCFA, p. 7044). Gave patients new rights, inspectors more enforcement power.

Proposed change. Required Patient Care Management System (PCMS) (based on PACE). Purpose: to enforce "more individualized patient-centered care planning" (HCFA, p. 7045). Required facilities to plan more "comprehensively" for the patient and set "time-limited goals" that inspectors could review and enforce.

Proposed change. Applied the proposed Conditions of Participation to intermediate-care facilities as well as skilled nursing facilities. Result expected by HCFA: "[tighter] wording, and the requirements more specific, than in the existing ICF standards" (HCFA, p. 7046).

Proposed change. Required physician to "evaluate the patient's condition as often as necessary," in addition to a visit at least every 30 days for the first 90 days and at least every 60 days after the patient has been in the facility for 90 days. Purpose: to obtain better care for patients.

Proposed change. Strengthened the role of the medical director. Purpose: to give medical director more control over attending physician's care patterns.

Proposed change. Would allow administrator (if state inspector approved) to discontinue consultant services after 1 year in the areas of medical records, dietitian, social services, and activities. Reason: to encourage administrators to improve their staffs.

The federal writers observed:

> The use of consultants has inadvertently created a subset of the long-term care industry. Originally, consultants were seen as backup resources for full-time staff who lacked required education, training, and experience. What has resulted instead is continued use of unqualified staff and a near total dependency on the consultant for professional judgment and the performance of routine activities that the facility should have the in-house capability to perform. (HCFA, p. 7047)

Proposed change. "Temporary pool personnel" would no longer be permitted to fill the position of charge nurse on the day shift or director of nursing services.

Proposed change. Eliminated the requirement for Medical Care Evaluation Studies under the Utilization Review requirements. Reason: "there are definite limitations to applying the Medical Care Evaluation study methodology to the long-term care setting" (HCFA, p. 7047). Their point: this model is useful for hospitals but not for nursing homes.

Proposed change. Required "a complete accounting system of patients' funds which prevents co-mingling of patient and facility monies" (HCFA, p. 7047).

Proposed change. Made "the pharmacist *and the nursing director* jointly responsible for developing a safe and accurate system of drug distribution" (HCFA, p. 7048). Also, to place a "5% limit on drug administration errors and a 4% limit on drugs which may be discarded" (HCFA, p. 7048). (There are no limits set in current Conditions of Participation.)

Proposed change. Reduced paperwork for surveyors and facilities by allowing construction waivers for periods of 2 and 5 years, instead of the current 1-year limit on all waivers.

Proposed change. Added a requirement for a 3-day supply of food and backup emergency power, heat, and water.

Proposed change. Defined "physician" as including a physician-directed team where direction need not be on-site, i.e., a physician extender could make the required patient visits. They noted, however, that "current Medicare law expressly prohibits this" (HCFA, p. 7049).

HCFA officials wrote that "most commenters [summer 1980] urged us to find ways to ease the burdens of regulation" (HCFA, p. 7044).

HCFA officials added

"Especially noteworthy about the comments received [in summer 1980] was the absence of the 'horror stories' of abuses which characterized the Senate hearings of the early 1970's. Acknowledging that conditions have been vastly improved, many commenters emphasized that the task for the 1980's should be to enhance the quality of life for the long-term care resident" (HCFA, p. 7043).

1987 AND BEYOND

The Institute of Medicine's 20-person panel issued a final 400-page report in the summer of 1986. The panel reported that it found the quality of care and quality of life in many nursing homes to be "unsatisfactory" and called for a stronger federal government regulation effort (Committee on Nursing Home Regulation, p. 21). The report proposed dropping the intermediate care category, using one standard (skilled) for all facilities. The panel members called for a rewriting of the Conditions of Participation adding new conditions emphasizing inspections based more on the quality of patient care actually received. Patients' rights, they argued, should be rewritten and given more visibility.

In response, four Congresspersons introduced a bill (the Medicaid

Nursing Home Quality Care Amendments of 1986, HR 5450) calling for (1) elimination of the distinction between skilled and intermediate facilities, (2) a revision of the survey procedures to include more emphasis on patient care actually received, (3) development of a resident assessment form to monitor quality of care, and (4) more federal financial support and participation in enforcing the Conditions of Participation (Waxman, p. 15).

One little known provision of HR 5450 was the elimination of the federal Medicaid legislative requirement that nursing home administrators be licensed. Deletion of the federal licensure requirement would leave it up to the individual states whether to require nursing home administrators be licensed.

Also in the summer of 1986, the federal Health Care Financing Administration (HCFA) introduced new forms emphasizing inspection for the quality of care actually being received by patients.

The 99th Congress adjourned before acting on HR 5450. The 100th Congress, which sits for the years 1987 and 1988, may consider similar legislative proposals that could modify the Conditions of Participation which follow.

In addition to reading the Conditions of Participation as given here, the reader may wish also to obtain a copy of the *HEW Interpretive Guidelines and Survey Procedures*. This volume, published by the American Health Care Association (AHCA), displays three columns side by side. The first column shows the standard, the second column the "interpretive guideline" for the states to use in imposing the standard, and the third column gives the actual procedures for the surveyors to use while inspecting a facility.

STANDARDS FOR CERTIFICATION AND PARTICIPATION IN MEDICARE AND MEDICAID PROGRAMS

This is Title 20 (of the Social Security Act), Chapter III—Social Security Administration, Department of Health, Education and Welfare (now administered by the Health Care Financing Administration, which was set up in 1974 to administer Medicare and Medicaid benefits in the renamed Department of Health and Human Services):

PART 405—FEDERAL HEALTH INSURANCE FOR THE AGED AND DISABLED; SKILLED NURSING FACILITIES

(this portion is Subpart F, some of paragraphs 405.604–405.685)

405.604. TERMS OF AGREEMENT

1. The term of an agreement may be for a period of **12 full calendar months** where the facility is in full compliance with the standards contained in Subpart K of this part (these standards follow, below).

2. Where the facility is not in full compliance with standards. . . the term of an agreement **may: be restricted to a term that ends no later than the 60th day following the end of the time period specified for the correction of deficiencies in a written plan which the Secretary (i.e., his/her representatives) has approved**; provided such term shall not exceed 12 full calendar months; or [several complicated provisos specifying steps the Secretary may take and protections afforded the facility according it due process are then given].

405.605. PROVIDER OF SERVICES; SCOPE OF TERM

. . . "provider of services" refers only to a hospital, **a skilled nursing facility**, or a home health agency. . .

405.606. ACCEPTANCE OF A PROVIDER AS A PARTICIPANT

1. [facility must voluntarily file **two application copies**]
2. [must **accept anyone approved as a program participant**]
3. If a participating hospital, skilled nursing facility, or agency has any restrictions on the types of services it will make available and/or the type of health conditions that it will accept, or has any other criteria relating to the acceptance of persons for care and treatment, it is expected that such restrictions or criteria, **if made applicable to program beneficiaries, will be applied in the same manner in which they are applied to all other persons seeking care and treatment** by such hospital, facility or agency. A provider's **admission policies** and practices that are **inconsistent with** the provider **agreement** objectives set forth in this paragraph **may be the basis for termination of participation**.

405.613. TERMINATION BY PROVIDER OF SERVICES

A provider may terminate. . .

1. **by filing with the Secretary a written notice** [giving a first of month date]
2. the provider also gives at least **15 days' notice to the public by publishing in one or more local newspapers** a statement of the date of termination of the provider agreement with the Secretary [and explains how this will affect individuals].

405.614. TERMINATION BY THE SECRETARY

Causes for termination (by the Secretary): if the provider:

1. **Is not complying substantially** with the provisions of Title XVIII and this Part 405, or with the provisions of the agreement entered into pursuant to 405.606, or
2. No longer meets the appropriate conditions of participation necessary to qualify as a...skilled nursing facility, or
3. **Fails to furnish information** as the Secretary finds to be necessary for a determination as to whether payments are due or were due.
4. **Refuses to permit examination of its fiscal or other records** by, or on behalf of, the Secretary as may be necessary for verification of information furnished as a basis for payment under the health insurance benefits program.

405.615. [PAYMENTS IF TERMINATION OCCURS]

[**Up to 30 days** of care may be reimbursed if a patient was admitted before the termination date].

405.616. REINSTATEMENT OF PROVIDER AS PARTICIPANT AFTER TERMINATION

[A facility may not reapply unless:]
...the Secretary finds that **the reason for the termination of the prior agreement has been removed AND that there is reasonable assurance that it will not recur. AND...the Secretary finds that such institution or agency has fulfilled (or has made arrangements satisfactory to the Secretary to fulfill) all of the statutory and regulatory responsibilities of its prior agreement with the Secretary.**

(We now turn from regulations that have focused on the contracts between the nursing facility and the government. All of the following sections constitute the Conditions of Participation as they apply to each facility that has a participation agreement with the government. They are contained in what is called "Subpart K—Conditions of Participation; Skilled Nursing Facilities.")

CONDITIONS OF PARTICIPATION; SKILLED NURSING FACILITY

(this portion is Subpart K, some of paragraphs 405.1101–405.1137)

405.1101. DEFINITIONS OF TERMS USED IN CONDITIONS OF PARTICIPATION FOR SKILLED NURSING FACILITIES

(a) Administrator of Skilled Nursing Facility   A person who:

1. **Is licensed** as required by State law; or
2. If the state does not have a Medicaid program, and has no licensure requirement, is a high school graduate or equivalent, has completed courses in administration or management approved by the appropriate state agency, and has 3 years of supervisory management experience in a skilled nursing facility or related health program; or [if administering a hospital in which an SNF is located, meets the requirements of 405.1021 (f) of the *Federal Register*.]

(b) Approved Drugs and Biologicals

Only such drugs and biologicals as are:

1. In the case of **Medicare:**
   (i) **Included (or approved for inclusion) in the United States Pharmacopoeia, National Formulary, or United States Homeopathic Pharmacopoeia**; or
   (ii) Included (or approved for inclusion) in AMA (American Medical Association) Drug Evaluations or Accepted Dental Therapeutics, except for any drugs and biologicals unfavorably evaluated therein; or (a) were furnished to the patient during prior hospitalization, and (b) **were approved for use during a prior hospitalization by the hospital's pharmacy and drug therapeutics committee**; and (c) are required for the continuing treatment of the patient in the facility.
2. In the case of **Medicaid:** were **approved by the State Title XIX agency.**

(c) Charge Nurse   A person who is:

1. Licensed by the State in which practicing as a
   (i) **Registered nurse**; or
   (ii) **Practical (vocational) nurse** who: Is a graduate of a State-approved school of practical (vocational nursing) and
2. **Is experienced** in nursing service administration and supervision, and in areas such as rehabilitative or geriatric nursing, or acquires such preparation through formal staff development programs.

(d) Controlled Drugs: drugs listed as being **subject to the Comprehensive Drug Abuse Prevention and Control Act of 1970.**

(e) Dietetic Service Supervisor   A person who:

1. Is a **qualified dietitian**; or
2. Is a graduate of a dietetic technician or dietetic assistant training program, corresponding or classroom, approved by the American Dietetic Association; or
3. Is a graduate of a State-approved course that provided **90** or more hours of classroom instruction in food service supervision and has experience as a supervisor in a health care institution with consultation from a dietitian; or
4. Has training and experience in food service supervision and management in a military service equivalent in content to paragraph (e) 2 or (e) 3 of this section.

(f) Dietitian **(qualified consultant)**   A person who:

1. **Is eligible for registration by the American Dietetic Association**
2. Has a **baccalaureate degree** with major studies in food and nutrition, dietetics, or food service management, has 1 year of supervisory experience in the dietetic service of a health care institution, and participates annually in continuing dietetic education.

(g) Director of Nursing Services

A registered nurse who is licensed by the State in which practicing and has **1 year of additional** education or experience in nursing service administration, as well as additional education or experience in such areas as rehabilitative or geriatric nursing, and participates annually in continuing nursing education.

(h) Drug Administration

An act in which a single dose of a prescribed drug or biological is given to a patient by an authorized person in accordance with all laws and regulations governing such acts. The **complete act** of administration entails **removing** an individual dose from a previously dispensed, properly labeled container (including a unit dose container) **verifying** it with the physician's orders, **giving** the individual dose to the proper patient, and promptly recording the time and dose given.

(i) Drug Dispensing

An act entailing the **interpretation** of an order for a drug or biological and, pursuant to that order, the proper **selection, measuring, labeling, packaging, and issuance** of the drug or biological for a patient or for a service unit of the facility.

(j) Existing Buildings

For the purposes of ANSI Standard No. A117.1 and minimum patient room size (see 405.1134 (c) and (e)) in skilled nursing facilities or parts thereof whose construction plans are approved and stamped by the appropriate State agency responsible therefor before the date these regulations become effective. (Some facilities do still exist with 3-ft-wide hallways and tiny patient rooms which were built and have been operating continuously since before these regulations became effective in 1974.)

(k) Licensed Nursing Personnel

Registered nurses or practical (vocational) nurses licensed by the State in which practicing.

(l) Medical Record Practitioner (i.e., permitted to serve as a consultant). A person who:

1. Is eligible for certification as a registered record administrator (**RRA**) OR an accredited record technician (**ART**), by the American Medical Record Association or
2. Is a graduate of a school of medical record science that is accredited jointly by the Council on Medical Education of the American Medical Association and the American Medical Record Association.

(m) Occupational Therapist (qualified consultant)   A person who:

1. Is a graduate of an occupational therapy curriculum accredited jointly by the Council on Medical Education of the American Medical Association and the American Occupational Therapy Association; or
2. Is eligible for certification by the American Occupational Therapy Association under its requirements in effect on the publication of this provision or
3. Has 2 years of appropriate experience as an occupational therapist, and has achieved a satisfactory grade on a proficiency examination approved by the Secretary, except that such determination shall not apply with respect to persons initially licensed after December, 1977. (A person who has 2 years' experience and passed the test before December 1977 may practice.)

(n) Occupational Therapy Assistant   A person who:

1. Is eligible for certification as a certified occupational therapy assistant (**COTA**) by the American Occupational Therapy Association under its requirements in effect February, 1974; or
2. (Same as for occupational therapist, i.e., has 2 years' experience and passes test up until, but not after, December 1977.

(o) Patient Activities Coordinator (can be a consultant).   A person who:

1. Is a qualified therapeutic recreation specialist; or

2. Has **2 years of experience** in a social or recreational program within the last 5 years, 1 year of which was full-time in a patient activities program in a health care setting; or
3. Is a qualified occupational therapist or occupational therapy assistant.

(p) Pharmacist   A person who:

1. **Is licensed** as a pharmacist by the State in which practicing, and
2. **Has training or experience** in the specialized functions of institutional pharmacy, such as residencies in hospital pharmacy, seminars on institutional pharmacy, and related training programs.

(q) Physical Therapist (may serve as a consultant).   A person who:

1. **Is licensed** as a physical therapist by the State in which practicing, and has graduated from a physical therapy curriculum approved by the American Physical Therapy Association, or by the Council on Medical Education and Hospitals of the American Medical Association, or jointly by the Council on Medical Education of the American Medical Association and the American Physical Therapy Association; or
2. (Prior to 1966 was a member of the American Physical Therapy Association, or in the American Registry of Physical Therapists, or had graduated from a 4-year physical therapy curriculum); or
3. (Until December 1977, had 2 years' experience and passed the test set by the Secretary); or
4. Was licensed or registered prior to January 1, 1966, and prior to January 1, 1970 had 15 years of full-time experience in the treatment of illness or injury through the practice of physical therapy in which services were rendered under the order and direction of attending and referring physicians. (Also, provisions are made for persons graduating outside the United States.)

(r) Physical Therapist Assistant   A person who:

1. **Is licensed** as a physical therapist assistant, if applicable, by the State in which practicing, and has **graduated** from a 2-year college level program approved by the American Physical Therapy Association; or
2. Is licensed and has 2 years of appropriate experience as a physical therapist assistant (and passes exam before December 31, 1977).

(s) Social Worker (may serve as a consultant).   A person who **is licensed**, if applicable, by the state in which practicing, **is a graduate** of a school of social work accredited or approved by the Council on Social Work Education, and has 1 year of social work experience in a health care setting.

(t) Speech Pathologist or Audiologist (may serve as a consultant).   A person who is licensed, if applicable, by the State in which practicing, and

1. **Is eligible** for a certificate of clinical competence in the appropriate area (speech pathology or audiology) granted by the American Speech and Hearing Association under its requirements in effect February, 1974; or
2. Meets the educational requirements for certification, and is in the process of accumulating the supervised experience required for certification.

(u) Supervision

Authoritative procedural guidance by a qualified person for the **accomplishment of a function or activity within his(/her) sphere of competence**, with initial direction and periodic inspection of the actual act of accomplishing the function or activity. Unless otherwise stated in regulations, the **supervisor must be on the premises if the person does not meet assistant-level qualifications specified in these definitions**.

(v) Therapeutic Recreation Specialist (may serve as a consultant).
A person who is licensed or registered, if applicable, by the State in which practicing, and is eligible for registration as a therapeutic recreation specialist by the National Therapeutic Recreation Society (Branch of National Recreation and Park Association) under its requirements in effect February, 1974.

405.1120. CONDITION OF PARTICIPATION: COMPLIANCE WITH FEDERAL, STATE AND LOCAL LAWS

The skilled nursing facility (must be) in compliance with applicable Federal, State, and local laws and regulations.

(a) Standard: Licensure

The facility, in any State in which State or applicable local law provides for licensing of facilities of this nature:

1. **Is licensed** pursuant to such law; or
2. If not subject to licensure, is approved by the agency of the State or locality responsible for licensing skilled nursing facilities as meeting fully the standards established for such licensing, and
3. Except that a facility which formerly met fully such licensure requirements, but is currently determined not to meet fully all such requirements, may be recognized for a period specified by the State standard-setting authority.

(b) Standard: Licensure or Registration of Personnel

Staff of the facility are licensed or registered in accordance with applicable laws.

(c) Standard: Conformity with Other Federal, State, and Local Laws

The facility (must be) **in conformity** with all Federal State, and local laws relating to **fire and safety, sanitation, communicable and reportable diseases, postmortem procedures, and other relevant health and safety requirements.**

405.1121. CONDITION OF PARTICIPATION: GOVERNING BODY AND MANAGEMENT

The skilled nursing facility (**must have**) an effective **governing body**, or designated persons so functioning, with full legal authority and responsibility for the operation of the facility.

The **governing body adopts and enforces** rules and regulations relative to health care and safety of patients, to the protection of their personal and property rights, and to the general operation of the facility.

The governing body **develops a written institutional plan** that reflects the operating budget and capital expenditures plan.

(a) Standard: Disclosure of Ownership

The facility supplies full and complete information to the survey agency as to the identity

1. of each person who has any direct or indirect ownership interest of **10% or more** in such skilled nursing facility or who is the owner (in part or in whole) of any mortgage, deed of trust, note, or other obligation secured (in whole or in part) by such skilled nursing facility or any of the property or assets of such skilled nursing facility.
2. in case a skilled nursing facility is organized as a corporation, of each officer and director of the corporation, and
3. in case a skilled nursing facility is organized as a partnership, of each partner, and **promptly reports any changes** which would affect the current accuracy of the information so required to be supplied.

(b) Standard: Staffing Patterns

The facility **furnishes to the State survey agency** information from payroll records setting forth the **average numbers and types of personnel** (in full-time equivalents) on each tour of duty **during at least 1 week of each quarter.** Such week will be selected by the survey agency.

(c) Standard: Bylaws

The **governing body adopts** effective **patient care policies and administrative policies** and bylaws, governing the operation of the facility, in accordance with legal requirements.

Such policies and bylaws are **in writing, dated, and made available** to all members of the governing body which ensures that they are operational, and reviews and revises them as necessary.

(d) Standard: Independent Medical Evaluation (Medical Review)

The **governing body adopts policies** to ensure that the facility cooperates in an effective program which provides for a regular program of independent medical evaluation and audit of the patients in the facility to the extent required by the programs in which the facility participates (including, **at least annually, medical evaluation of each patient's need for skilled nursing facility care**).

(e) Standard: Administrator

The **governing body appoints** a qualified administrator who:
is responsible for

the overall **management** of the facility

enforces the rules and regulations relative to the level of health care and safety of patients, and to the protection of their personal and property rights,

and **plans and organizes and directs** those responsibilities delegated to him (/her) by the governing body.

Through meetings and periodic reports, the administrator **maintains ongoing liaison** among the governing body, medical and nursing staffs, and other professional and supervisory staff of the facility,

and **studies and acts upon** recommendations made by the utilization review and other committees.

In the absence of the administrator, an employee is **authorized, in writing,** to act on his (/her) behalf.

(f) Standard: Institutional Planning

The **institutional plan:**

1. Provides for an **annual operating budget** which includes all anticipated income and expenses related to items which would, under generally accepted accounting principles, be considered income and expense items (except that nothing in this paragraph shall require that there be prepared, in connection with any budget, an item-by-item identification of the components of each type of an anticipated expenditure or income).

2. Provides for **a capital expenditures plan for at least a 3-year period** (including the year to which the operating budget described in

paragraph (1) of this section is applicable), which includes and identifies in detail, the anticipated sources of financing for, and the objectives of, each anticipated expenditure in excess of **$100,000** related to the acquisition of land, the improvement of land, buildings, and equipment, and the replacement, modernization, and expansion of the buildings, and equipment which would, under generally accepted accounting principles, be considered capital items,

3. Provides for **review and updating at least annually**, and
4. **Is prepared**, under the direction of the governing body of the institution, **by a committee** consisting of representatives of the governing body, the administrative staff, and the organized medical staff (if any) of the institution.

(g) Standard: Personnel Policies and Procedures

The **governing body, through the administrator, is responsible for**

implementing and maintaining written personnel policies and procedures that support sound patient care and personnel practices:

personnel records (that are) current and available for each employee and contain sufficient information to support placement in the position to which assigned;

written policies for control of communicable disease which are, in effect to ensure that **employees with symptoms or signs of communicable disease or infected skin lesions** are not permitted to work;

a **safe and sanitary environment** for patients and personnel exists; and that

incidents and accidents to patients and personnel are reviewed to identify health and safety hazards; and that

employees are provided, or referred for, **periodic health examinations**, to ensure freedom from communicable disease.

(h) Standard: Staff Development

An **ongoing educational program** is planned and conducted for the development and improvement of skills of all the facility's personnel, including training related to problems and needs of the aged, ill, and disabled.

Each employee receives appropriate orientation to the facility and its policies, and to his (/her) position and duties.

Inservice training includes at least:
— prevention and control of infections,
— fire prevention and safety,
— accident prevention,
— confidentiality of patient information, and

— preservation of patient dignity, including protection of his (/her) privacy and personal and property rights

Records are **maintained** which indicate the **content of, and attendance at,** such staff development programs.

(i) Standard: Use of Outside Resources

If the facility does not employ a qualified professional person to render a specific service to be provided by the facility, there **(must be) arrangements** for such a service provided by an outside resource—a person or agency that will render direct service to patients or act as a consultant to the facility.

The responsibilities, functions, and objectives, and the terms of agreement, including financial arrangements and charges of each such outside resource are (to be) **delineated in writing and signed** by an authorized representative of the facility and the person or agency providing the service.

Agreements pertaining to services must specify that **the facility assumes professional and administrative responsibility** for the services rendered.

The outside resource, when acting as a consultant, apprises the administrator of recommendations, plans for implementation and continuing assessment through **dated, signed reports, which are (to be) retained** by the administrator for follow-up action and evaluation of performance.

(j) Standard: Notification of Changes in Patient Status

The facility (must have) appropriate written policies and procedures relating to **notification of the patient's attending physician and other responsible persons** in the event of an accident involving the patient, or **other significant change** in the patient's physical, mental, or emotional status, or patient charges, billing, and related administrative matters.

Except in a **medical emergency**, a patient is not transferred or discharged, nor is treatment altered radically, **without consultation** with the patient, or if he is incompetent, without prior notification of next of kin or sponsor.

(k) Standard: Patient's Rights

The **governing body of the facility (must establish) written policies** regarding the rights and responsibilities of patients and, through the administrator, is responsible for development of, and adherence to procedures implementing such policies.

These policies and procedures **(must be) made available** to patients, to any guardians, next of kin, sponsoring agency(ies), or representative payees selected pursuant to section 205 (j) of the Social Security Act and Subpart Q of Part 404 of this chapter, and to the public.

The **staff** of the facility is (to be) trained and involved in the implementation of these policies and procedures.

These patients' rights policies and procedures must ensure that **for each patient** admitted to the facility:

1. RULES AND REGULATIONS   Each patient is fully **informed, as evidenced by the patient's written acknowledgment**, prior to or at the time of admission and during stay, of these rights and of all rules and regulations governing patient conduct and responsibilities;
2. CHARGES FOR SERVICES   Each patient is fully informed, prior to or at the time of admission and during stay, of services available in the facility, and of related charges including **any charges for services not covered** under titles XVIII or XIX of the Social Security Act, or not covered by the facility's basic per diem rate;
3. MEDICAL TREATMENT   Each patient is fully **informed, by a physician, of his (/her) medical condition unless medically contraindicated** (as **documented** by a physician in his medical record) and is afforded the **opportunity to participate** in the planning of his (/her) medical treatment and to refuse to participate in experimental research;
4. TRANSFER AND DISCHARGE   Is transferred or discharged only for medical reasons, or for his welfare or that of other patients, or for non-payment for his stay (except as prohibited by titles XVIII or XIX of the Social Security Act), and is given **reasonable advance notice** to ensure orderly transfer or discharge, and **such actions are documented** in the medical record;
5. CITIZENSHIP   Is encouraged and assisted, throughout the period of stay, to exercise his (/her) rights as a patient and as a citizen, and to this end **may voice grievances and recommend changes** in policies and services to facility staff and/or to outside representatives of his (/her) choice, **free from restraint, interference, coercion**, discrimination, or reprisal;
6. FINANCES   **May manage** his (/her) personal financial affairs, or is given at least a quarterly accounting of financial transactions made on his (/her) behalf should the facility accept his (/her) **written delegation of this responsibility to the facility** for any period of time in conformance with State law;
7. ABUSE, RESTRAINT   Is free from mental and physical abuse, and free from chemical and (except in emergencies) physical restraints **except as authorized in writing by a physician for a specified and limited period of time**, or when necessary to protect the patient from injury to himself or to others;
8. CONFIDENTIALITY   Is assured confidential treatment of his (/her) personal and medical records, and **may approve or refuse their release** to any individual outside the facility, except, in case of his

(/her) transfer to another health care institution, or as required by law or third-party payment contract;

9. PRIVACY   Each patient is treated with consideration, respect, and full recognition of his dignity and individuality, including privacy in treatment and in care for his (/her) personal needs;

10. WORK   **Is not required to perform services** for the facility that are not included for therapeutic purposes in his (/her) plan of care;

11. COMMUNICATION   May associate and communicate privately with persons of his (/her) choice, and send and receive his (/her) **personal mail unopened**, unless medically contraindicated (as documented by his/her personal physician in his/her medical record);

12. SOCIAL ACTIVITIES   May meet with, and participate in activities of, social, religious and community groups at his (/her) discretion, unless medically contraindicated (as documented by his/her physician in his/her medical record);

13. POSSESSIONS   May retain and use his (/her) personal clothing and possessions as space permits, unless to do so would infringe upon rights of other patients, and unless medically contraindicated (as documented by his/her physician in his/her medical record);

14. MARRIAGE   If married, is assured privacy for visits by his/her spouse; if both are in-patients in the facility, they are **permitted to share a room**, unless medically contraindicated (as documented by the attending physician in the medical record);

15. GUARDIANSHIP (added later)   All rights and responsibilities specified in the preceding paragraphs, "Rules and Regulations," "Charges for Services," "Medical Treatment," and "Transfer and Discharge" as they pertain to a patient adjudicated incompetent in accordance with State law, a patient who is found, by his or her physician, to be medically incapable of understanding these rights, or a patient who exhibits a communication barrier, **devolve** (go to) to such patient's guardian, next of kin, sponsoring agency(ies) or representative payee. However, **the facility and its employees may not assume these rights**.

405.1122. CONDITION OF PARTICIPATION: PATIENT CARE POLICIES

The skilled nursing facility (must have) written patient care policies to govern the continuing skilled nursing care and related medical or other services provided.

(a) Standard: Development and Review of Patient Care Policies

The facility (must have) policies which are developed with the advice of (and with **provision for review of such policies at least annually**, by) a group of professional personnel including:

— one or more physicians and
— one or more registered nurses

to govern the skilled nursing care and related medical or other services it provides.

The **policies (must be) available to**

— admitting physicians
— sponsoring agencies
— patients and
— the public and reflect awareness of and provision for meeting the total medical and psychosocial needs of patients including
— admission transfer and discharge planning and
— the range of services available to patients including frequency of physician visits by each category of patients admitted.

These policies (must) also include provisions to protect patients' personal and property rights. Medical **records and minutes of staff and committee meetings (must) reflect** that

— patient care is being rendered in accordance with the written patient care policies, and
— that utilization review committee recommendations regarding the policies are reviewed and necessary steps taken to ensure compliance.

(b) Standard: Execution of Patient Care Policies

The facility (must have) a physician, a registered nurse, or a medical staff **designated in writing**, to be responsible for the execution of such policies.

If the responsibility for day-to-day execution of patient care policies has been delegated to a registered nurse, the facility (must make) available an **advisory physician** from whom she (/he) receives medical guidance.

Medical Direction:

The facility **(must retain), pursuant to a written agreement**, **a physician**, licensed under State law to practice medicine or osteopathy, to serve as medical director on a part-time or full-time basis as is appropriate for the needs of the patients and the facility.

If the facility has an organized medical staff, the medical director is designated by the medical staff with approval of the governing body.

A medical director may be designated for **a single facility or multiple facilities** through arrangements with a group of physicians, a local medical society, a hospital medical staff, **or through another similar arrangement**.

The medical director is responsible for the overall coordination of the medical care in the facility to ensure the adequacy and appropriateness of the medical services provided to patients and to maintain surveillance of the health status of employees. (See 405.1911(b) regarding waiver of the requirement for a medical director.)

(c) Standard: Coordination of Medical Care

Medical direction and coordination of medical care in the facility are provided by a medical director. The **medical director is responsible for the development of written bylaws, rules and regulations which are approved by the governing body** and include delineation of the responsibilities of attending physicians. Coordination of medical care includes liaison with attending physicians to ensure their writing **orders promptly upon admission of a patient, and periodic evaluation** of the adequacy and appropriateness of health professionals and supportive staff and services.

(d) Standard: Responsibilities to the Facility

The medical director is responsible for surveillance of the **health status of the facility's employees**.

Incidents and accidents that occur on the premises are reviewed by the medical director to identify hazards to health and safety.

The administrator is given appropriate information to help ensure a safe and sanitary environment for patients and personnel.

The medical director is responsible for the execution of patient care policies in accordance with 405.1121(1).

405.1123. CONDITION OF PARTICIPATON: PHYSICIAN SERVICES

Patients in need of skilled nursing or rehabilitative care are **admitted to the facility only upon recommendation, and remain under the care of a physician**.

To the extent feasible, each patient or his (/her) sponsor designates a personal physician.

(a) Standard: Medical Findings and Physicians' Orders at the Time of Admission

There (must be) made available to the facility, **prior to or at the time of admission**, patient information which includes

— current medical findings, diagnoses and
— orders from a physician for immediate care of the patient.

Information about the **rehabilitation potential** of the patient and a

summary of prior treatment (must be) made available to the facility at the time of admission **or within 48 hours thereafter**.

(b) Standard: Patient Supervision by Physician

The facility (must have) a policy that the health care of every patient be under the supervision of a physician who, based on a medical evaluation of the patient's immediate and long-term needs, prescribes a planned regimen of total patient care.

Each attending physician is required to make arrangements for the medical care of his (/her) patients in his (/her) absence.

The medical evaluation of each patient (must be) based on **a physical examination done within 48 hours of admission unless such examination was performed within 5 days prior to admission**.

The patient (must be) seen by his (/her) attending physician at least **once every 30 days for the first 90 days following admission**.

The patient's total program of care (including medications and treatments) (must be) reviewed during a visit by the attending physician **at least once every 30 days for the first 90 days, and revised as necessary**.

A progress note (must be) written and signed by the physician **at the time of each visit, and he (/she) must sign all his (/her) orders**.

Subsequent to the 90th day following admission, an **alternate schedule** for physician visits may be adopted where the attending physician determines and so justifies in the patient's medical record that the patient's condition does not necessitate visits at 30-day intervals. This alternate schedule **does not apply** for patients who require specialized rehabilitative services, in which case the review must be in accordance with 405.1126(b) (which requires 30-day review of specialized rehabilitative services). **At no time may the alternate schedule exceed 60 days between visits**.

If the physician decides upon an alternate schedule of visits of more than 30 days for a patient:

— in the case of a Medicaid benefits recipient, the **facility notifies** the State Medicaid agency of the change in schedule, including justification and

— the **utilization review committee** or the medical review team (see 405.1121(d)) promptly **reevaluates** the patient's need for monthly physician visits as well as his (/her) continued need for skilled nursing facility services (see 405.1137(d), review of cases of extended duration).

— **if** the utilization review committee or the medical review team does not concur in the schedule of visits at intervals of more than 30 days, the alternate schedule is not acceptable.

(c) Standard: Availability of Physicians for Emergency Patient care

The facility (must have) **written procedures**, available **at each nurses' station**, that provide for having a physician available to furnish necessary medical care in case of emergency.

405.1124. CONDITION OF PARTICIPATION: NURSING SERVICES

The skilled nursing facility (must) provide **24 hour service by licensed nurses, including the services of a registered nurse at least during the day tour of duty 7 days a week**. There (must be) an organized nursing service with a sufficient number of qualified nursing personnel to meet the total nursing needs of all patients in the facility.

(a) Standard: Director of Nursing Services

The director of nursing services (must be) a qualified **registered nurse, employed full-time** who has, **in writing**, administrative authority, responsibility, and accountability for the functions, activities, and training of the nursing services staff, and **serves only one facility** in this capacity.

If the director of nursing services has other institutional responsibilities, a qualified registered nurse (must serve) as her (/his) assistant so that there is the **equivalent of a full-time director of nursing services** on duty.

The director of nursing services is responsible for the development and maintenance of:
— nursing service objectives
— standards of nursing practice
— nursing policy and procedure manuals
— written job descriptions for each level of nursing personnel
— scheduling of daily rounds to see all patients
— methods for coordination of nursing services with other patient services
— recommending the number and levels of nursing personnel to be employed
— nursing staff development.

(b) Standard: Charge Nurse

A registered nurse, or a qualified licensed practical (vocational) nurse, is designated as charge nurse by the director of nursing services for each tour of duty, and is responsible for supervision of the total nursing activities in the facility during each tour of duty.

The director of nursing services **(cannot) serve** as charge nurse in a facility with an average daily total occupancy of 60 or more patients.

The **charge nurse delegates** responsibility to nursing personnel for the direct **nursing care of specific patients** during each tour of duty, on the basis of

— staff qualifications
— size and physical layout of the facility
— characteristics of the patient load
— the emotional social and nursing care needs of patients.

(c) Standard: 24-Hour Nursing Service

The facility (must) provide **24-hour nursing service** which is sufficient to meet nursing needs in accordance with the patient care policies developed as provided in 505.1121(1) (see above).

The policies **(must) insure**:

— that each patient receives treatments, medications, and diet as prescribed
— rehabilitative care as needed
— proper care to prevent decubitus (open skin) ulcers and deformities
— is kept comfortable, clean, well-groomed
— protected from accident, injury, and infection
— encouraged, assisted, and trained in self-care and group activities.

Nursing personnel—including at least one registered nurse on the day tour of duty **7 days a week**—, licensed practical nurses, nurse's aides, orderlies, and ward clerks (must be) **assigned duties consistent with**

— their education and experience
— the characteristics of the patient load
— the kinds of nursing skills needed to provide care to the patients.

Weekly time schedules (must be) maintained and indicate the number and classification of nursing personnel, **including relief personnel**, who worked on each unit for each tour of duty.

(d) Standard: Patient Care Plan

In coordination with other patient care services to be provided, **a written patient care plan for each patient** (must be) developed and maintained by the nursing service consonant with (i.e., in accordance with) the attending physician's plan of medical care, and (be) implemented upon admission.

The plan (must) indicate:

— **care** to be given
— **goals** to be accomplished and
— **which professional service** is responsible for each element of care.

The patient care plan (must be) reviewed, evaluated and **updated as necessary** by all professional personnel involved in the care of the patient.

(e) Standard: Rehabilitative Nursing Care

Nursing personnel (must be) trained in rehabilitative nursing, and the facility **(must have) an active program of rehabilitative nursing care** which is an integral part of nursing service and is directed toward assisting each patient to achieve and maintain an **optimal** level of self care and independence.

Rehabilitative nursing care services (must be) **performed daily** for those patients who require such service, and (must be) recorded routinely.

(f) Standard: Supervision of Patient Nutrition

Nursing personnel (must be) **aware of** the nutritional needs and food and fluid intake of patients, and **assist promptly** where necessary in the feeding of patients.

A procedure (must be) established to inform the dietetic service of physicians' diet orders and of patients' dietetic problems.

Food and fluid intake of patients (must be) observed, and deviations from the normal recorded and reported to the charge nurse and the physician.

(g) Standard: Administration of Drugs

Drugs (can be) administered **(only) by**:

— physicians
— licensed nursing personnel or
— other personnel who have completed a State-approved training program in medication administration.

Procedures (must be) established by the pharmaceutical services committee to ensure that

— drugs to be administered are checked against physicians' orders
— that the patient is identified prior to administration of a drug
— that each patient has an individual medication record
— that the dose of drug administered to that patient is properly recorded therein by the person who administered the drug.

Drugs and biologicals (must be):

— administered as soon as possible after doses are prepared
— be administered by the **same person** who prepared the doses for administration (except under single-unit-dose package distribution systems).

(h) Standard: Conformance with Physicians' Drug Orders

Drugs (must be) administered in accordance with written orders of the attending physician.

— drugs not specifically limited as to time or number of doses when ordered (must be) controlled by **automatic stop orders** or other methods in accordance with written policies

— physicians' **verbal orders** for drugs (must be) given only to a licensed nurse, pharmacist, or physician

— and are immediately recorded and signed by the person receiving the order. (Verbal orders for Schedule II drugs [habit-forming drugs] are permitted only in the case of a bona fide emergency situation.)

— (verbal) orders (must be) **countersigned by the attending physician within 48 hours**

— the attending physician (must be) notified of an automatic stop order prior to the last dose so that he (/she) may decide if the administration of the drug or biological is to be continued or altered.

(i) Standard: Storage of Drugs

Procedures for storing and disposing of drugs and biologicals (must be) established by the pharmaceutical services committee.

In accordance with State and Federal laws:

— all drugs and biologicals (must be) stored in locked compartments under proper temperature controls and

— only authorized personnel can have access to the keys.

Separately locked, permanently affixed compartments (must be) provided for storage of controlled drugs listed in Schedule II of the Comprehensive Drug Abuse Prevention and Control Act of 1970 and other drugs subject to abuse (except under single-unit-package drug distribution systems in which the quantity stored is minimal and a missing dose can be readily detected).

An **emergency medication kit** approved by the pharmaceutical services committee (must be) kept readily available.

405.1125. CONDITION OF PARTICIPATION: DIETETIC SERVICES

The skilled nursing facility (must) provide a **hygienic dietetic service** that

— meets the daily nutritional needs of patients
— ensures that special dietary needs are met, and
— provides palatable and attractive meals.

A facility that has a **contract with an outside food management company** may be found in compliance with this condition provided the facility and/or company meets the standards listed herein.

(a) Standard: Staffing

Overall supervisory responsibility for the dietetic service (must be) assigned to a **fulltime qualified dietetic service supervisor**.

If the dietetic service supervisor is not a qualified dietitian he (/she) functions with frequent, regularly scheduled **consultation** from a person so qualified.

In addition, the facility (must) employ sufficient supportive personnel competent to carry out the functions of the dietetic service.

Food service personnel (must be) on duty daily over a period of **12 or more hours**.

If consultant dietetic services are used, the consultant's visits (must be) at appropriate times, and of sufficient duration and frequency

— to provide continuing liaison with medical and nursing staffs
— (to provide) advice to the administrator
— (to provide) patient counseling
— (to provide) guidance to the supervisor and staff of the dietetic service
— (to provide) approval of all menus, and
— to participate in development or revision of dietetic policies and procedures and
— planning and conducting inservice education programs.

(b) Standard: Menus and Nutritional Adequacy

Menus (must be) planned and followed to meet **nutritional needs** of patients in accordance with:

— **physicians' orders and,**
— to the extent medically possible, in accordance with the recommended dietary allowances of the Food and Nutrition Board of the National Research Council, National Academy of Sciences.

(c) Standard: Therapeutic Diets

Therapeutic diets (when needed) (must be) prescribed by the attending physician.

Therapeutic menus (must be) **planned in writing**, and prepared and served as ordered, with supervision or consultation from the dietitian and advice from the physician whenever necessary.

A current therapeutic diet manual approved by the dietitian (must be) readily available to attending physicians and nursing and dietetic service personnel.

(d) Standard: Frequency of Meals

At least 3 meals or their equivalent (must be)

— served daily
— at regular hours
— with **not more than a 14-hour span between a substantial evening meal and breakfast**.

To the extent medically possible (i.e. unless the physician prohibits it) **bedtime nourishments** (must be) offered routinely to all patients.

(e) Standard: Preparation and Service of Food

Foods (must be) prepared by methods that conserve nutritive value, flavor and appearance, and are attractively served at the proper temperatures and in a form to meet individual needs.

If a patient refuses food served, appropriate substitutes of similar nutritive value (must be) offered.

(f) Standard: Hygiene of Staff

Dietetic service personnel (must be) **free of communicable diseases** and practice hygienic food-handling techniques.

In the event food service employees are assigned duties outside the dietetic service, these duties (must not) interfere with the sanitation, safety, or time required for dietetic work assignments.

(g) Standard: Sanitary Conditions

Food (must be) procured from sources approved for considered satisfactory by Federal, State, or local authorities, and stored, prepared, distributed, and served under sanitary conditions.

Waste (must be) disposed of properly.

Written reports of inspections by State and local health authorities (must be) **on file at the facility, with notation made of action taken** by the facility to comply with any recommendations.

405.1126. CONDITION OF PARTICIPATION: SPECIALIZED REHABILITATIVE SERVICES

In addition to rehabilitative nursing, the skilled nursing facility (must) provide or arrange for, under written agreement, specialized rehabilitative services by qualified personnel, e.g.,

— **physical therapy**
— **speech pathology and audiology**
— **occupational therapy**

as needed by patients to improve and maintain functioning.

These services (must be) provided **upon the written order of the patient's attending physician.**

Safe and adequate space and equipment (must be) available, commensurate with the services offered.

If the facility does not offer such services directly, it does not admit nor retain patients in need of this care unless provision is made for such services under arrangement with qualified outside resources under which **the facility assumes professional and financial responsibilities for the services rendered**.

(a) Standard: Organization and Staffing

Specialized rehabilitative services (must be) provided in accordance with accepted professional practices, by qualified therapists or by qualified assistants or other supportive personnel under the supervision of qualified therapists.

Other rehabilitative services also may be provided, but must be in a facility where all rehabilitative services are provided through an organized rehabilitative service under the supervision of **a physician qualified in physical medicine** who determines the goals and limitations of these services and assigns duties appropriate to the training and experience of those providing such services.

Written administrative and patient care policies and procedures (must be) developed for rehabilitative services by appropriate therapists and representatives of the medical, administrative, and nursing staffs.

(b) Standard: Plan of Care

Rehabilitative services (must be) provided under a written plan of care, initiated by the attending physician, and developed in consultation with appropriate therapist(s) and the nursing service.

Therapy (must be) provided ONLY upon written orders of the attending physician.

A report of the patient's progress (must be) communicated to the attending physician **within 2 weeks** of the initiation of specialized rehabilitatve services.

The patient's progress (must be) thereafter reviewed regularly, and the plan of rehabilitative care (must be) evaluated as necessary, **but at least every 30 days, by the physician and the therapist(s)**.

(c) Standard: Documentation of Services

The physician's orders, the plan of rehabilitative care, services rendered, evaluations of progress, and other pertinent information (must be) **recorded in the patient's medical record and dated and signed by the physician ordering the service and the person who provided the service**.

(d) Standard: Qualifying to Provide Outpatient Physical Therapy Services

If the facility provides outpatient physical therapy services, it (must) meet the applicable health and safety regulations pertaining to such services.

405.1127. CONDITION OF PARTICIPATION: PHARMACEUTICAL SERVICES

The skilled nursing facility (must) provide appropriate methods and procedures for the dispensing and administering of drugs and biologicals.

Whether drugs and biologicals are obtained from community or institutional pharmacists or stocked by the facility, **THE FACILITY is responsible**

— for providing such drugs and biologicals for its patients, insofar as they are covered under the programs
— **and** for ensuring that pharmaceutical services are provided in accordance with accepted professional principles and appropriate Federal, State and local laws.

(a) Standard: Supervision of Services

The pharmaceutical services (must be) under the general supervision of a qualified **pharmacist who is responsible to the administrative staff** for developing, coordinating, and supervising all pharmaceutical services.

The pharmacist (if not a full-time employee) (must) devote a sufficient number of hours, based upon the needs of the facility, during regularly scheduled visits to carry out these responsibilities.

The pharmacist (must) **review the drug regimen of each patient at least monthly, and report any irregularities to the medical director and administrator**.

The pharmacist (must) submit a **written report at least quarterly** to the pharmaceutical services committee on the status of the facility's pharmaceutical service and staff performance.

(b) Standard: Control and Accountability

The pharmaceutical service (must have) procedures for control and accountability of all drugs and biologicals throughout the facility.

Only approved drugs and biologicals (may be) used in the facility, and are dispensed in compliance with Federal and State laws.

Records of receipt and disposition of all controlled drugs (must be) maintained in sufficient detail to enable an accurate reconciliation.

The pharmacist determines that drug records are in order and that an **account of all controlled drugs is maintained and reconciled.**

(c) Standard: Labeling of Drugs and Biologicals

The labeling of drugs and biologicals (must be) based on currently accepted professional principles, and include the appropriate accessory and cautionary instructions, as well as the expiration date when applicable.

(d) Standard: Pharmaceutical Services Committee

A pharmaceutical services committee (or its equivalent) (must) **develop written policies and procedures for**:

— safe and effective drug therapy
— distribution, control, and use.

The committee (must be) comprised of at least

— the pharmacist
— the director of nursing services
— the administrator
— one physician.

The committee (must)

— oversee pharmaceutical service in the facility
— make recommendations for improvement
— monitor the service to ensure its accuracy and adequacy.

The committee (must)
— **meet at least quarterly and**
— **document its activities, findings, and recommendations**.

405.1128. CONDITION OF PARTICIPATION: LABORATORY AND RADIOLOGIC SERVICES

The skilled nursing facility (must) provide for promptly obtaining required laboratory, X-ray, and other diagnostic services.

(a) Standard: Provision for Services

If the facility provides its own laboratory and X-ray services, these (must) meet the applicable conditions established for certification of hospitals.

If the facility itself does not provide such services, arrangements (must be) made for obtaining these services from

— a physician's office
— a participating hospital or skilled nursing facility
— a portable X-ray supplier
— an independent laboratory which is approved to provide these services under the program.

All such services are provided ONLY on the orders of the attending physician, who is notified promptly of the findings.
The facility (must) assist the patient, if necessary, in arranging for transportation to and from the source of service.

Signed and dated reports of a clinical laboratory, X-ray, and other diagnostic services (must be) filed with the patient's medical record.

(b) Standard: Blood and Blood Products

Blood handling and storage facilities (must be) safe, adequate, and properly supervised.

If the facility provides for maintaining and transfusing blood and blood products, it (must) meet the conditions established for certification of hospitals.

If the facility does not provide its own facilities, but does provide transfusion services alone, it (must) meet at least the requirements under (the appropriate law).

405.1129. CONDITION OF PARTICIPATION: DENTAL SERVICES

The skilled nursing facility (must) have satisfactory arrangements to **assist patients to obtain routine and emergency dental care**.

(a) Standard: Advisory Dentist

An advisory dentist (must) participate in the staff development program for nursing and other appropriate personnel, **and recommend** oral hygiene policies and practices for the care of patients.

(b) Standard: Arrangements for Outside Services

The facility (must) **have a cooperative agreement** with a dental service and **maintain a list** of dentists in the community for patients who do not have a private dentist.

The facility (must) **assist the patient, if necessary**, in arranging for transportation to and from the dentist's office.

405.1130. CONDITION OF PARTICIPATION: SOCIAL SERVICES

The skilled nursing facility (must) have satisfactory arrangements for identifying the medically related social and emotional needs of the patient.

It is not mandatory that the skilled nursing facility itself provide social services in order to participate in the program.

If the facility does not provide social services, it (must) have **written procedures for referring patients** in need of social services to appropriate social agencies.

If social services are offered by the facility, they (must be) provided under a clearly defined plan, by qualified persons, to assist each patient to adjust to the social and emotional aspects of his (/her) illness, treatment, and stay in the facility.

(a) Standard: Social Service Functions

Medically related social and emotional needs of the patient (must be) **identified and services provided to meet them**, either by qualified staff of the facility, or by referral, based on established procedures, to appropriate social agencies.

If financial assistance is indicated, arrangements (must be) made promptly for referral to an appropriate agency.

The patient and his (/her) family or responsible person (must be) fully informed of the patient's personal and property rights.

(b) Standard: Staffing

If the facility offers social services, a member of the staff of the facility (must be) designated as responsible for social services.

If the designated person is not a qualified social worker, **the facility (must have) a written agreement** with a qualified social worker or recognized social agency for consultation and assistance on a **regularly scheduled basis**.

The social services (must) have sufficient supportive personnel to meet patient needs.

Facilities (must be) adequate for social service personnel, easily accessible to patient and medical and other staff, and ensure privacy for interviews.

(c) Standard: Records and Confidentiality

Records of pertinent social data about personal and family problems medically related to the patient's illness and care, and of action taken to meet his needs, (must be) maintained in the patient's medical record.

If social services are provided by an outside resource, a record (must be) maintained of each referral to such resource.

Policies and procedures (must be) established for ensuring the **confidentiality of all patients' social information**.

405.1131. CONDITION OF PARTICIPATION: PATIENT ACTIVITIES

The skilled nursing facility (must) provide for an **activities program, appropriate to the needs and interests of each patient** to encourage

— self care
— resumption of normal activities
— maintenance of an optimal level of psychosocial functioning.

(a) Standard: Responsibility for Patient Activities

A member of the facility's staff (must be) designated as responsible for the patient activities program.

— if he (/she) is not a qualified patient activities coordinator, he (/she) functions with frequent, regularly scheduled consultation from a person so qualified.

(b) Standard: Patient Activities Program

Provision (must be) made for an ongoing program of meaningful activities

— appropriate to the needs and interests of patients
— designed to promote opportunities for engaging in normal pursuits, including religious activities of their choice, if any.

Each patient's activities program (must be) approved by the patient's attending physician as not in conflict with the treatment plan.
The activities (must be) so designed as to promote the

— physical
— social, and
— mental well-being of the patients.

The facility (must) make available adequate space and a variety of supplies and equipment to satisfy the individual interests of patients.

405.1132. CONDITION OF PARTICIPATION: MEDICAL RECORDS

The facility (must) maintain clinical (medical) records on all patients in accordance with accepted professional standards and practices.
The medical records service (must) have sufficient staff facilities, and equipment to provide medical records that are

— completely and accurately documented
— readily accessible and
— systematically organized to facilitate retrieving and compiling information.

(a) Standard: Staffing

Overall supervisory responsibility for the medical record service (must be) **assigned to A FULL TIME EMPLOYEE of the facility.**
The facility (must) also employ sufficient supportive personnel competent to carry out the functions of the medical record service.
If the medical record supervisor is not a qualified medical record practitioner, this person (must) function with **consultation** from a person so qualified.

(b) Standard: Protection of Medical Record Information

The facility (must) safeguard medical record information against loss, destruction, or unauthorized use.

(c) Standard: Content

The medical record (must) contain sufficient information to:

— identify the patient clearly
— justify the diagnosis and treatment, and
— document the results accurately.

All medical records (must) contain the following general categories of data:

— documented evidence of assessment of the needs of the patient
— establishment of an appropriate plan of treatment
— the care and the services provided
— authentication of hospital diagnoses (discharge summary, report from patient's attending physician, or transfer form)
— identification data and consent forms
— medical and nursing history of patient
— report of physical examination(s)
— diagnostic and therapeutic orders
— observations and progress notes
— reports of treatments and clinical findings
— discharge summary, including final diagnosis and prognosis.

(d) Standard: Physician Documentation

Only physicians (are permitted to) enter or authenticate in medical records opinions that require medical judgment (in accordance with medical staff bylaws, rules, and regulations, if applicable).
Each physician must sign his (/her) entries into the medical record.

(e) Standard: Completion of Records and Centralization of Reports

Current medical records and those of discharged patients (must be) completed promptly.
All clinical information pertaining to a patient's stay **(must be) centralized** in the patient's medical record.

(f) Standard: Retention and Preservation

Medical records (must be) retained for a period of time **not less than**:

— **that determined by the respective State statute**
— the **statute of limitations** in the State, or
— **five** years from date of discharge in the absence of a State statute, or
— in the case of a minor, 3 years after the patient becomes of age under State law.

(g) Standard: Indexes

Patient's medical records (must be) indexed according to

— name of patient and
— final diagnosis to facilitate acquisition of statistical medical information and retrieval of records for research or administrative action.

(h) Standard: Location and Facilities

The facility (must) maintain adequate facilities and equipment, conveniently located, to provide efficient processing of medical records (reviewing, indexing, filing, and prompt retrieval).

405.1133. CONDITION OF PARTICIPATION: TRANSFER AGREEMENT

The skilled nursing facility (must) have in effect a transfer agreement with one or more hospitals approved for participation under the programs (i.e., Medicare or Medicaid programs) which provides the basis for effective working arrangements under which inpatient hospital care or other hospital services are available promptly to the facility's patients when needed. A facility that has been unable to establish a transfer agreement with the hospital(s) in the community or service area after documented attempts to do so is considered to have such an agreement in effect.

(a) Standard: Patient Transfer

A hospital and a skilled nursing facility shall be considered to have a **transfer agreement in effect if,** by reason of a written agreement between them or in case the two institutions are under common control by reason of a written undertaking by the person or body which controls them, there is reasonable assurance that

— transfer of patients will be effected between the hospital and the skilled nursing facility, ensuring **timely admission**, whenever such transfer is medically appropriate as determined by the attending physician, and
— there will be **interchange of medical and other information** necessary or useful in the care and treatment of individuals transferred between the institutions, or in determining whether such individuals can be adequately cared for otherwise than in either of such institutions, and
— security and accountability for patients' personal effects are provided on transfer.

405.1134. CONDITION OF PARTICIPATION: PHYSICAL ENVIRONMENT

The skilled nursing facility (must be) constructed, equipped, and maintained to protect the health and safety of patients, personnel, and the public.

(a) Standard: Life Safety from Fire

The skilled nursing facility (must) meet such provisions of the **Life Safety Code of the National Fire Protection Association** as are applicable to nursing homes

— except that in consideration of a recommendation by the State survey agency, the Secretary may waive, for such periods as deemed appropriate, specific provisions of such Code which, if rigidly applied, world result in unreasonable hardship upon a skilled nursing facility, BUT ONLY IF such waiver will not adversely affect the health and safety of the patients
— and except the [Secretary determines that a state has an effective code in force].

Where waiver permits the participation of an existing facility of two or more stories which is not at of least **2-hour fire resistive construction**, blind, non-ambulatory, or physically handicapped patients are **not (to be) housed above the street level floor unless the facility** is of **1-hour protected noncombustible construction** (as defined in National Fire Protection Association Standard No. 220 21st Ed, 1967), fully sprinklered 1-hour protected ordinary construction, or fully sprinklered 1-hour protected woodframe construction.

Nonflammable medical gas systems, such as oxygen and nitrous oxide, installed in the facility (must) comply with applicable provisions of National Fire Protection Association Standard No. 56B (Standard for the Use of Inhalation Therapy) 1968 and National Fire Protection Association Standard No. 56F (Nonflammable Medical Gas Systems) 1970.

(b) Standard: Emergency Power

The facility (must) provide **an emergency source of electrical power** necessary to protect the health and safety of patients in the event the normal electrical supply is interrupted.

The emergency electrical power system must supply power **adequate at least for**

— lighting in all means of egress
— equipment to maintain fire detection, alarm and extinguishing systems; and
— life support systems.

Where life support systems are used, emergency electrical service (must be) provided by an emergency generator located on the premises.

(c) Standard: Facilities for Physically Handicapped

The facility (must be) accessible to, and functional for, patients, personnel, and the public.

All necessary accommodations (must be) made to the needs of persons with

— semiambulatory disabilities
— sight and hearing disabilities
— disabilities of coordination
— other disabilities

in accordance with the American National Standards Institute (ANSI) Standard No A117.1 American Standard Specifications for Making Buildings and Facilities Accessible to, and Usable by, the Physically Handicapped. [Secretary may waive.]

(d) Standard: Nursing Unit

Each nursing unit has at least the following basic service areas

— nurses' station
— storage and preparation area(s) for drugs and biologicals
— utility and storage rooms that are adequate in size, conveniently located, and well lighted to facilitate staff functioning.

The nurse's station (must be) equipped to register patients' calls through a communication system from patient areas, including:

— patient rooms
— patient toilet
— patient bathing area.

(e) Standard: Patient Rooms and Toilet Facilities

Patient rooms (must be) designed for:

— adequate nursing care and
— the comfort and
— privacy of patients

and have no more than 4 beds [12 in facilities for the mentally retarded].
Single patient rooms (must) measure **100 square feet**, and multipatient rooms (must) provide a minimum of **80 square feet** per bed. [Secretary may waive.]
Each room (must be) equipped with or be conveniently located near, adequate toilet and bathing facilities.
Each room (must)

— **have direct access to a corridor and outside exposure**
— **have the floor at or above grade level.**

(f) Standard: Facilities for Special Care (Isolation Room(s))

Provision (must be) made for isolating patients as necessary in

— **single rooms**
— **ventilated to the outside**
— **with private toilet and handwashing facilities**.

Procedures in aseptic and isolation techniques (must be) **established in writing and followed** by all personnel.

Such areas (must be) identified by **appropriate precautionary signs**.

(g) Standard: Dining and Patient Activities Rooms

The facility (must) **provide one or more** clean, orderly, and appropriately furnished rooms of adequate size designated for patient dining and for patient activities.

The areas (must be) well-lighted and well-ventilated. (If a multi-purpose room is used for dining AND patient activities, there (must be) sufficient space to accommodate **all** activities and prevent their interference with each other.

(h) Standard: Kitchen and Dietetic Service Area

The facility (must have) kitchen and dietetic service areas adequate to meet food service needs.

These areas must be arranged, and equipped for sanitary refrigeration, storage, preparation, and serving of food as well as for dish and utensil cleaning, and refuse storage and removal.

(i) Standard: Maintenance of Equipment, Building, and Grounds

The facility (must) establish a written preventive maintenance program to ensure that equipment is operative and that the interior and exterior of the building are clean and orderly.

All essential mechanical, electrical, and patient care equipment (must be) maintained in safe operating condition.

(j) Standard: Other Environmental Considerations

The facility must provide

— functional, sanitary, and comfortable environment for patients, personnel, and public
— adequate and comfortable lighting levels in all areas
— maintain a comfortable room temperature
— (have) procedures to ensure water to all essential areas in the event of loss of normal water supply
— adequate ventilation through windows or mechanical means or a combination of both
— corridors (must be) equipped with firmly secured handrails on each side.

405.1135. CONDITION FOR PARTICIPATION: INFECTION CONTROL

The skilled nursing facility (must) **establish an infection control committee** of representative professional staff with responsibility for overall infection control in the facility.

(a) Standard: Infection Control Committee

The infection control committee is composed of members of:

- **the medical staff**
- the nursing staff
- administration
- dietary
- the pharmacy
- housekeeping
- maintenance
- other services.

The committee establishes policies and procedures for

- investigating
- controlling
- preventing infections in the facility, and monitors staff performance to ensure that the policies and procedures are executed.

(b) Standard: Aseptic and Isolation Techniques

Written effective procedures in aseptic and isolation techniques (must be) followed by all personnel.

Procedures (must be) reviewed and revised annually for effectiveness and improvement.

(c) Standard: Housekeeping

The facility (must) employ sufficient housekeeping personnel and provide all necessary equipment to maintain a safe, clean, and orderly interior.

A full-time employee (must be) designated responsible for the services and for supervision and training of personnel.

Nursing personnel (may not) be assigned housekeeping duties.

A facility that has a contract with an outside resource for housekeeping services may be found to be in compliance with this standard provided the facility and/or outside resource meets the requirements of the standard.

(d) Standard: Linen

The facility (must have) available at all times a quantity of linen essential for proper care and comfort of patients.

Linens (must be) handled, stored, processed, and transported in such a manner as to prevent the spread of infection.

(e) Standard: Pest Control

The facility (must be) maintained free from insects and rodents through operation of a pest control program.

405.1136. CONDITION OF PARTICIPATION: DISASTER PREPAREDNESS

The skilled nursing facility (must have) **a written plan, periodically rehearsed**, with procedures to be followed in the event of an internal or external disaster and for the care of casualties (patients and personnel) arising from such disasters.

(a) Standard: Disaster Plan

The facility (must have) **an acceptable written plan in operation, with procedures to be followed** in the event of fire, explosion, or other disaster.

The plan (must be) developed and maintained with the assistance of qualified fire, safety, and other appropriate experts and include procedures for:

— prompt transfer of casualties and records
— instructions regarding the location and use of alarm systems and signals, and of fire-fighting equipment
— information regarding methods of containing fire
— procedures for notification of appropriate persons and
— specifications of evacuation routes and procedures.

(b) Standard: Staff Training and Drills

All employees (must be) trained, as part of their employment orientation, in all aspects of preparedness for any disaster.

The disaster program (must) include orientation and ongoing training and drills for all personnel in all procedures so that each employee promptly and correctly carries out his (/her) specific role in case of a disaster.

405.1137. CONDITION OF PARTICIPATION: UTILIZATION REVIEW

The skilled nursing facility (must) carry out utilization review of services provided in the facility at least to **inpatients who are entitled to benefits under the programs** (Medicare, Medicaid).

Utilization review has as its overall objectives both

— the maintenance of high quality patient care and
— assurance of appropriate and efficient utilization of facility services.

There are two elements to utilization review:

— medical care evaluation studies that identify and examine patterns of care provided in the facility, and
— review of extended duration cases which is concerned with efficiency, appropriateness, and cost effectiveness of care.

[The Secretary may require Medicaid, i.e., Title 19, procedures if he/she wishes.]

(a) Standard: Written Plan of Utilization Review Activity

The facility (must) have a **written, currently applicable utilization review plan, approved by the governing body and the medical director** or organized medical staff (if applicable), which includes at least the following:

— procedures for medical care evaluation studies and for dissemination and follow-up of study findings and committee recommendations
— **definition of the period(s)** of extended duration and procedures for review of individual cases of extended duration
— **a method for identifying patients other than by name (e.g., medical record number)**
— provision for maintaining written records of committee activities.

(b) Standard: Composition and Organization of Utilization Review Committee

The committee or group responsible for utilization review (must be) composed of

— **two or more physicians**, and
— optionally, other professional personnel.

ALL medical determinations are made by the physician members of the committee.

NO physician (can) review any case in which he (/she) was professionally involved.

(c) Standard: Medical Care Evaluation Studies

Medical care **evaluation studies (must be) performed** to promote the most effective and appropriate use of available health facilities and services consistent with patient needs and professionally recognized standards of health care.

Studies, which could include assessment of findings resulting from periodic medical review, (should) emphasize identification and analysis of patterns of patient care and changes indicated to maintain a consistent high quality of services.

Each medical care evaluation study (whether medical or administrative in emphasis) (should) identify and analyze factors related to the patient care rendered in the facility, and serve as the basis for recommendations for change beneficial to patients, staff, the facility and the community.

Studies, on a sample or other basis, (should) include but need not be limited to,

— admissions
— duration of stay
— professional services including drugs and biologicals furnished.

At least one study (must) be in progress at any given time.

(d) Standard: Review of Cases of Extended Duration

Periodic review (must be) made of

— **each current inpatient skilled nursing facility beneficiary case of continuous duration** to determine whether further inpatient stay is necessary. **Reviews may also** be applied to patients not covered by the program, and/or to cases where duration of stay has not yet reached the definition(s) of extended duration.

The plan may specify a different number of days for different diagnostic classes of cases, or may use the same number of days for all cases. In any event, the period(s) specified (must) bear a reasonable relationship to current average length-of-stay statistics, and **not exceed 21 days from admission.**

An exception to this 21-day limit may be made where the specific diagnostic class of cases has average lengths of stay exceeding 21 days, in which instances the plan specifies the extended duration period for each specific diagnostic class.

In cases for which advance approval of payment has been made, the period(s) of extended duration may be defined as that period for which payment has been approved.

After the initial review, reviews for medical necessity for further inpatient stay (must be) made **at least every 30 days for the first 90 days and at least every 90 days thereafter.**

A review (must be) made and a final determination regarding the patient's further care reached no later than **7 days** following the time period specified as the period of extended duration in the utilization review plan.

(e) Standard: Admission or Further Stay Not Medically Necessary

Final determination regarding the necessity for admission or for further stay, including stay beyond the period of extended duration, **is limited to physician members of the committee, and may be made by**

— the full physician complement
— a subcommittee
— or a **single committee physician.**

When a single committee physician has decided that admission is not medically necessary or is inappropriate, or that further stay is no longer medically necessary, **further concurrence** (must be) obtained as specified in the plan **to include at least a second committee physician within the 7-day period**.

If committee members determine from an extended duration review or a medical care evaluation study, that further stay is not medically necessary,

— the attending physician is consulted or given the opportunity for consultation, and
— notification is made **in writing within 48 hours** by the committee to the
— administration
— the attending physician, and
— the patient or his (/her) representative.

(f) Standard: Administrative Responsibilities

The administrative staff of the facility (must be) kept directly and fully informed of committee activities to facilitate support and assistance.

The administrator (must) study and act upon recommendations made by the committee, coordinating such functions with appropriate staff members.

(g) Standard: Utilization Review Records

Written records of committee activities (must be) maintained.

Appropriate reports, signed by the committee chairman, (must be) made regularly to

— the medical staff
— administrative staff
— governing body
— sponsors, if any.

MINUTES of each committee meeting (must be) maintained and include at least:

— name of committee
— date and duration of meeting
— names of committee members present and absent
— description of activities presently in progress to satisfy the requirements for medical care evaluation studies, including the
— subject and reason for study
— dates of commencement and expected completion
— summary of studies completed since the last meeting
— conclusions

— follow-up on implementation of recommendations made from previous studies and
— summary of extended duration cases reviewed, including
— the number of cases
— case identification numbers
— admission and review dates
— decisions reached
— basis for each determination and action taken for each case not approved for extended care.

(h) Standard: Discharge Planning

The facility (must) maintain a centralized, coordinated program to ensure that each patient has a planned program of continuing care which meets his (/her) postdischarge needs.

The facility (must) have in operation an organized discharge planning program.

The utilization review committee, in its evaluation of each extended duration case, (must) have available to it the results of such discharge planning, and information on alternative available community resources to which the patient may be referred.

The administrator (must) delegate responsibility for discharge planning, in writing, to one or more members of the facility's staff, with consultation, if necessary, OR (he/she) (must) arrange for this service to be provided by a health, social, or welfare agency.

The facility (must) maintain written discharge planning procedures which describe

— how the discharge coordinator will function, and his (/her) authority and relationships with the facility's staff
— the time period in which each patient's need for discharge planning is determined, preferably within 7 days after the day of admission
— the maximum time period after which a reevaluation of each patient's discharge plan (will be) made
— local resources available to the facility, the patient, and the attending physician to assist in developing and implementing individual discharge plans
— **provisions for periodic review and reevaluation of the facility's discharge planning program**.

At the time of discharge, the facility (must) provide those responsible for the patient's postdischarge care with an appropriate summary of information about the discharged patient to ensure the optimal continuity of care.

The discharge summary **(must) include at least current information relative to**

— diagnoses
— describing rehabilitation potential
— summarizing the course of prior treatment
— documenting physician orders for the immediate care of the patient, and
— pertinent social information.

4.5 Management and Labor Legislation and Regulations

What rights do nursing home administrators have when employees in the facility are seeking to form a union? What rights do the employees have?

This section provides a framework to enable the reader to answer these questions.

4.5.1 Early Management– Labor Relations in the United States

During most of the earlier years of its history, the government of the United States strongly supported management in its dealings with employees. It was not until 1935 that American workers won government sanction of the right to form trade unions.

The passage of the National Labor Relations Act (better known as the Wagner Act) in 1935 was the first nationwide American labor legislation to favor the growth of trade unions. This was the culmination of a long slow process.

MANAGEMENT PREFERENCES

Most managers would prefer not to have to deal with organized labor. Unionization is perceived as intensifying the difficulty of the administrator's responsibilities. There is a natural tendency for what organizational theorists call the "we–they" phenomenon to occur in the relationship between labor and management. Workers often perceive their interests as different from those of managers, whose task is to operate cost-effectively, that is, to produce the best results for the least cost.

The administrator would be happy to pay nurses and nurse's aides the premium wages that will attract the most competent workers available, but pressures to keep costs down do not permit this. As discussed in Part 2, the result is that most nursing home workers, especially the nurse's aides, and the kitchen and housekeeping staffs are paid at prevailing rates in the particular geographical area, which are usually close to the required minimum wage levels. Understandably, these workers seek to increase their personal incomes and obtain the best working conditions on their jobs. Tensions between managers and workers are inevitably built into the situation. How do they deal with them? What are the manager's rights? What rights do employees have?

Individual states have reserved all powers to themselves that are not expressly given to the federal government. Similarly, management has, in effect, reserved all powers to itself that have not expressly been given to workers, usually by the government.

THE COLONIAL PERIOD

So powerful were the managers in the Colonial period that workers contented themselves with forming "fraternal unions" to help each other in coping with personal economic adversity, but certainly not to act collectively for improved working conditions and more pay (U.S. Department of Labor, pp. 1–104). Employers were able to prevent effective unionization. They could, at their own discretion, fire any worker seeking to organize a union, refuse to negotiate with any union representative, and require each new employee to sign a "yellow dog" contract, by which they agreed not to join a union (Chruden & Sherman, p. 345).

During the 19th century the U.S. courts consistently sided with management. In 1806 a federal court ruled that workers who sought to combine to exert pressure on managers were participating in a "conspiracy in restraint of trade," which in effect meant that such grouping was to be treated as criminal activity (Ivancevich & Glueck, p. 533). The first hint of rights for workers did not appear until 1842, when the Massachusetts Supreme Court ruled that unions that did not resort to illegal tactics were not guilty of criminal conspiracy (Chruden & Sherman, p. 345). Still, managers could fire any worker at will for union activity, impose yellow-dog contracts, and when all else failed, obtain a court injunction against threatened strikes. The managers still retained nearly all of the power (Ivancevich & Glueck, p. 533). Despite this, the union movement grew. By 1886 skilled workers such as machinists, bricklayers, and carpenters formed the American Federation of Labor (AFL).

It was not until 1935 that another major labor force, the Congress of Industrial Organizations (CIO), emerged (Raskin, pp. 12–32) and in 1955 merged with the American Federation of Labor. It was a slow process because the government did not substantially back labor until the Wagner Act was passed in 1935.

The federal government had actually given American workers some negotiating rights earlier in the century in order to keep the nation's railroads running. The Railway Labor Act of 1926 was the first federal legislation sanctioning union organization and the right to bargain collectively with management (Chruden & Sherman, p. 353).

The first national effort to define workers' and managers' respective rights came just 6 years later. In 1932 the Norris-LaGuardia Act, also called the Anti-Injunction Act, limited the powers of federal courts to side with management through issuing injunctions, i.e., court decrees stopping or limiting union efforts to picket, boycott, or strike. Yellow-dog contracts, in which a prospective employee promised not to form or join a union, were prohibited (Ivancevich & Glueck, p. 534).

4.5.2 Major 20th-Century Legislation Affecting Employer–Employee Relationships

THE WAGNER ACT, 1935

The Wagner Act of 1935 is the landmark bill that, for the first time in federal legislation, defined the rights of workers (Boling et al., p. 185). The Wagner Act limited the freedom of employers to give their views on proposed unionization. The Wagner Act also guaranteed employee bargaining rights: "Employees shall have the right to self-organization, to form, join, or assist labor organizations, to bargain collectively through representatives of their own choosing, and to engage in concerted activities, for the purpose of collective bargaining or other mutual aid or protection" (Chruden, p. 354).

PROPORTION OF WORKERS IN UNIONS

In 1933 there were 3 million unionized workers in this country. By 1947 they numbered 15 million, representing about 31% of the work force. Union membership increased until about 1956, then declined until 1963, when it resumed a slow growth. In 1980, about 20 million workers were in unions—approximately 20% of the total work force and 28% of nonagricultural workers (Ivancevich & Glueck, p. 547).

Well under 50% of nursing home employees are union members (Boling et al., p. 185). Unionization of hospital workers is in proportion with the national level: in 1976, 23% of hospitals had collective bargaining agreements with one or more unions (Williams & Torrens, p. 157).

The period from 1935 to 1947 was one of dramatic growth in union membership. The power given to unions through the Wagner Act resulted in what Congress in 1947 viewed as abuses. This led to the Taft-Hartley Act, which placed limitations on unions, just as the Wagner Act had placed limitations on managers 12 years earlier.

THE TAFT-HARTLEY ACT, 1947

The provisions of the Taft-Hartley Act unions were prohibited from the following actions (Ivancevich & Glueck, p. 534; Chruden & Sherman, p. 355):

1. Restraining or coercing employees in the exercise of their right to join a union or not (unless an agreement existed with management that every worker must be a union member). Union members could not physically prevent other workers from entering a facility, nor act violently toward non-union employees, nor threaten employees for not supporting union activities.

2. Causing an employer to discriminate against an employee for antiunion activity, nor could unions force employers to hire only workers acceptable to the union.

3. Bargaining with an employer in bad faith. They could not insist on negotiating "illegal" provisions, such as the administration's prerogative to appoint supervisors.

4. Participating in secondary boycotts or jurisdictional disputes. Unions may not picket a nursing home in an attempt to force it to apply pressure

on a subcontractor (e.g., a food service contractor) to recognize a union, nor can a union force an employer to do business only with others, such as suppliers, who are unionized; nor can one unon picket for recognition when another union is already certified for a nursing home.

5. Charging excessive or discriminatory membership fees. They may not charge a higher initiation fee to employees who did not join the union until after a union contract was negotiated.

6. Coercing or restraining employers in the selection of the parties to bargain on management's behalf. The manager is free to hire the best labor lawyer available to represent the facility.

7. Forcing managers to hire employees when they are not needed (called featherbedding).

However, when the Wagner Act was amended by this pro-management Labor–Management Relations Act of 1947 (the Taft-Hartley Act), certain employees' rights were retained (Ivancevich & Glueck, p. 535). Managers may not

1. Interfere with, restrain, or coerce employees in the exercise of their rights. They may not, for example, give wage increases timed to discourage employees from joining a union or threaten loss of their jobs for employees who vote for a union.

2. Interfere with or attempt to dominate any labor organization, or contribute financial or other support to a labor organization. For example, they cannot take an active part in union affairs or permit a nursing home supervisor to participate actively in a union, or show favoritism toward one union over another union.

3. Discriminate in hiring or giving tenure to employees or set any terms for employment so as to encourage or discourage union membership. For example, they cannot fire an employee who urges others to join a union or demote an employee for union activity.

4. Fire or discriminate against any employee who files charges or gives testimony under the Wagner Act.

5. Refuse to bargain collectively with the duly chosen representatives of its employees. For example, the nursing home administrator must provide financial data to a union if the facility claims to be experiencing financial losses, must bargain on mandatory subjects such as hours and wages, and must meet with union representatives duly appointed by a certified bargaining unit.

An important consideration for nursing home administrators is the denial of legal protection to supervisors seeking to form their own unions, thus keeping the management roles of these persons (typically department heads in nursing homes) clearly managerial in function and identification.

Probably the single most important provision of the Taft-Hartley Act for nursing home administrators is the *restoration of the right of managers to express their views regarding unions and unionizing efforts*. This means that administrators are free to express their opinions about their employees voting for a union in the work place and judgments about unions in general. They are still prohibited from threatening, coercing, or bribing employees concerning their union membership or their decision to join or not to join a union.

THE NATIONAL LABOR RELATIONS BOARD

A major aspect of the Taft-Hartley Act was its creation of the National Labor Relations Board (NLRB), which plays a dominant role in U.S. labor–management relations. It has the following responsibilities (Chruden & Sherman, p. 355):

1. To determine what the bargaining unit or units within an organization shall be. (A unit contains those employees who are to be represented by a particular union and are covered by the agreement with it.)
2. To conduct representation elections by secret ballot for the purpose of determining which, if any, union shall represent the employees within a unit.
3. To investigate unfair labor practices charges filed by unions or employers and to prosecute any violations revealed by such investigations.

The Board is empowered to initiate action against illegal strikes or unfair labor practices by unions. According to D.W. Twomey (1980), in a typical month as many as 4,000 new cases are filed with the NLRB.

One of the more controversial features of the Taft-Hartley Act is a provision allowing the President of the United States, through the Office of the Attorney General, to seek an injunction for a period of 80 days against strikes or walkouts affecting the nation's welfare or health. Some labor leaders have called this "slave labor" (Chruden & Sherman, p. 356).

THE LANDRUM-GRIFFIN ACT, 1959

Officially designated the Labor-Management Reporting and Disclosure Act of 1959, the Landrum-Griffin Act seeks to protect the interests of the individual union member against possible union abuses. Specifically the Act gives to each union member the following rights (Ivancevich & Glueck, p. 536):

1. Nominate candidates for union office
2. Vote in union elections
3. Attend union meetings
4. Examine required annual financial reports by the union to the Secretary of Labor.

In addition, employers were required to report any payments or loans made to unions—the officers or any members—to eliminate what were called "sweetheart contracts," under which union officials and the managers benefited, but the rank and file of union members did not.

SPECIAL DISPUTE-SETTLING RULES FOR NURSING HOME AND HOSPITAL ADMINISTRATORS

The NLRB had jurisdiction over health care institutions. However, until 1974 the Board was expressly forbidden by the original Taft-Hartley law to hear cases in the nonprofit sector. Since the vast majority of nursing homes and hospitals operated in the 1950s and 1960s were nonprofit, this meant that most of the health care industry were not subject to these labor laws.

In 1973 Congress began talking of having the law apply to not-for-profit nursing homes and hospitals. Nursing homes and hospitals pressed for the following benefits (American Hospital Association, 1976; Rosmann, pp. 64–68):

1. Special protection against strikes
2. Priority for rapid NLRB action on disputes
3. Mandatory mediation requirements
4. Limit on the number of bargaining units to one each for professional, technical, clinical, and maintenance and service workers.

The nursing homes and hospitals got most of what they wanted.

In 1974 Congress amended the Taft-Hartley Act to bring nursing homes and hospitals under its regulations (1974 Non-Profit Hospital Amendments, Public Law 93-360) (Wilson & Neuhauser, p. 89). However, special provisions were made (Pointer & Metzger, pp. 41–60):

1. A nursing home, hospital, or union must give to the other party 90 days notice of a desire to change an existing contract; this is 30 days more notice than required of others.
2. The Federal Mediation and Conciliation Service (FMCS) must be given 30 days notice if an impasse occurs in bargaining for an initial contract after the union is first recognized.

3. *A nursing home or hospital union may not picket or strike without 10 days prior notice, in order to allow the facility to make provisions for continuity of care.* (No prior notice is required of other unions).
4. The FMCS may appoint a board of inquiry to mediate the dispute if it decides a strike would imperil the welfare or health of the community. Neither the nursing home nor the union is obliged to accept the board's recommendations, but they must provide any witnesses or information sought by the Board.

For-profit nursing homes benefited from the 1974 amendment to the Taft-Hartley Act because of the four special labor relations rules cited above (Miller, p. 49).

THE BARGAINING UNIT

Labor unions must seek recognition as representing the majority of persons in a specific bargaining unit of a nursing home. As indicated above, nursing homes and hospitals sought to limit the number of bargaining units in negotiations to professional, technical, clinical, and maintenance and service workers.

During most of the decade after the 1974 amendments to the Taft-Hartley Act, the NLRB ruled that in nursing homes and hospitals, service and maintenance workers, clerical staff, licensed practical nurses, registered nurses, and security guard units constitute appropriate bargaining units (Miller, pp. 49–50).

In August 1984 the NLRB issued a new ruling. In the case of St. Francis Hospital (Memphis, Tennessee) v. International Brotherhood of Electrical Workers Local 474, the NLRB ruled that a group of 39 maintenance workers did not constitute an appropriate bargaining unit. Health care workers now must represent either "all professionals" or "all nonprofessionals" rather than the particular interest groups allowed during the previous decade.

The effect of this NLRB ruling is to make union organization of nursing facility employees much more difficult. A far more diverse group of workers must be approached than before for purposes of union representation in elections. The Service Employees International Union has argued that this makes it extremely difficult for health care workers to unionize (*Washington Report on Medicine & Health*, Perspectives, October 1, 1984).

Decisions favoring either labor or management are reflections of the political administrations in power. Nursing homes and hospitals had originally wanted to keep the number of bargaining units to no more than four. The NLRB, under more liberal administrators in Washington, according to Miller, had permitted five. Under the more management-oriented Reagan administration, the number of allowable bargaining units was cut back to two, which could ease matters considerably for nursing home administrators.

NONUNION WORKERS

At least 75% of the total labor force in this country is not unionized. What of their rights?

Over the years the federal government has enacted legislation establishing and protecting the rights of workers in general. Two of these laws are the Civil Rights Act of 1964 and, subsequently, the Equal Employment Opportunities Act of 1972.

CIVIL RIGHTS ACT, 1964

Title VII of the Civil Rights Act of 1964 prohibited employers and others from discriminating against employees on the basis of race, color, religion, sex, or national origin.

Title VII also prohibits discrimination with regard to any employment condition including hiring, firing, promotion, transfer, and admission to training programs.

THE EQUAL EMPLOYMENT OPPORTUNITIES ACT, 1972

The Equal Employment Opportunities Act (EEOA) amended Title VII of the Civil Rights Act. EEOA strengthened enforcement of the original Act and expanded its coverage to additional groups, such as state and local government workers and private employment of more than 15 persons.

What Is Discrimination?

Congress did not define discrimination in its legislation. Over the years the courts have established three definitions:

1. During World War II, discrimination was defined as *harmful actions* motivated by personal animosity toward the group of which the target person was a member.
2. Later this was redefined as *unequal treatment*. Accordingly, a practice is illegal if it applies different standards or different treatment to different groups of employees or applicants. For example, minorities may not be kept in less desirable departments (different treatment); rejecting women with preschool-age children is not permissible

(different standards). Point: the administrator may impose any
standards so long as they are applied equally to all groups or
individuals.

3. In Griggs v. Duke Power Co. (1971) the U.S. Supreme Court defined
   employment discrimination as *unequal impact.* In this case Duke
   Power was using employment tests and educational requirements that
   screened out a greater proportion of blacks than whites (Ivancevich &
   Glueck, p. 67). This is also called adverse impact.

Adverse impact is often measured (for the purposes of Title VII cases)
when the selection rate for a protected minority group is less than 80% of
the selection rate for a majority group.

Although the practice in the Duke Power case was not motivated by
prejudice against blacks, and the tests were all applied equally, they had
the result of adverse impact, i.e., unequal impact on blacks. The job
involved was that of shoveling coal into a furnace. Duke failed to prove
that passing employment tests and requiring a level of education related to
success on the job. The burden of proof is on the employer to show that a
hiring standard is job-related.

Minority groups that are specifically protected under the Civil Rights
Act are blacks, Hispanics, American Indians, Alaskan natives, and Asian-
Pacific Islanders.

Discrimination Based on Sex

What is discrimination based on sex? Few situations exist that justify
discrimination based on sex. Employment of a wet nurse is justifiable, of a
woman to model women's clothes, of a woman as a locker room attendant
for other women. It is not clear that any job in the nursing home justifies
discrimination based on sex.

The Pregnancy Discrimination Act, 1978

The 1964 Civil Rights Act was amended in 1978 to end discrimination
against pregnant women. The Act makes it illegal to discriminate on the
basis of pregnancy, childbirth, or related medical conditions in hiring,
promoting, suspending, or discharging women who are pregnant. In
addition, the employer is required by this act to pay medical and hospital
costs for childbirth to the same extent it pays for hospital costs and medical
care for other conditions.

Enforcing the EEOC Laws

The Equal Employment Opportunity Commission (EEOC) was established by the 1964 Civil Rights Act. The Commission was empowered to

interpret the Act and resolve charges brought under it. The 1972 amendments gave the Commission additional authority to bring lawsuits against employers in the federal courts.

Even so, the Commission still cannot issue directly enforceable orders, as do other agencies such as the Environmental Protection Agency. Hence, the EEOC cannot order an employer to discontinue discriminatory practices, nor can it order back pay to victims of discrimination. It must seek action through the courts.

The average backlog of cases for the EEOC runs approximately 20,000. It is not possible to handle all of them, of course. Only a small percentage of charges are eventually resolved by EEOC or by the courts (Ivancevich & Glueck, p. 74). Nevertheless, legal history is being made by the EEOC, and its presence is felt in employment practices.

EEOC Procedures

Step 1. The EEOC has the power to require employers to report employment statistics on federal forms.

Step 2. If the EEOC feels charges are justified, it authorizes its preinvestigation division to review the complaints.

Step 3. The investigation division then interviews all parties concerned.

Step 4. If there is substance to the case, the EEOC seeks an out-of-court settlement.

Step 5. If the parties cannot be reconciled, the EEOC can sue the employer.

In cases settled by court decisions, the courts have required such actions as back pay, reinstatement of employees, immediate promotion of employees, hiring quotas, abolition of testing programs, creation of special training programs. Some settlements have cost in the millions of dollars.

Laws Affecting Federal Contractors and Subcontractors

Several laws and executive orders govern hiring and job practices of firms that hold federal contracts of over $50,000. While it is unlikely that any nursing facility would be directly affected by these regulations, many contractors doing construction work for them are subject to these regulations.

Executive Order 11246

This order by the President of the United States requires written affirmative action programs of all contractors with 50 or more employees and $50,000 or more in federal contracts.

To enforce this order, the Office of Federal Contract Compliance Programs (OFCCP) was established. This agency was later given responsibility for administering laws protecting veterans and handicapped persons as well.

Vietnam Era Veterans Readjustment Act, 1974

This act requires firms with more than $10,000 in federal contracts to have affirmative action programs for employment and advancement of Vietnam veterans.

Age Discrimination Employment Act, 1973

This act was amended in 1978 and protects persons aged 40 to 70 against job discrimination. It is intended to prevent employers from replacing older employees with younger ones, whether to achieve a younger average age of workers or to avoid paying pension benefits.

Not all persons are protected, however. Greyhound Bus Corporation obtained a ruling permitting them to hire no one over the age of 40 as a bus driver. They argued that persons 40 and over have slower reaction times, thus reducing safety to passengers. Is this an example of "agism?"

The Vocational Rehabilitation Act of 1973

This act requires federal government contractors to have affirmative action programs for the handicapped. It is enforced by the OFCCP. The Act also provides a measure of federal support for programs to assist in training the handicapped. By 1980 approximately half of the 15 million Americans of working age deemed to be handicapped had been able to find employment (Ivancevich & Glueck, p. 82).

4.5.3 Regulation of Compensation

Most states and the federal government have passed laws that regulate compensation for work done.

Federal jurisdiction covers only those *workers engaged in producing goods for interstate and foreign commerce.* Technically, the federal government does not have authority to regulate worker compensation within states.

More than 40 states have their own wage and hour laws and also regulate other conditions of employment, such as hours allowed per week before overtime must be paid.

The practical effect of having both federal and state regulations governing compensation is that both prevail. In reality, the federal laws are applied to most workers regardless of whether or not they are producing goods for interstate or foreign commerce. This breadth of application of the federal wage laws is achieved by including persons whose work is (loosely defined) closely related to any production for interstate or foreign commerce.

On a day-to-day basis, this means that nursing home employee compensation and other work conditions must meet both federal and state regulations. Any facility claiming exemption from federal laws might be restricted to admitting patients and hiring employees who were full-time residents of that state. In sum, the government would find some reason to apply federal law to that situation.

States usually have laws restricting women to fewer hours of work per week than men do. Although these regulations may not be enforced, it is important to be aware of the compensation and work regulations in one's own locality.

The original goals of federal wage and hour regulations were (a) to encourage the spreading of work among as many wage earners as feasible and (b) to establish a floor for wages for any worker regardless of the job. Requiring a rate 1½ times the regular pay rate for all overtime has helped to accomplish spreading the work. Requiring a minimum wage for all persons has accomplished the second goal.

There are three federal laws that regulate compensation: The Fair Labor Standards Act, the Walsh-Healy Act, and the Davis-Bacon Act.

FAIR LABOR STANDARDS ACT (Wage and Hour Act)

The Fair Labor Standards Act was originally passed in 1938, but like the Social Security Act of 1935, it has been amended many times. The four primary foci of the Act are (a) minimum wage rates, (b) overtime, (c) child labor, and (d) equal rights.

Minimum Wage Rates

When first instituted, the minimum wage was 25 cents per hour. Over the decades it has risen nearly 15-fold as the value of the dollar has declined.

The minimum wage must be calculated on the actual earning rate before any additional payments are added. For example, the employee works 46 hr a week. He/she received the minimum wage for the first 40 hr and is paid at 1½ times that rate for the additional 6 hr. The manager is not permitted to average in the 1½ times the regular pay rate earned on hours above 40 in a week to reduce the wage back to the equivalent of the minimum wage for all hours worked in a week.

Minimum wage rates are especially important to nursing homes because many, if not most, nursing homes pay nurse's aides and housekeeping and maintenance employees at or just above the minimum wage.

Overtime

If bonuses are paid over some other period—a month or a quarter, for example—the base for overtime wage must be recalculated to add any additional remuneration to the base rate for that period in calculating the time-and-a-half rate for all hours worked over 80 in each 2-week period.

Whenever compensatory time is given for overtime hours worked, the employee must be given 1½ hr off for every hour of overtime worked.

Management personnel are not covered by these rules but are normally paid a salary with no specific hours set. Although a 40-hr work week is the norm, they are expected to work until they accomplish their assignments. Management staff may or may not, at the discretion of the administration, be paid overtime.

Due to their exemption from coverage by the Fair Labor Standards Act, management personnel are referred to as exempt employees. Nonmanagement employees are considered nonexempt.

Congress amends this act frequently, so it is important to check with the Department of Labor to keep abreast of current and upcoming regulations and changes. Changes in the minimum wage rate can be especially important for planning the upcoming budget if an increase in minimum wage is to occur during that planning period.

Child Labor

Minors under 16 may not be employed except under a temporary permit issued by the Department of Labor. Many states have regulations concerning the employment of persons between ages 16 and 18 in certain industries, such as nursing homes, where the worker can be exposed to disease or other hazardous conditions.

Equal Rights

In 1963 the Fair Labor Standards Act was amended by the Equal Pay Act. Under that amendment,

No employer shall discriminate between employees on the basis of sex by paying wages to employees less than the rate at which he pays wages to employees of the opposite sex for equal work on jobs which require equal skill, effort and responsibility, and similar working conditions. (quoted in Chruden & Sherman, p. 453)

Progress has been slow in this area. U.S. Department of Labor, Bureau of Labor Statistics, studies have shown that women earn about 59 cents for every dollar men earn in comparable positions (*U.S. Working Women*, p. 29).

The equal-pay provision of the Fair Labor Standards Act is of special concern to nursing home operators, who may employ both male and female nurses, male and female aides, and male and female maintenance and laundry persons.

THE WALSH-HEALY ACT

The Walsh-Healy Act was originally passed in 1936. It applies to workers employed on government contract work in excess of $10,000. Its significance for the nursing home is that the Secretary of Labor sets prevailing wages in each area of the United States. This affects the cost of construction and other activities in the geographical area in which the nursing facility is located. This act is often called the Public Contracts Act.

THE DAVIS-BACON ACT

Passed in 1931, the Davis-Bacon Act requires minimum wage rates for persons employed on federal public works projects. Again, this act does not directly affect operations of the nursing home.

4.5.4 Workman's Compensation: Assistance for On-the-Job Injuries

Workman's compensation laws are based on the principle that employees themselves should not have to pay costs associated with injuries that occur at work. On-the-job injuries, the lawmakers have reasoned, are a cost of doing business and should be passed on to the consumer.

In New Jersey, Texas, and South Carolina, worker compensation insurance is voluntary. In all other states it is compulsory for employers to participate in a state sponsored or state approved program.

Under most state laws, workers are paid a percentage of their regular wages while recovering from an injury on the job. States normally set limits to benefits and specify how long they must be paid.

Hospitalization and other medical costs are also normally covered by worker compensation insurance funds. There are usually death benefits for the worker's family. States establish commissions that handle any claims that are in dispute. Generally, the result is little cost to the injured worker and reasonably rapid assistance.

States typically take one of two basic approaches to funding worker's compensation insurance. Sometimes the state operates its own insurance system in which employers are usually obliged to participate. In other states, employers are allowed either to self-insure or to join a private insurance company program.

One characteristic of most worker accident compensation plans is that the amount the employer must pay per month is experience-based. Under this system, *employers with good safety records pay less than those with large numbers of claims.* In some states, benefits to the injured worker are reduced if the worker is willfully negligent in following safety procedures.

4.5.5 Unemployment Compensation

Employees who participate in the Social Security Act program are eligible for unemployment compensation when they are laid off by their employer. Nearly all nursing home employees are covered by the Social Security Act.

Unemployment compensation is available for up to 26 weeks through the state employment agency if the worker registers and is willing to accept any suitable comparable work offered through the agency.

Unemployment compensation is funded by a federal payroll tax based on the wages of each employee up to a certain maximum. The federal government turns these monies over to the states for disbursement.

A separate record is kept for each employer. Once a company has paid an amount equivalent to the required reserve, its rate of taxation is reduced. In practical application, this means that nursing facilities with few unemployment compensation claims against them pay at a lower tax rate than those with a large number of such claims.

Experience has shown that, even when employees are discharged or let go for valid reasons (unrelated to lack of work), unless the facility has extremely good documentation on the circumstances of the dismissal, the employee may be successful in claiming unemployment compensation. When this happens, the costs of the unemployment compensation paid by the state are allocated to that individual nursing facility's account.

4.5.6 Federal Laws Determining Retirement

Before 1979 the employer could set retirement age for the staff. Beginning January 1, 1979, an amendment to the Age Discrimination in Employment Act prohibited mandatory retirement under the age of 70 for persons in private employment. Beginning in 1987, the age limit was removed. Workers may now work to any age provided they can perform the job. There are some exceptions, such as facilities with fewer than 20 employees, but the practical effect is that no employees can be forced to retire against their wishes solely on the basis of age.

During the 1960s Congress investigated pensions for American workers and discovered that for a variety of reasons, up to one-half of American workers covered by pension plans would never receive any benefits. The largest problem was a failure of businesses to fund their pension plans adequately. For the worker the basic problem was loss of any pension benefits when leaving the company for almost any reason before retirement.

THE EMPLOYEE RETIREMENT INCOME SECURITY ACT, 1975

In reaction Congress passed the Employee Retirement Income Security Act (ERISA) of 1975. This act sets minimum funding levels for pension funds, requires certification every 3 years of the actuarial soundness of the plan, and requires vesting of the employee's equity in the pension fund. *Employers are not required under ERISA or any other law to provide a private pension fund for their employees.*

ERISA set up a number of detailed rules governing pension plans. A facility may not, for instance, establish requirements of more than 1 year of service or an age greater than 25, whichever comes later. ERISA was successful in setting rules that protect the employee and greatly increase the likelihood that the employee will eventually receive the retirement benefits promised under the pension plan.

There is, however, one major drawback to the ERISA legislation: its rules are so demanding that many employers choose not to offer pension plans. Many employers withdrew their plans rather than try to comply with the law when it went into effect.

PENSION BENEFIT GUARANTY CORPORATION

Among its regulations ERISA set up the Pension Benefit Guaranty Corporation, which is supported by premiums from employers to assure that employees will eventually receive retirement funds. Companies that decide to withdraw from the plan must make substantial payments into the Corporation before being permitted to do so. This and other elements of the Act create hardships for employers who otherwise are committed to providing pension benefits for employees.

One unfortunate result is that many employees are being given their accumulated "retirement" benefits when they leave the organization. This avoids having to deal with the ERISA legislation. Studies have shown that few of these benefits find their way back into retirement options such as reinvestment in an Individual Retirement Account (IRA).

4.6 Work-Place Safety: The Occupational Safety and Health Act (1970)

ORIGIN AND PASSAGE

For the first 7 decades of the 20th century state governments were responsible for safety in the work place. During that period organized labor became less and less satisfied with enforcement of state laws, variation in laws among the states, and often absence of safety laws. In the half-decade before the passage of federal legislation, job-related accidents were causing up to 2.5 million disabilities and 14,000 deaths annually (U.S. Department of Labor, p. 1).

After 3 years of intense lobbying by employees and the unions, Congress passed the Occupational Safety and Health Act (OSHA) in 1970 (Public Law 91-596). OSHA applies to nearly all employees and includes all of those working in nursing homes.

FEDERAL IMPLEMENTATION

Two federal agencies have been set up to implement OSHA. The Act is administered by the Occupational Safety and Health Administration in the Department of Labor. The National Institute of Occupational Safety and Health (NIOSH) was established to conduct research and develop standards.

A major goal of the Act has been to turn work-place safety enforcement back to the states with a strengthened work-safety law. States have been encouraged to establish their own inspection programs and industrial safety laboratories in three stages. State laws must, however, be consistent with OSHA regulations.

In addition to meeting all standards set, OSHA imposes on each employer a *general duty* to provide each employee a safe work place, free from recognized hazards, causing or likely to cause death or serious physical harm.

THREE OSHA IMPACT AREAS

OSHA directly affects the operations of nursing care facilities in three main areas:

1. Meeting the standards set by OSHA
2. Cooperating in OSHA inspections of the facility
3. Keeping the necessary records on accidents and illnesses that are job related

SOURCES OF STANDARDS

OSHA standards may originate from a variety of sources. The Secretary of Labor may issue and revise standards at will. This may be done on the Secretary's own initiative, on recommendation of the National Institute of Occupational Safety and Health, or at the urging of interested parties such as labor unions or groups of affected employees.

Adopting Standards of Other Groups

OSHA has adopted several national consensus standards that were developed by other groups, including the National Fire Protection Association's *Life Safety Code* and the *Standards for the Physically Handicapped* of the American National Standards Institute.

DEFINITION OF "STANDARD"

OSHA safety standards are "practices, means, operations or processes, reasonably necessary to provide safe...employment" (Ivancevich & Glueck, p. 595). Each employer is responsible for knowing the OSHA standards for his/her facility (either federal or a combination of federal and state).

The original standards required 350 pages of small print in the *Federal Register*. Subsequent years have witnessed the publication of supplementary volumes of standards. Some annual volumes have been over 700 pages in length. Even so, each manager is responsible for knowing applicable standards and is subject to both fines and imprisonment if found to be in violation of standards.

SOME OSHA REQUIREMENTS

OSHA bulletins have listed the following as among OSHA's requirements:

Employers

Each employer must furnish a work place free from recognized hazards that are causing or are likely to cause death or serious harm to employees and shall comply with OSHA standards. Employers are responsible for informing employees about OSHA standards, displaying the OSHA poster that informs employees of their rights and responsibilities, and compiling annual figures on work-related illnesses and accidents.

Employees

Each employee shall obey all OSHA requirements. However, the facility is held responsible for worker violation of OSHA standards. The employer has the choice of letting such a worker go, but there are no punishments for the worker who willfully ignores OSHA requirements. Willful disregard of OSHA rules is, however, grounds for termination permitted under federal law.

Any employee may lodge a complaint with OSHA. The complaint must be in writing and signed with a description of the hazardous condition. The complaint is submitted (signed) to the OSHA regional director and to the employer (unsigned, if the employee wishes).

Inspections

OSHA inspectors will visit at times of their own choosing, or at the invitation of an employer, union, or employee. Employees requesting an inspection need not be identified.

The employer and the employees must each designate a representative to accompany the OSHA inspector(s). If the employees do not do so, the OSHA compliance officer must consult several employees during the visit. This officer must hold an opening conference to discuss the scope and reason for the inspection and a concluding conference in which findings are presented to the employer.

Employers must not discriminate against any employee(s) who asks for an OSHA safety or health inspection. Any employee may file a complaint with the nearest OSHA office within 30 days for any alleged discimination.

OSHA inspectors examine *the premises* for compliance with regulations and *the records* of illnesses and injuries to employees.

Citations

Citations may be issued at the end of the inspection itself *or* later by mail. Any citation issued must be posted at or near the site of violation for 3 days or the duration of the violation, whichever is longer. One citation must be issued for *each* serious and nonserious violation found and a time limit specified for its correction.

OSHA compliance officers may categorize employer violations as

1. *imminent danger* (can close operations down)
2. *serious* (calls for a major fine)
3. *nonserious* (a violation in which a direct and immediate relationship exists between the condition and occupational health but not such as to cause death or serious physical harm)
4. *de minimus* (small violation)—a notification is given, but no fine; a violation of a standard that is not directly or immediately related to occupational safety or health

In every case, a time period is specified within which the violation must be corrected. A fine of $1,000 per day per citation may be assessed after the time limit set for abatement (correction) of the violation.

Fines

Fines, some mandatory, are to be imposed for the following:

1. *willful or repeated violations:* up to $10,000 per violation (mandatory); may double after first conviction
2. *serious violation:* mandatory penalty up to $1,000 for each violation
3. *nonserious violation:* optional penalties up to $1,000 each
4. *failure to correct within proposed time period:* up to $1,000 per day
5. *willful violation causing death:* up to $10,000 and/or 6 months in jail
6. *falsifying records or statements:* up to $10,000 and/or 6 months in jail

Employers have the right to appeal fines or citations within the OSHA structure *or* in the courts. Notice of contest must be filed within 15 days.

RECORD KEEPING

The area that most directly affects nursing home administrators on a day-to-day basis is keeping standardized records of illnesses and injuries from which ratios must be calculated. This record is OSHA Form 200, "Log and Summary of Occupational Injuries and Illnesses," which must be kept by each facility.

Accidents and illnesses that *do not* have to be reported are those that require only first aid and do not result in any work time lost. Accidents and illnesses that *do* have to be reported are those that result in death(s), disabilities that cause the employee to miss work, and injuries that require treatment by a physician. Fatal or serious multiple cases (five or more hospitalized) must be reported to the OSHA regional director orally, by phone or telegraph, within 48 hr. Other cases must be recorded within 6 days and reported on routine forms as requested by OSHA.

Occupational illness is a definition of special relevance to the nursing home setting. *An occupational illness is any abnormal condition or disorder, other than one resulting from an occupational injury, caused by exposure to environmental factors associated with employment.* It includes acute and chronic illnesses or diseases that may be caused by inhalation, absorption, ingestion, or direct contact (Chruden & Sherman, p. 524).

OSHA defines an occupational injury as any injury, such as a cut, fracture, sprain, amputation, that results from a work accident or from an exposure involving a single accident in the work environment (Chruden & Sherman, p. 524).

Each time a recordable case is entered in the log mentioned above, a "Supplementary Record of Occupational Injuries and Illnesses" (OSHA Form 101) must be completed, giving information on what the employee was doing, which part of the body was affected, and the identity of the employee.

OSHA Form 102, "Summary of Occupational Injuries and Illnesses," must be submitted annually and posted where employees can easily see it, e.g., above the time clock.

THE CURRENT AND EMERGING SITUATION

Completing, submitting, and posting accident and illness forms as required will remain a continuing requirement for nursing home administrators, but the inspection issue is another matter. The U.S. Supreme Court has ruled that OSHA inspectors can be barred from a facility if the inspectors do not have a search warrant (Ivancevich & Glueck, p. 596). The courts, however, have been cooperative in issuing warrants on request from OSHA. President Reagan focused on OSHA as one of the areas in which government bureaucracy was weighing too heavily on employers. He reduced funding for OSHA, which resulted in a 20% reduction in inspections and in the number of inspectors ("Deregulation," pp. 50–53). Enforcement of OSHA standards varies in intensity from state to state, since states now must fund a larger portion of inspection activity.

In recent years OSHA has begun to emphasize voluntary compliance. In place of inspections with resulting citations, OSHA has stressed educational programs in which safety inspectors do a "dry run" for an employer, advising of any "violations" and providing an opportunity for correction before any official inspection.

Since OSHA was enacted, fatalities in the work force are estimated to have decreased by 10% and total injuries to have decreased by 15% (Ivancevich & Glueck, p. 601).

4.7 Facility and Services Expansion: Federal Health Planning Regulations

Health planning in 20th-century America has moved through three phases. During the first half of the century it was mainly the concern of voluntary private groups. In the 1960s and 1970s health planning leadership was assumed by the federal agencies. In the 1980s the states have gradually assumed responsibility for health planning.

PHASE 1: PRIVATE VOLUNTARY HEALTH PLANNING

The Local Health Council Movement

A need for coordinating planning of health organizations in the public and private sectors was first felt by consumers. Concern about overlapping and duplication of services, lack of data collection efforts, and a desire to lobby for health legislation proposals brought a number of private citizens together in the early 1920s in the local health council movement. By 1950 there were approximately 1,200 local health councils meeting in 32 of the 48 states.

Many professional health administrators were equally concerned about lack of coordination and increasing costs in hospitals during those years and this gave rise to a number of hospital planning associations.

The Hill Burton Act

A new phase in health planning began shortly after the passage in 1946 of the Hill Burton Act, which, over the next several decades, was to fund the building of hundreds of hospitals, long-term care facilities and other related structures across the country.

Increasing Federal Involvement

During the 20 years following World War II, the federal government became actively involved, for the first time, in financial support of almost every aspect of health care, from sponsoring research, building hospitals, and providing health care to the poor and elderly to actually paying for the education of nurses and physicians.

PHASE 2: FEDERALLY DOMINATED HEALTH PLANNING

Comprehensive Health Planning Act, 1966

In 1966, seeking to rationalize health planning and to give consumers a meaningful role in health care policymaking, the federal government passed its first health planning law: Public Law 89-749, the Comprehensive Health Planning Act.

This legislation mandated that all participating states set up state and local health planning entities called Comprehensive Health Planning Agencies (CHPs). The hospital planning associations often served as the nuclei for these agencies. Consumers were to constitute 51% of the boards and have an active voice in program planning.

Professional Overrepresentation. Within 5 years it became evident that the Comprehensive Health Planning Agencies were all too often dominated by concerned health professionals. To counteract this trend, a new health planning law was passed in 1974, defining a "consumer" much more narrowly so as to assure that professionals were not overrepresented on the local and state health planning agency boards.

The National Health Planning and Resources Development Act, 1974

Public Law 93-641, the National Health Planning and Resources Development Act of 1974, was intended to rationalize health planning in the U.S. To accomplish this, 213 local offices, called Health Systems Agencies, were established. In many cases, the former Comprehensive Health Planning

Agencies won the contracts to become the new Health Systems Agencies (HSAs).

Each local Health Systems Agency was made responsible for estimating the health needs in its geographical area for the prospective 5 years. Based on this plan, the Agency would attempt to determine whether the health care needs of its area were being met. It is this process that so directly affects nursing home operations in many states.

Certificate of Need.   If the local health planning agency believes that there are insufficient nursing home beds in the area, it may be willing to issue what is called a Certificate of Need, which is often referred to as a CON.

If the local health planning agency considers that there are enough or perhaps too many nursing home beds in the geographical area, it may refuse to issue a Certificate of Need. In effect, the agency may deny permission to build new long-term care beds in that geographical region.

Capital Project Review.   A second area in which local Health Systems Agencies may affect nursing home administrators and owners is through review of capital projects. Each Health Systems Agency is responsible for reviews of requests by nursing homes and other health providers to make capital expenditures for building new facilities or renovating existing structures.

PHASE 3: HEALTH PLANNING AS A STATE LEVEL ACTIVITY

Deemphasis of the Federal Role

President Reagan opposed the federal government's heavy involvement in health planning from his first day in office. During the early years of his first administration he consistently sought to have the federal health planning program dismantled because he felt that it was more properly a state government function. Congress formally killed PL # 93-641 as of October 1, 1986.

Health planning is now a state activity.

Increased Reliance on States

Certificate of Need requirements is now an activity at the state level ("The state of health planning," 1984).

Certificate of Need thresholds now vary from one state to another. Some are tightening up the granting of Certificates of Need for new construction or new long term-care beds at the same time that others are allowing all state Certificate of Need requirements to lapse. For example, California decided to suspend its Certificate of Need requirements on January 1, 1987. Montana has enacted similar legislation.

The net effect of these changes on long-term care providers is that the building of new facilities or adding of beds is becoming more and more a determination of the individual state governments.

4.8 Voluntary Operating Standards: Joint Commission on Accreditation of Hospitals

Long-term care facilities that meet certain requirements are eligible to apply for accreditation from the Joint Commission on Accreditation of Hospitals (JCAH). Accreditation by JCAH is voluntary, and less than 10% of long-term care facilities have sought it. Until recently those who did tended to be part of or associated with hospitals.

Some states are beginning to accept JCAH accreditation in lieu of state and/or federal inspections for meeting the federal and/or state conditions of participation (Miller, p. 5039). The Omnibus Reconciliation Act of 1980 removed the federal requirement for annual surveys, thus clearing the way for a 2- or 3-year accreditation period such as JCAH offers (Miller, p. 5040).

ORIGINS OF JCAH

The JCAH had its origins in a program for hospital evaluation established in 1918 by the American College of Surgeons (JCAH, 1983, p. ix). Its current 22-member board consists of representatives from the American College of Physicians, the American College of Surgeons, the American Dental Association, the American Hospital Association, and the American Medical Association (*Facts about JCAH*).

JCAH MEMBERSHIP

In 1984, 7,400 facilities and programs were JCAH members, including 75% of acute-care general hospitals in the United States (*Facts about JCAH*).

ELIGIBILITY TO APPLY FOR JCAH ACCREDITATION

An eligible long-term care facility is one that is either hospital based or freestanding and established "for inpatient care, that has an organized medical staff, medical staff equivalent, or medical director, and that provides continuous nursing service under professional nurse direction" (*JCAH Eligibility Criteria*, p. 1).

The facility must also have been under the same ownership for at least 6 months, have a current unrestricted state license, and operate without restriction by reason of race, color, sex, or national origin. It must, in addition, submit a completed JCAH application with all information requested.

JCAH ACCREDITATION PROCESS

The JCAH offers a concise manual summarizing all JCAH accreditation requirements. After the application is accepted and processed, a survey team consisting of an administrator, a registered nurse, and a social worker visit the facility. The survey team report is evaluated by the JCAH headquarters staff and a recommendation from the staff is forwarded to the Accreditation Committee of the JCAH Board of Commissioners, who make the final decision. This entire process is normally completed in a total of 90 days and costs anywhere from $6,000 to $10,000, depending on the number of team members and the number of days they are at the facility.

The JCAH survey team examines for meeting the following standards (JCAH, 1983, p. v):

- Building and grounds safety
- Dental services
- Dietetic services
- Functional safety
- Governing body and management
- Infection/environment control
- Laboratory, radiologic, and other diagnostic services
- Medical records

- Medical services
- Nursing services
- Patient/resident activities
- Patient/resident care management
- Patient/resident rights and responsibilities
- Pharmaceutical services
- Quality assurance
- Rehabilitation services
- Social services
- Spiritual services
- Transfer agreements

CRITICISMS OF THE JCAH STANDARDS

After criticism that their standards were too structural and not sufficiently patient oriented (Jonas, p. 411), the JCAH placed additional emphasis on "the development, implementation, and ongoing reassessment of a multidisciplinary plan of care for each patient/resident [as] an essential feature of resident care" (JCAH, 1983, foreword). In late 1986 JCAH announced that by 1991 it expects to have an accreditation process based primarily on the quality of care received by patients in hospitals and long term care facilities.

JCAH standards are not significantly different from the federal Conditions of Participation for Skilled Nursing Facilities. If anything, JCAH standards may be somewhat more stringent in some areas and tend to be rather medically oriented. It is for this reason that certain states will accept JCAH accreditation in lieu of state inspections.

REFERENCES TO PART FOUR

American Hospital Association. (1976). *Taft Hartley Amendments: Implications for the health care field. Report of a symposium.* Chicago: Author.

American National Standards Institute. (1980). *American national standard specifications for making buildings and facilities accessible to and usable by physically handicapped people* (ANSI A117.1-1980). New York: ANSI.

Boling, T.E., Vrooman, D.M., & Sommers, K.M. (1983). *Nursing home management.* Springfield, IL: Charles C Thomas.

Chruden, J.J., & Sherman, A.W., Jr. (1980). *Personnel management: The utilization of human resource* (6th ed.). Dallas, TX: South-Western Publishing.

Committee on Nursing Home Regulation, Institute of Medicine. (1986). *Improving the Quality of Care in Nursing Homes.* Washington, DC: National Academy Press.

Freymann, J.G. (1980). *The American health care system: Its genesis and trajectory* Huntington, NY: Robert E. Krieger Publishing.

Health Care Financing Administration (HCFA). (1982). Conditions of participation for skilled nursing and intermediate care facilities (a proposed rule), 42 CFR Parts 405, 442, and 483, March 19, 1980. In D.B. Miller (Ed.), *Long term care administrators desk manual* (pp. 7042–7076). Greenvale, NY: Panel Publishers.

Hogstel, M.O. (1983). *Management of personnel in long-term care.* Bowie, MD: Robert J. Brady Co.

Ivancevich, J.M., & Glueck, W.F. (1983). *Foundations of personnel: Human resource management* (rev. ed.). Plano, TX: Business Publications.

Joint Commission on Accreditation of Hospitals. (1979). *Accreditation manual for hospitals, 1980.* Chicago: JCAH.

Joint Commission on Accreditation of Hospitals. (1982a). *Facts about JCAH.* Chicago: JCAH.

Joint Commission on Accreditation of Hospitals. (1983). *Accreditation manual for long term care facilities/84.* Chicago: JCAH.

Joint Commission on Accreditation of Hospitals. (1983a). *JCAH eligibility criteria.* Chicago: JCAH.

Jonas, S. (1981). *Health care delivery in the United States* (2nd ed.). New York: Springer Publishing Co.

Kart, C.S. (1981). *The realities of aging* Boston: Allyn and Bacon.

Lathrop, J. K. (1985). *Life safety code® handbook.* Quincy, MA: National Fire Protection Association.

Miller, D.B. (Ed.). (1982). *Long term care administrator's desk manual.* Greenvale, NY: Panel Publishers.

Miller, D.B., & Barry, J.T. (1979). *Nursing home organization and operation.* Boston: CBI Publishing.

National Fire Protection Association, Inc. (1985). *Life safety code 1985.* (NFPA 101 ANSI/NFPA 101).

A deregulation report card. (1982, Jan. 11). *Newsweek*, pp. 50–53.

Pointer, D., & Metzger, N. (1975). *The National Labor Relations Act: A guidebook for health care facility administrators* . New York: Spectrum Publications.

Raskin, A.H. (1981, December). From sitdowns to solidarity: Passage in the life of American labor. *Across the Board*, pp. 12–32.

Rogers, W.W. (1980). *General administration in the nursing home* (3rd ed.). Boston: CBI Publishing.

Rosenfeld, L.S., Gaylord, S.A., & Allen, J.E. (1983). *Introduction to long-term care for the aging.* Chapel Hill, NC: The University of North Carolina Independent Study by Extension.

Rosmann, J. (1975). One year under Taft-Hartley. *Hospitals, 49*(24), 64–68.

Smith, D.B. (1981). *Long-term care in transition: The regulation of nursing homes.* Washington, DC: Association of University Programs of Health Administration Press.

Staff. (1984, Oct. 1). Perspectives. *Washington Report on Medicine and Health*, 1–4.

The State of Health Planning. (1984, Oct. 22). *Medicine and Health*, INSERT, 4 pp.

Twomey, D.W. (1980). *Labor law and legislation.* Cincinnati: South-Western Publishing.

U.S. Department of Health, Education and Welfare. (1975). *Interpretive guidelines and survey procedures.* Washington, DC: American Health Care Association. (Originally published in the *Federal Register*, January 17, 1974).

U.S. Department of Labor. (1976). *Brief history of the American labor movement.* (Bulletin 1000). Washington, DC: U.S. Government Printing Office.

U.S. Department of Labor, Bureau of Labor Statistics. (1977). *U.S. Working women: A databook.* Washington, DC: U.S. Government Printing Office.

U.S. Department of Labor, Occupational Safety and Health Administration. (1976). *All about OSHA.* Washington, DC: U.S. Government Printing Office.

Vladeck, B.C. (1980). *Unloving care: The nursing home tragedy.* New York: Basic Books.

Waxman, Congressman H.A. (1986). Consensus Calls for Nursing Home Reform. *Provider 12*(11), 15–16.

Williams, S.J., & Torrens, P.R. (1980). *Introduction to health services.* New York: John Wiley and Sons.

Wilson, F.A., & Neuhauser, D. (1982). *Health services in the United States* (2nd ed.). Cambridge, MA: Ballinger.

PART FIVE

Patient Care

5.1 The Aging Process

How many Americans die of old age each year? Depending on the definitions used, the answer could range from more than 1 million persons to no one. Our answer is "no one." Old age is not a disease process.

It used to be customary to say that a person died of old age. This is too imprecise an observation about the cause of death of an aged person. It seems more functional to approach disease and disabilities and causes of death among older persons as one approaches these concerns in younger persons: to look for causes and seek either cure or relief.

Each older person, just like every younger person, dies of specific causes. Generally, one or more of the body systems (which are described below) becomes overwhelmed for some specific reason, such as a disease or an injury to the person, and death results.

RESEARCH ON AGING

Two groups of persons who study aging individuals are identified by two different titles. Physicians who specialize in treating older persons are called *geriatricians*. Professionals who study the problems of the aging population in society, and normally are not physicians, are called *gerontologists*.

How much have the geriatricians and gerontologists learned about aging? With the development of clinical medicine over the past century, attention to diseases of aging persons and the aging process itself have become increasingly active areas of scientific investigation. Much has been learned, and some of this knowledge will be discussed below. However, a good deal of uncertainty remains.

Because much of the "knowledge" about the aging process is still being tested and is not yet well established, we have heavily documented the material we present so that the reader can refer to orginal sources.

GENERAL OBSERVATIONS

One observation that seems safe to make is that aging is highly individualized. In the typical nursing home there are persons whose chronological age is 90, yet their physiological appearance and strong activity level are more characteristic of a 60-year-old person. Similarly, there are patients in their 60s and 70s in the same facility who appear to be more aged than the 90-year-old patient.

The extent to which this is due to genetic inheritance or is influenced by an individual's life-style and health behaviors remains a subject of debate.

A few additional general observations can be made about aging, none of them entirely safe, because for every such observation the reader may be able to think of persons who are valid exceptions.

Take, for example, observations of Alexander Leaf in *Scientific American* (pp. 44–52). Leaf compared persons aged 75 with persons aged 30 and found that among those he studied, a person of age 75 has

92% of the former brain weight
84% of the former basal metabolism
70% of the former kidney filtration rate
43% of the former maximum breathing capacity

Those are impressive figures. What do they mean? Does the progressive loss of cortical neurons (brain cells) mean that older persons are that much less smart? Apparently not. There is little substantial clinical evidence that reduction of mental competence accompanies reduction in brain weight.

If Leaf's data are correct—that, on average, when a person reaches age 75 the brain weighs about 10% less, the body is burning calories at a reduced rate, the kidneys are filtering about three-fourths as fast, and the lungs process oxygen more slowly, what is the significance? Certainly this may be important for the physician and the pharmacist concerned about drug tolerance and dosages, but these data do not make the 75-year-old individual any more or less of a person than the 30-year-old.

The main import of Leaf's data may be to confirm that, in general, aging is a continuous process that may begin at birth, that aging is a gradual decline of at least some systems of the body that proceed at different rates in different individuals.

5.1.1 Overview of Some Appearance and Functional Changes Believed to Be Associated with Aging

The following observations are discussed at greater length under the headings of the ten body systems described. By way of gaining an overall perspective, these phenomena can be observed.

Change in collagen. Collagen is connective tissue that loses elasticity over time and appears to account for sagging of the skin often observed in the aging person. Sagging can occur around the eyes and jaws and can affect the general body tone of the muscles, especially in the arm.

Reduced reserve. Leaf's observation that the lungs' capacity to process oxygen may be reduced by age 75 to less than half their previous capacity tends to be true of several other body systems. One researcher believes that after age 20 the heart muscle, too, loses strength every year at the rate of 0.85% (Starr, p. 771). Another concludes that at-rest heart output at age 75 is no more than 70% of at-rest heart output at age 30 (Leaf, p. 44).

Gradual changes in the immune system. Normally, the body rejects foreign cells, but as the body ages, one theory holds that a progressive weakening of the immune response increases susceptibility to respiratory and other illnesses.

Temperature response changes. A reduction of capacity to maintain body temperature within a narrow range appears to lead to a diminished shivering and sweating response, allowing the body temperature of some older individuals to range dangerously. This can lead to the elderly dying in heat waves and cold waves that do not so adversely affect younger persons. Ten percent of people over 65, or 2.5 million Americans, are believed to be vulnerable to hypothermia (lowered body heat) due to reduced heat production by the body.

Postural imbalances. The balancing mechanisms appear to function less well, resulting in some persons aged 65 and over being progressively at risk of tripping.

Decalcification of the bones. Many older persons are at increased risk of bones breaking, especially if they fall.

Decreases in bowel function control. As the central nervous system tends to function less and less well in some older persons, the ability to control the bowels lessens.

Frequent anorexia. Anorexia (loss of appetite) among some elderly leads to skipping meals and a reduced level of nutrition.

Skin. With the loss of some subcutaneous fat an older person may feel colder, and the skin may wrinkle. Some pigment (color) cells of the skin enlarge with age, resulting in the pigmented plaques often seen on the skin of aged persons.

Decreased bone and muscle mass. This process among some elderly individuals can result in stooped posture, reduced height, loss of muscle power, misshaped joints, and limitations in mobility.

Renal system. The bladder of some persons appears to reduce to less than half its former capacity, and micturition, the desire to urinate, appears delayed until the bladder is at near capacity instead of triggering at one-half of capacity.

Hearing and vision. Both hearing and vision appear to become reduced among many aged persons.

5.1.2 Theories of Aging

Because no one really knows why people age, there are several theories instead of one generally accepted explanation.

A Limit to the Number of Cell Divisions?

Leonard Hayflick, a Stanford University researcher, has found that normal human fibroblasts (embryonic cells that give rise to connective tissue), when cultured *in vitro* (in a test tube or other artificial environment), undergo only a limited number of divisions, usually about 50, before they die. His hypothesis is that the life span of a normal human cell is a programmed event under genetic control (Hayflick, pp. 614–636). He obtained support for his theory by showing that cells from adult human tissue undergo about 20 divisions before they die.

An Answer in Cancer Research?

Cancer cells appear to be able to continue reproducing indefinitely. If this is so, what causes noncancerous cells to lose their ability to divide? Some researchers think that the answer to cancer cell divisions may hold information that will indicate what limits the normal human cell's ability to continue dividing.

A Loss in Genetic Programming?

Bernard Strehler, while doing research at the University of California, hypothesized that age-related changes in cell metabolism are a programmed loss of the genetic material found in the DNA molecule (the molecule of heredity in most organisms).

Random Mutations?

Marott Sinex, when at the Boston University Medical School, proposed that random mutations of cells may produce aging by causing damage to DNA molecules. His theory is that as mutations (changes) accumulate in the body cells the cells progressively lose their ability to reproduce and perform their original functions (Sinex, 1977).

An Autoimmune Explanation?

Several researchers (see Blumenthal, H.T., pp. 3–5) suggest that a progressive failure of the body's immune system, which consists of white blood cells and various antibodies that are our first line of defense against diseases (discussed below), lead to autoimmune responses in older persons. Their idea is that "copying errors" in repeated cell divisions lead to cells that are progressively not recognized by the body, triggering the immune system to attack these cells, thinking foreign cells have invaded.

Wear and Tear?

Some theorists have suggested that the body simply wears out, or that vital parts wear out, similar to what occurs in machines.

Failure of Collagen?

Collagen (discussed below) is a protein fiber that is distributed in the walls of the blood vessels, the heart, and the connective tissue. Is age accompanied by a reduction in the elasticity of this protein, possibly leading to heart muscle inefficiency and, because of stiffness, to reduced cell permeability, making cell nutrition more difficult?

Regardless of which, if any, of these explanations of the aging process turns out to be correct, the nursing home administrator must deal with the effects of aging in planning the care of patients in the facility.

In the sections below we further explore some of the possible important relationships between diseases and aging found in the typical nursing home population. Before turning to an exploration of these relationships, however, the following section, which presents and defines a number of medical and related terms, is offered. The section is divided into four vocabulary-building topics: (a) a list of medical and related specialists, (b) therapeutic action of some drugs, (c) abbreviations commonly used in patient charting, and (d) a series of the more common prefixes and suffixes.

5.2 Medical and Related Terms

5.2.1 Common Medical Specializations

"Specialization" is typically a three-year training program taken beyond medical school curriculum and required internships. By professional custom, physicians normally place only "M.D." after their names, omitting any reference to certification they may hold as a "specialist."

Allergist—a physician who treats and diagnoses reactions and sensitivities to various substances such as foods, pollens, and dust.

Anesthesiologist—a physician who supervises and administers anesthesia during surgery and other medical procedures.

Cardiologist—a physician who specializes in the diagnosis and treatment of heart diseases.

Chiropodist—see Podiatrist.

Dermatologist—a physician who diagnoses and treats diseases of the skin.

Endocrinologist—a physician who specializes in disorders affecting the endocrine (ductless gland) system. This system includes the pituitary, thyroid, pancreas, and adrenal glands, which secrete hormones into the blood stream.

Exodontist—a dentist who specializes in the extraction of teeth.

Gastroenterologist—a physician who treats and diagnoses diseases of the digestive tract.

General surgeon—a physician who specializes in operative procedures to treat illnesses or various injuries.

Geriatrician—a physician who concentrates on the treatment of elderly persons. (A *gerontologist* is a professional who studies the problems of the aging population in society and normally is not a medical doctor.)

Gynecologist—a physician who specializes in diseases of the female reproductive organs.

Internist—a physician who specializes in diagnostic procedures and treatment of nonsurgical cases.

Neurologist—a physician who diagnoses and treats diseases of the brain, nervous system, and spinal cord.

Obstetrician—a physician who specializes in the care and treatment of childbearing women.

Ophthalmologist—a physician who diagnoses and treats eye diseases and disorders, performs eye surgery, refracts the eyes, and prescribes corrective eye glasses and lenses.

Optician—a technician, not a physician, trained to grind lenses and to fit eye glasses.

Optometrist—a professional person, not a physician, who is trained to give limited eye care involving testing vision, correcting focusing errors, and prescribing corrective lenses.

Oral surgeon—a dentist specializing in surgical techniques for correcting deformities and injuries and treating diseases in or adjacent to the mouth.

Orthodontist—a dentist who specializes in treating and correcting malformations of the jaw and teeth.

Orthopedist—a physician who specializes in diseases and injuries to bones, muscles, joints, and tendons. An orthopedic surgeon is a physician who specializes in surgical procedures relating to the bones, muscles, joints, and tendons.

Osteopath—a doctor of osteopathy, not a medical doctor, who uses methods of diagnosis and treatment that are similar to those of a medical doctor but who places special emphasis on the interrelationship of the musculoskeletal to the other body systems.

Pathologist—a physician who specializes in examination of body tissues under laboratory conditions. Research pathologists who do not provide laboratory services for human tissue examinations may hold a Ph.D. degree or the D.V.M. (Doctor of Veterinary Medicine) degree.

Pediatrician—a physician who specializes in diagnosis and treatment of diseases of children and adolescents.

Periodontist—a dentist specializing in treating diseases of the gums.

Plastic surgeon—a physician who practices restorative surgery.

Podiatrist—a trained professional, who is not a medical doctor, concerned with care of the feet, including clipping of toenails for diabetics, and who treats ailments such as corns and bunions.

Proctologist—a physician specializing in the diagnosis and treatment of the large intestine, particularly the anus and rectum.

Psychiatrist—a physician who specializes in the diagnosis and treatment of mental disorders.

Psychoanalyst—a psychiatrist who specializes in the use of psycho-analytic technique of therapy.

Psychologist—one, not a physician, who studies the function of the mind and behavioral patterns and administers psychological tests.

Radiologist—a physician specializing in the use of X-ray and similar medical diagnostic machines in treatment and diagnosis of injuries and other medical problems.

Urologist—a physician specializing in the diagnosis and treatment of diseases of the kidney, bladder, and reproductive organs.

5.2.2 Therapeutic Actions of Drugs

Analgesic—reduces pain, e.g., aspirin.

Antacid—neutralizes the acid in the stomach, e.g., Maalox.®

Antianemic—used in treatment of anemia, e.g., liver extract.

Antibiotic—destroys microorganisms in the body, e.g., penicillin.

Anticoagulant—depresses (slows) the clotting of blood.

Antidote—used to counteract poisons.

Antiseptic—slows down growth of bacteria, but does not kill all of the bacteria, e.g., hydrogen peroxide.

Antispasmodic—relieves smooth muscle spasm, e.g., Valium.®

Antitoxin—neutralizes bacterial toxins in infections, e.g., tetanus anti-toxin.

Astringent—used to constrict skin and mucous membranes by with-drawing water, e.g., alum.

Carminative—an agent that reduces flatulence (gas) in the stomach or intestinal tract.

Cathartic—laxative, purgative, inducing bowel movements, e.g., Cascara Sagrada.

Caustic—destroys tissue by local application, e.g., silver nitrate.

Chemotherapeutics—chemicals uses to treat illness, e.g., sulfanilamide for streptococcal infection.

Coagulant—stimulates clotting of the blood.

Diaphoretic—used to induce perspiration.

Disinfectant—destroys pathogenic organisms, e.g., Zephiran®chloride.
Diuretic—stimulates elimination of urine, often used with medications prescribed to reduce hypertension, e.g., diazide.
Emetic—induces vomiting, e.g., warm salt water.
Emollient—used to soften and soothe tissue, e.g., cold cream, petroleum jelly.
Expectorant—used to induce coughing, an agent that increases bronchial secretion and facilitates its expulsion (coughing), e.g., Robitussin®.
Hypertensive—helps raise blood pressure.
Hypnotic—assists patients to fall alseep, e.g., Nembutal®.
Miotic—constricts the pupil of the eye.
Mydriatic—dilates the pupils of the eye.
Sedative—relieves anxiety and emotional tensions, e.g., Seconal®.
Tonic or **stimulant**—used to stimulate body activity, e.g., Eldertonic® or Ritalin®.
Vasoconstrictor—causes blood vessels to narrow or constrict.
Vasodilator—expands or dilates blood vessels.
Vitamins—used in replacement therapy, e.g., vitamin C.

5.2.3 Abbreviations

aa.	of each
Abd.	abdomen
Ad. lib.	as much as desired, at pleasure
Adm.	admission
a.c.	before meals
A/G	albumin/globulin ratio
aq.	water
aq. dist.	distilled water
A.S.H.D.	arteriosclerotic heart disease
amp.	ampule
amt.	amount
ax.	auxilliary
B.E.	barium enema
b.i.d.	twice a day
B.M.R.	basal metabolic rate
BP or B/P	blood pressure
BRP	bathroom privileges

C.	centigrade
Ca.	carcinoma
caps.	capsules
cath.	catheter
c̄.	with
c.c.	cubic centimeter
C.B.C.	complete blood count
cf.	compare
comp.	compound
C.O.L.D.	chronic obstructive lung disease
	same as
C.O.P.D.	chronic obstructive pulmonary disease
C.N.S.	central nervous system
C.S.F.	cerebrospinal fluid
C.V.A.	cerebral vascular accident
D.& C.	dilatation and curettage
d/c	discontinued
decub.	lying down
Diab.	diabetic
Diag. or **Dx.**	diagnosis
Diff.	differential blood count
Dil.	dilute
Disc.	discontinue
Disch. or **D/C**	discharge
dr.	dram
dx	diagnosis
E.E.G	electroencephalogram
E.K.G. or **E.C.G.**	electrocardiogram
exam.	examination
fl. or **fld.**	fluid
F.U.O.	fever of unknown origin
Fx.	fracture
G.B.	gallbladder
G.I.	gastrointestinal
gm.	gram
gr.	grain
gt. gtts.	drop (s)
H. or **hr.**	hour
h.s.	at bedtime

hypo.	hypodermically
I.M.	intramuscular
inf.	infusion
I.V.	intravenous
K.U.B.	kidney-ureter-bladder
l.	liter
lab.	laboratory
Lat.	lateral
lb	pound
liq.	liquid
mg	milligram
min	minute
ml	milliliter
mm	millimeter
M.N.	midnight
N.	noon
no.	number
noct.	at night
N.P.O.	nothing per mouth
N. & V.	nausea and vomiting
pt	pint
o.d.	right eye
o.s.	left eye
o.u.	each eye
O.T.	occupational therapy
oz	ounce
p.	pulse
p.c.	after meal
PEARL	pupils equal and reactive to light
p.o.	by mouth
p.r.n.	as needed
prog.	prognosis
PROM	passive range of motion
P.T.	physical therapy
P.X.	physical examination
q.d.	every day

q.h.	every hour
q.h.s.	each bedtime
q.i.d.	four times a day
q.n.	every night
q.o.d.	every other day
q.s.	sufficient quantity
R.B.C.	red blood cells
ROM	range of motion
Rx.	prescription
s̄.	without
sol.	solution
S.O.B.	shortness of breath
s.o.s.	one dose, if necessary
spec.	specimen
S.S.	soap solution
s.s.	half
stat.	immediately
surg.	surgery
T.	temperature
tab.	tablet
TB	tuberculosis
t.i.d.	three times a day
tinct.	tincture
T.O.	telephone order
TPR or T.P.R.	temperature, pulse, and respiration
u.	unit
ung.	ointment
URI	upper respiratory infection
UTI	urinary tract infection
vol.	volume
V.O.	verbal order
v.s.	vital signs
W.B.C.	white blood cells
W/C	wheel chair
wt.	weight

5.2.4 Prefixes

a-, an- *without*, e.g., anorexia (loss of appetite).

ab- *from, off, away*, e.g., abnormal (not normal).

ad- *toward, to, at*, e.g., additive (a substance added to another substance to improve its appearance or nutritional value).

adeno- *gland*, e.g., adenoma, a benign (noncancerous) epithelial (surface-covering) tumor in which the cells form recognizable glandular structures.

ambi- *both*, e.g., ambilateral (relating to both sides).

ana- *up, toward*, e.g., anabolism (building up metabolism).

angio- *to a vessel*, e.g., angiofibrosis (the hardening of a vessel wall).

ante- *in front of, before*, e.g., ante cibum (before a meal).

antero- *in front of*, e.g., anteromedian (in front and toward the middle).

anti- *against*, e.g., antibacterial (preventing the growth of bacteria).

apo- *away from, off*, e.g., apocleisis (aversion to eating).

arterio- *pertaining to the arteries*, e.g., arteriogram (X ray of arteries).

arthro- *relation to the joints*, e.g., arthropathy (any disease affecting the joints).

auto- *self, same*, e.g., autoanalysis (analysis by a person of his/her own disorder).

bi- *two*, e.g., bilateral (relating to two sides).

bio- *relation to life*, e.g., biopsy (the process of removing tissue from living patients for a diagnostic examination).

brady- *slow*, e.g., bradycardia (a slow hearbeat).

broncho- *relating to the trachea or windpipe*, e.g., bronchoedema (swelling of the mucosa of the bronchial tube).

carcino- *pertaining to cancer*, e.g., carcinogen (any cancer producing substance) or carcinoma (a malignant neoplasm or cancer).

cardio- *pertaining to the heart*, e.g., cardioplegia (paralysis of the heart).

cata- *downward, against*, e.g., catabolism (the breaking down in the body of complex chemical compounds into simpler ones, often accompanied by the liberation of energy).

celio- *pertaining to the abdomen*, e.g., celiectomy (excision of the stomach) or celiocentesis (puncture into the abdominal cavity).

cephalo- *head*, e.g., cephalogram (an X-ray image of the structures of the head).

cervico- *neck or cervix*, e.g., cervicovesical (pertaining to the urinary bladder and the cervix).

chiro- *pertaining to the hand*, e.g., chiroplasty (plastic surgery on the hand).

chole- *pertaining to bile*, e.g., cholecystotomy (incision into the gall-bladder).

circum- *around*, e.g., circumcorneal (around or about the cornea of the eye).

com-, con- *with, together*. e.g., complication (a disease or adverse condition associated with another disease or adverse condition).

contra- *against, opposite*, e.g., contraindicated (not recommended, advised against).

counter- *against, opposite*, e.g., counteraction (action of a drug or agent opposed to that of some other drug or agent).

cranio- *pertaining to the head*, e.g., cranioplasty (any plastic operation on the skull).

cysto- *pertaining to the bladder*, e.g., cystitis (inflammation of the urinary bladder) or cystocele (hernia of the bladder).

cyto- *relation to a cell*, e.g., cytolysis (the dissolution of a cell).

de- *down, away from*, e.g., defibrillation (the arrest of fibrillation, i.e., irregular or rapid randomized contractions of the cardiac muscle restored to normal rhythm).

derm- *pertaining to the skin*, e.g., dermatitis (inflammation of the skin).

dextro- *toward or on the right side*, e.g., dextrocardiogram (the part of the electrocardiogram that is derived from the right ventricle of the heart).

di- *double, twice*, e.g., diarthric (relating to two joints).

dia- *through, apart*, e.g., diagastric (through the stomach).

dys- *painful, difficult*, e.g., dysphasia (difficulty in talking) or dyspnea (difficulty in breathing).

ecto- *out, away from*, e.g., ectoderm (the outermost layer of the skin).

em-, en- *in*, e.g., embolic (pushing or growing in).

encephalo- *condition in the brain or head*, e.g., encephalomyolitis (an acute inflammation of the brain and spinal cord) or encephalosclerosis (a hardening of the brain).

endo- *within, inner*, e.g., endocarditis (inflammation of the endocardium or lining membrane of the heart) or endoscope (an instrument for the examination of the interior of a body canal or hollow area).

entero- *relating to the intestines*, e.g., enterocolitis (inflammation of the mucous membrane of both small and large intestines).

epi- *above, upon, over*, e.g., epidermitis (inflammation of the epidermis or the superficial layer of the skin).

eu- *good*, e.g., euphoria (a feeling of well-being, commonly exaggerated and not necessarily well founded) or eupnea (easy, free respiration).

fibro- *pertaining to fiber*, e.g., fibrocarcinoma (a cancer with fibrous elements).

gastro- *stomach,* e.g., gastrostomy (the establishment of an artificial opening into the stomach, usually for feeding purposes).

glyco- *relationship to sweetness (sugar)* e.g., glycogen, the chief carbohydrate storage material in animals formed by and largely stored in the liver and, to a lesser extent, in the muscles.

gyn-, gyno- *pertaining to a female,* e.g., gynecology (the science of diseases of women, especially those of the genital tract).

hema-, hemo- *pertaining to the blood,* e.g., hemorrhage (bleeding, a flow of blood) or hematuria (blood in the urine).

hemi- *half,* e.g., hemialgia (pain affecting one entire half of the body) or hemiplegia (paralysis of one side of the body).

hepato- *liver,* e.g., hepatitis (inflammation of the liver).

histo- *relationship to tissue,* e.g., histolysis (disintegration of the tissue).

hydro- *pertaining to water,* e.g., hydrocyst (a cyst or sore with clear, watery contents).

hyper- *excessive,* e.g., hyperesthesia (abnormal acuteness of sensitivity to touch, pain, or other stimuli).

hypno- *relating to sleep,* e.g., hypnotherapy (the treatment of disease by inducing prolonged sleep).

hypo- *deficiency, lack of,* e.g., hypochondria (a false belief that one is suffering from some disease).

hystero- *relating to the uterus,* e.g., hysterogram (an X ray of the uterus).

ileo- *relating to the ileum (remote end of the small intestine),* e.g., ileocolitis (inflammation of the mucous membrane of both ileum and colon).

infra- *below, beneath,* e.g., infracardiac (beneath the heart, below the level of the heart).

inter- *between,* e.g., intercostal (between two ribs).

intra- *within,* e.g., intracutaneous (within the substance of the skin) or intraoral (within the mouth).

intro- *in, into,* e.g., introgastric (leading or passed into the stomach, e.g., a nasogastric tube for feeding).

kerato- *relating to the cornea, or horny tissue,* e.g., keratoconjunctivitis (inflammation of the conjunctiva at the border of the cornea of the eye).

labio- *relating to the lip,* e.g., labiocervical (pertaining to the lip and to the neck).

macro- *large, long,* e.g., macrocyte (a giant red cell).

mast- *relating to the breast,* e.g., mastectomy (amputation of the breast).

mega- *large, oversize,* e.g., megacardia (enlargement of the heart).

meta- *after, beyond, transformation,* e.g., metastasis (the shifting of a disease).

micro- *small,* e.g., microinfarct (a very small infarct, i.e., death of tissue due to lack of blood supply, due to obstruction of circulation in capillaries or small arteries).

multi- *many*, e.g., multicellular (composed of many cells).

myel- *pertaining to the spinal cord*, e.g., myeloplegia (spinal paralysis).

myo- *relating to muscle*, e.g., myotrophy (muscular atrophy) or myocardial infarction (death of some heart muscle due to lack of blood supply, a heart attack).

necro- *relating to death*, e.g., necrocytosis (death of cells).

nephro- *pertaining to the kidney*, e.g., nephritis (inflammation of the kidney).

odont- *relating to the teeth*, e.g., odontalgia (a toothache).

omo- *pertaining to the shoulder*, e.g., omodynia (pain in the shoulder joint).

ophthalmo- *relating to the eye*, e.g., opthalmoplegia (paralysis of the motor nerves of the eye).

opto- *relating to vision*, e.g., optometer (an instrument for determining the refraction of the eye).

ortho- *straight*, e.g., orthograde (walking or standing in a straight or upright position).

osteo- *pertaining to the bones*, e.g., osteoporosis (reduction in the quantity of bone or atrophy of skeletal tissue).

oxy- *sharp, acute*, e.g., oxyesthesia (a condition of increased acuity of sensation).

pachy- *thick*, e.g., pachylosis (a condition of roughness, dryness, and thickening of the skin).

pan- *all*, e.g., pancarditis (diffuse inflammation of the heart).

para- *beyond, beside*, e.g., paralysis (loss of the ability to move).

patho- *disease*, e.g., pathogenesis (the origin or development of a disease).

per- *through*, e.g., perfusion (the act of pouring over or through, especially the passage of a fluid through the vessels of a specific organ).

peri- *around*, e.g., peribronchitis (inflammation of the tissues surrounding the bronchial tubes).

phlebo- *relating to a vein*, e.g., phlebitis (inflammation of a vein).

pneumo- *lung*, e.g., pneumonia (inflammation of the lung).

poly- *many, much*, e.g., polyarthritis (inflammation of several joints).

procto- *relating to the anus*, e.g., proctoscope, a short tubular instrument with illumination for inspecting the rectum. A *sigmoidoscope*, a foot-long tube, is used to examine the sigmoid (shaped like the letter *C*) colon, i.e., left colon from the descending colon to the rectum. A *colonoscope*, which is the longest, is used to examine the entire colon.

pseudo- *false*, e.g., pseudodementia (a condition of indifference to one's surroundings without actual mental impairment).

psycho- *pertaining to the mind*, e.g., psychotherapy (counseling help).

pyo- *signifying pus*, e.g., pyoderma (any infection of or on the skin that contains pus, i.e., a collection of white blood cells and other materials generated by the immune response).

rachi- *spine*, e.g., rachiocampsis (curvature of the spine).

rhino- *nose*, e.g., rhinoplasty (a repair of the nose).

sub- *under*, e.g., subcutaneous (under the skin).

tachy- *rapid*, e.g., tachycardia (rapid beating of the heart).

thermo- *heat*, e.g., thermophobia (morbid fear of heat).

uni- *one*, e.g., unicellular (composed of one cell).

vaso- *vessel*, e.g., vasoconstriction (narrowing of the blood vessels) or vasodilation (widening of the blood vessels).

5.2.5 Suffixes

-ac *pertaining to*, e.g., cardiac (pertaining to the heart).

-algia *pain*, e.g., neuralgia (nerve pain).

-cele *hernia, i.e., protrusion of a portion of an organ or tissue through an abnormal opening*, e.g., rectocele (herniation of the rectum).

-centesis *surgical puncture*, e.g., paracentesis (a puncture of the body cavity for removing fluid).

-clasis *breaking*, e.g., thromboclasis (the breaking up of a blood clot).

-clysis *washing, irrigation*, e.g., enteroclysis (enema of the intestines).

-coccus *berry-shaped, round bacterium*, e.g., dermococcus (round bacteria found in the skin).

-cyte *cell*, e.g., hematocyte (any blood cell).

-ectasia *dilation, stretching*, e.g., gastrectasia (dilation of the stomach).

-emesis *vomiting*, e.g., hyperemesis (excessive vomiting).

-emia *denoting a condition of the blood*, e.g., glycemia (sugar in the blood).

-ectomy *excision (cutting out) of*, e.g., tonsillectomy (cutting out of the tonsils).

-genesis *condition of producing*, e.g., carcinogenesis (the origin or production of cancer).

-itis *inflammation*, e.g., dermatitis (inflammation of the skin).

-lith *stone*, e.g., nephrolith (kidney stone).

-lysis *breakdown*, e.g., hemolysis (the destruction of red blood cells).

-malasia *softening*, e.g., osteomalasia (a disease characterized by gradual softening and bending of the bones).

-megaly *enlargement*, e.g., cardiomegaly (enlargement of the heart).

-odynia *painful condition*, e.g., cardiodynia (pain in the heart).

-oma *tumor*, e.g., carcinoma (a malignant tumor).

-opsy *to view*, e.g., biopsy (the process of removing tissue from a living patient for diagnostic examination).

-orexia *appetite, desire*, e.g., anorexia (lack of appetite).

-orrhagia *bursting forth of blood*, e.g., gastrorrhagia (hemorrhage from the stomach).

-orrhaphy *suture*, e.g., gastrorrhaphy (the suture of a perforation of the stomach).

-orrhea *flow, discharge*, e.g., gastrorrhea (excessive secretion of gastric juice or mucus by the stomach).

-ostomy *to make a new opening*, e.g., colostomy (the establishment of an artificial anus by an opening into the colon).

-otomy *incision, to cut into*, e.g., nephrotomy (an incision into a kidney).

-pathy *disease*, e.g., neuropathy (any nerve disease) or angiocardiopathy (disease of the heart and blood vessels).

-penia *deficiency*, e.g., leukopenia (any situation in which the total number of leukocytes—white blood cells—in the circulating blood is less than normal).

-pepsia *digestion*, e.g., dyspepsia (indigestion or upset stomach).

-pexy *fixation, to put into place*, e.g., nephropexy (the operative fixation of a floating kidney).

-phagia *eating, swallowing*, e.g., dysphagia (difficulty in swallowing).

-phasia *speech*, e.g., aphasia (loss of the power of speech).

-phobia *fear*, e.g., claustrophobia (fear of being closed in a small space).

-plasty *surgical repair*, e.g., thoracoplasty (reparative or plastic surgery to the chest).

-pnea *breath*, e.g., polypnea (very rapid breathing).

-rhythmia *rhythmical*, e.g., arrhythmia (any variation from the normal rhythm of the heart).

-sclerosis *hardening*, e.g., arteriosclerosis (hardening of the arteries).

-spasm *sudden violent involuntary contraction of muscles*, e.g., myospasm (spasm of a muscle).

-stasis *stopping, controlling*, e.g., cholestasis (an arrest in the flow of bile from the liver).

-stenosis *tightening, stricture*, e.g., arteriostenosis (narrowing of the size or caliber of an artery).

-taxis *order, arrangement*, e.g., thermotaxis (regulation of the temperature of the body).

-tripsy *crushing*, e.g., lithotripsy (the crushing of a stone in the kidney by a new machine, called a lithotripter, that uses sound waves to break stones into minute particles, which can then be passed in the urine).

-trophy *development, nourishment*, e.g., hypertrophy (an overgrowth or increase in the bulk of a body part or organ).

-uria *urine*, e.g., albuminuria (the presence of protein in urine, chiefly albumin; albumin is any protein that is soluble in water).

5.3 The Aging Process As It Relates to Diseases Common to the Nursing Home Population

It is useful for the administrator to be familiar with the rudiments of biological processes and human anatomy and to be able to recognize the parts of the body that are affected by the aging process. In this way the administrator will be better able to appreciate the special problems with which the facility must cope.

All physical processes in the body undergo some changes as a result of aging, including a slowing down, a decrease in the overall energy reserve, breakdown of some of the body functions, and an alteration of some individual cell structures, which ultimately affects the functioning of some body tissues and organs as well.

The systems referred to are groups of structures that perform a specialized function for the body. Below is a list of ten systems of the body processes and structures as they are most commonly categorized. They are presented to reflect also the prevalence of diseases affecting them in the nursing home population.

It is important to remember that these systems are highly interrelated and that most nursing home residents typically suffer from multiple chronic diseases that may affect combinations of body systems.

1. **Blood circulation**—the basic processes and structures that enable the body to transport oxygen to the cells and tissues.

2. **Breathing**—the process by which the body obtains oxygen from the environment and distributes it throughout the body.
3. **Nervous system**—responsible for controlling all of the body functions and assuring that they are functioning properly; these are the regulatory activities.
4. **Digestion**—the process by which the body breaks down food into a form in which the nutrients may be used by the individual cells.
5. **Nutritional needs**—needs of the body for nutrients.
6. **External and internal defense mechanisms**—the skin and an internal immune system, which play important roles in protecting the body from any harmful invasions.
7. **Musculoskeletal system**—the bones, muscles, cartilage, tendons, and joints used in movement.
8. **Urinary system**—the way in which the body relieves itself of fluid and chemical waste products.
9. **Reproductive system**—sexuality in the elderly.
10. **Emotional and mental well-being**—the psychological status.

5.3.1 Blood Circulation

The circulatory system, also called the cardiovascular system, may be thought of as an elaborate pumping mechanism (Rosendorff, p. 1). It is powered by the heart, which pumps the blood throughout the body within a network of blood vessels (arteries and veins).

ARTERIES

Arteries are the vessels that carry blood rich in nutrients away from the heart to the remainder of the body cells.

Nutrients obtained from the food are processed in the digestive tract. Combined with oxygen, nutrients permit individual cells to perform the chemical reactions that produce energy.

Oxygen is a colorless, odorless, gaseous chemical element that is found in the air. Oxygen is most plentiful in the arteries, which divide into smaller and smaller branches until they become capillaries. These capillaries are the smallest blood vessels and form a network connecting the smallest arteries to the smallest veins (see Figure 5-1). It is here at the capillaries that the function of oxygenation occurs.

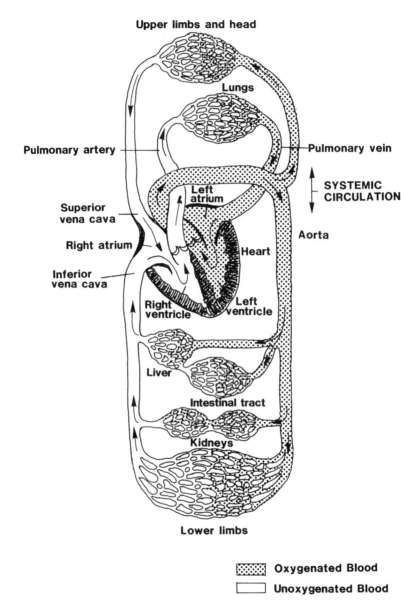

Upper limbs and head

Lungs

Pulmonary artery

Pulmonary vein

SYSTEMIC CIRCULATION

Left atrium

Superior vena cava

Aorta

Right atrium

Heart

Inferior vena cava

Right ventricle

Left ventricle

Liver

Intestinal tract

Kidneys

Lower limbs

☷ **Oxygenated Blood**

☐ **Unoxygenated Blood**

FIGURE 5-1. Representation of the circulatory and oxygenation process.

Oxygenation is the transfer of oxygen from the blood cells at the capillary level into the necessary tissues in exchange for carbon dioxide. Carbon dioxide is also a gas. It is produced as a waste product of the chemical reactions in the cells.

VEINS

The blood cells carry carbon dioxide through the vein network and back to the heart. Veins return blood that is carrying carbon dioxide back to the heart through the superior (from upper body) and inferior (lower body) vena cava (see Figure 5-1).

The blood then enters the right side of the heart. When a sufficient amount of blood has collected, the right ventricle of the heart contracts, actually squeezing its contents into the artery that leads to the lungs (*pulmonary artery*).

LUNGS

Within the lungs the carbon dioxide that has been collected by the veins is discarded and exchanged for oxygen. The carbon dioxide is then exhaled into the air as the breath is expelled. It has followed the reverse of the oxygen pathway until it is removed from the body. This is a simplification of the respiratory process (breathing), which will be discussed further in the next section.

The newly oxygenated blood returns to the heart through the pulmonary vein. The blood is then channeled into the left side of the heart. When enough blood has collected, this blood is then pumped forcefully out of the heart into the *aorta*. The aorta is the largest artery from which all the smaller arteries branch off, carrying blood that is rich in oxygen throughout the rest of the body again. This process occurs with every heartbeat.

THE HEART

The heart itself is a complex organ. It is a muscle composed of various types of cells to facilitate the pumping process. The heart requires oxygen to function and is supplied by a network of coronary arteries that stem from the aorta (see Figure 5-2).

The inner structure of the heart is also very complex, with four distinct chambers and a valve network that regulates blood flow.

CELL CHANGES

Any substantial change in these structures or the circulatory process itself can eventually affect all the body cells. The significance, then, of the oxygenation process is that when the health of cells has deteriorated, it is

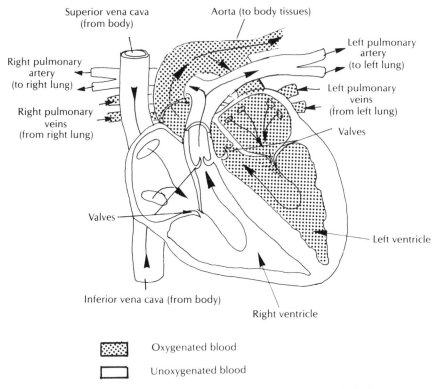

Superior vena cava
(from body)

Aorta (to body tissues)

Left pulmonary
artery
(to left lung)

Right pulmonary
artery
(to right lung)

Left pulmonary
veins
(from left lung)

Right pulmonary
veins
(from right lung)

Valves

Valves

Left ventricle

Inferior vena cava (from body)

Right ventricle

Oxygenated blood

Unoxygenated blood

FIGURE 5-2. Schematic representation of blood flow through the heart.

usually due to a change in the cardiovascular system that interferes with the supply of nutrients to the cells and with the supply of oxygen. This in turn damages the tissues and organs in the body, leading to the decline of other major processes.

AGING EFFECTS

The extent to which the aging process plays a role in this deterioration is still being argued. It is known that the cardiovascular system (heart and blood vessels) is not designed to last indefinitely. Many of the cells are not capable of dividing and remain part of the system for long periods of time.

A theory of aging that directly relates to the heart functions focuses on collagen, which is a protein that surrounds every muscle fiber within each muscle cell. The amount of collagen produced seems to increase with age, resulting in a stiffening or hardening of the tissues that contain cells with this substance (Kart, Metress, & Metress, p. 172; Kenny, p. 48) In the blood vessels this process is referred to as *arteriosclerosis* (literally, a hardening of the arteries).

Decreased Elasticity

A specific age-related change in the heart includes a lessening of the force of contraction (pumping) due to the decreased elasticity of muscle. *Elasticity* is the ability of the heart muscle to stretch and return to normal size spontaneously. When this property has been decreased in the heart muscle, the heart becomes stretched. This loss of elasticity reduces the force of contractions by the heart (pumping), which ultimately diminishes the amount of blood pumped by the heart (also termed cardiac output).

Decreased Cardiac Output

The reduced cardiac output is also due to an increased resistance to blood flow within the blood vessels and a loss in the heart's ability to compensate by beating faster. This added resistance to the blood flow within blood vessels may be a direct result of arteriosclerosis (hardening of the arteries) or more specifically atherosclerosis (one type of arteriosclerosis).

A change in any one of these components will affect the other two. If the amount of blood circulated is reduced, the organs and tissues will receive fewer nutrients and less oxygen, resulting in some cells dying (if deprived for more than 3 to 5 min).

It is estimated that in the elderly the blood flow to the kidneys is reduced by as much as 50%, and to the brain by as much as 20%, due to these same processes (Kenney, p. 51). These changes can explain changes in other systems associated with aging.

Blood Pressure Changes

There is much debate among scientists about the role of the aging process and its effect on blood pressure. In many elderly persons the blood pressure does increase. This increased pressure may be attributed to the stiffness of large arteries (arteriosclerosis) and *peripheral vascular resistance* (the resistance in the blood vessels throughout the body) that are commonly associated with the aging process. Other studies of individuals in isolated areas reveal no changes in blood pressure levels for the elderly. Some investigators feel there is a strong association of social and environmental factors contributing to the presence of high blood pressure in any individual (*hypertension*).

Blood vessel changes due to this progressive stiffening have suggested that they become like rigid tubes (Finch & Hayflick, p. 286). This promotes the resistance to blood flow throughout the body (peripheral vascular resistance) and may exacerbate an already adversely affected heart function and increased blood pressure.

The vein walls tend to weaken with increased collagen deposits, resulting in their twisting and forming winding pathways that can lead to such conditions as varicose veins. The capillary walls become thickened, thus decreasing their ability to exchange oxygen with the cells. This thickening also contributes to the overall decrease in perfusion of (flow of nutrients into) the tissues and organs.

SIX COMMON CARDIOVASCULAR DISEASES

Cardiovascular disease is the major cause of death in the elderly population. The primary diagnosis of approximately 40% of nursing home residents is some problem associated with heart disease (Hing, p. 14). The distinction between changes related to the aging process and those related to disease is a fine one. This dilemma becomes clear with the discussion of arteriosclerosis.

Arteriosclerosis

Normally, arteries are smooth inside and can stretch to permit the passage of more blood and oxygen when needed. With arteriosclerosis, the blood vessels are not as responsive as they previously were. Everyone has arteriosclerosis to some degree. Almost half of all nursing home residents manifest disease changes due to chronic arteriosclerosis. Two forms of this condition (*atherosclerosis* and *aortic stenosis*) account for much of the heart disease in the elderly.

Aortic Stenosis. The term describes a narrowing of the aorta, which is the major artery leading from the heart and channeling the oxygenated blood supply to the rest of the body. This stenosis, or narrowing of the vessel, increases the workload specifically for the left ventricle of the heart, since it now has to pump harder to overcome the obstructive resistance to blood flow.

The increased workload eventually is felt by the entire heart, and when combined with the normal changes attributed to the aging process, this disease places considerable stress on the cardiovascular system. It can result in congestive heart failure, which will be discussed at the end of this section.

For many elderly patients, the cause of the disease is either the result of scarring from a childhood outbreak of rheumatic fever or calcified deposits found lining the blood vessels.

Some of the **symptoms** of aortic stenosis are difficulty in breathing, dizziness, high blood pressure, chest pain, and symptoms associated with congestive heart failure.

Treatment can consist of surgical correction, rest to decrease the workload on the heart, and medication therapy.

Atherosclerosis. In this the most common form of arteriosclerosis, there is a progressive buildup of fat deposits on the inner lining of blood vessel walls. The disease does not usually manifest itself until the blood vessel becomes completely obstructed or shows a markedly decreased ability to facilitate blood flow. The symptoms can be found affecting the body anywhere that an initial pathology (a disease-related change in a tissue or organ) may be present; this usually includes the main arteries.

Cerebrovascular Disease

This disease manifests itself through restricted blood flow to the brain, caused by occlusions within the carotid arteries that supply blood to the brain. One of the most important causes of strokes is atherosclerosis.

Nursing home residents who may be predisposed to cardiovascular disease are those with high blood pressure, previous history of heart disease, and overweight (Birchenall & Streight, p.188). The specific symptoms of the disease depend on the affected location in the brain. *Transient ischemic attacks* (also termed "mini-strokes") are caused by a temporarily diminished blood supply to the brain.

Signs of cerebrovascular disease can be slurred speech, blurred vision, dizziness, numb hands and fingers, and mental confusion. Some of these symptoms could be easily attributed to the "aging process" rather than this underlying disease pathology.

A much more severe consequence of cerebrovascular disease is a *stroke*, or cerebrovascular accident (CVA). This occurs when the lack of oxygen for a much larger area of the brain causes permanent damage. Again, the resulting damage will depend on the area of the brain affected and may range from temporary loss of taste or smell to paralysis of many of the body parts.

Peripheral Vascular Disease

This actually describes a group of diseases that affect the veins, arteries, and other blood vessels of the extremities (Birchenall & Streight, p. 202). The symptoms are a result of decreased blood flow to the affected area. The most frequent symptom is *intermittent claudication*, which is a complex of **symptoms** including the following:

- pain on movement of an extremity
- pain that is chronic in a localized area
- cold, numb feet
- changes in skin integrity, such as ulcers or infections that are slow to heal

Treatment can include encouraging walking and exercise, attention to foot care, and assuring that the extremities are kept warm.

Coronary Artery Disease

Also known as chronic ischemic heart disease, here the heart muscle itself suffers from a lack of oxygen due to blockages in the coronary arteries that usually supply it.

The currently popular coronary artery bypass graft surgery is a common treatment for persons with severe blockages who do not respond to medical therapy. Since this is major surgery, some nursing home residents would not be considered good surgical risks for such treatment.

Symptoms can include chest pain—commonly called angina—which results from a lack of oxygen to certain areas of the heart muscle. Pain may be located anywhere in the chest, especially in the left arm or neck. This symptom is commonly found in patients over 60 years of age (Kleiger, p. 68).

Myocardial infarction (MI) (literally meaning heart muscle death) results when a large enough area of the heart muscle does not receive oxygen for a period of time. With a massive myocardial infarction, the heart can no longer continue to act as a pump and may completely stop beating. There is a greater chance that patients over 60 years old will die from a heart attack than will younger patients (Kleiger, p. 68).

The phases in coronary artery disease range from diffuse, incomplete blockages throughout the arteries, to one or more large blockages that occlude more of the blood flow.

Symptoms can range from none at all to various types of angina or, most serious, to a complete cessation of heart activity that occurs after MI or complete heart block.

Treatments vary. Initially, patients without severe manifestations of the disease can be treated conservatively with restrictions of sodium and fat from their diet. Medications commonly used in the nursing facility are nitroglycerin and propranolol.

Nitroglycerin, the most common medication prescribed for patients with angina, is administered sublingually, the patient holding the pill under the tongue. This drug lowers the blood pressure by dilating the blood vessels, including the coronary arteries, to decrease resistance to blood flow. Other medications, such as Isordil and Nitrol Paste, provide the same relief but are longer-acting.

Propranolol hydrochloride (Inderal) is referred to as a beta blocker because of its action in blocking body chemicals that act to increase the heart rate. This acts to slow the heart down, thereby decreasing blood pressure, and lowering the amount of oxygen required by the heart muscle.

There are also a variety of antiarrhythmic medications available, which are prescribed in accordance with the particular type of arrhythmia diagnosed.

A common result of prolonged or diffuse coronary artery disease is the inability of the heart to initiate contractions independently. When this occurs another type of treatment is often prescribed: permanent pacemaker. The pacemaker is a mechanical device implanted under the skin with its wires attached to the heart muscle to provide a continuous flow of electrical impulses that stimulate the heart to contract with a steady rhythm.

High Blood Pressure

High blood pressure, also called hypertension, is usually considered to be present when the blood pressure measurement is consistently greater than 160/95.

The numbers 160/95 are a measurement of the amount of pressure the blood exerts on the walls of the arteries. The first number (160) measures the maximum pressure (systolic) exerted when the heart is fully contracted near the end of the stroke output of the left ventricle. The second number (here 95) measures the minimum or diastolic pressure occurring when the heart ventricles are in the period of dilation or fully relaxed. This must be monitored for each individual to account for height and weight variations.

There are two types of this disease: (a) *essential hypertension* and (b) *secondary hypertension*. The cause of essential hypertension is unknown, and therefore the disease is without a complete cure, but it can be successfully controlled by medication. Secondary hypertension in the elderly results from other underlying diseases, including anemia, fever, endocrine disease or hormonal disruption, arteriosclerosis and/or kidney disease (Rubin, p. 309). These diseases place a greater demand on the heart and may cause the blood pressure to increase during the disease episode or permanently.

The effects of continued high blood pressure, regardless of the cause, may be harmful to various organs within the body, especially the heart, brain, kidney, and eyes. When a person has high blood pressure, the heart must automatically pump harder to circulate the blood throughout the body. As the heart works harder and harder to compensate, eventually it begins to fail after being overworked for such long periods of time. This in turn reduces the blood flow to the vital organs, damaging their functioning as well.

Some **signs** of hypertension are prolonged, elevated blood pressure greater than 160/95, or the individual's norm, and prolonged presence of risk factors such as overweight, smoking, high salt intake.

Treatments typically used include prescribing weight loss and diet therapy, including restricted salt intake. The goal of medication therapy is to use as few drugs as possible. Some of the most common medications used in a nursing facility include diuretics, nitroglycerin, and propranolol.

Diuretics are frequently used to get rid of the excess fluids in the body to decrease the workload of the heart by decreasing the blood volume that it must pump. Vasodilators such as nitroglycerin are used to dilate blood vessels and therefore decrease the amount of resistance against which the heart must work. Cardiac drugs such as propranolol may also be used to relieve the workload of the heart by decreasing its rate of contractions or pumping.

Congestive Heart Failure

This is not a disease, but is actually a complex set of many symptoms associated with an impaired performance of the heart. A progressively weakening heart results in an increasing inability of the heart to pump enough oxygen to the various tissues of the body. This failure results in a congestion of blood being backed up in the circulatory system. This backup causes fluids to leak out of the bloodstream into the various tissues and organs, most notably the lungs. Taken together, these constitute the disease process called congestive heart failure (CHF).

The cause of congestive heart failure may be a variety of diseases or conditions, most notably arteriosclerosis, coronary artery disease, uncontrolled high blood pressure and/or a problem with one of the heart valves, heart attack, alcoholism, or chronic exposure to agents harmful to the body tissues.

The **symptoms** usually are seen in other organs and can be classified according to whether the heart failure primarily affects the left or right side of the heart.

Right-sided failure of the heart:

- edema: a build-up of fluids outside of the blood vessels that forces fluid into the tissues; occurs mostly in the ankles.
- gradual loss of energy
- anorexia (loss of appetite for food)

- constipation
- weight gain (because kidneys cause the body to keep too much sodium and water)
- grayish or blue color of the skin due to decreased blood flow

Left-sided failure of the heart:

- frequent coughing or wheezing
- shortness of breath (dyspnea) a result of the blood backing up into the lungs thus decreasing the amount of space in the lungs available to hold air. This is one of the definitive signs of CHF and usually occurs after exercise (Anderson, p. 136)
- confusion and loss of memory are severe symptoms that suggest the disease has progressed far enough to damage the brain tissue.

Treatment generally consists of rest; monitoring weight to guard against sudden changes; diet therapy, including reducing salt intake and encouraging potassium intake with foods like bananas and oranges; and oxygen therapy to improve the oxygen content of red blood cells, since there is less and less exchange area available in the lungs.

Technological advances are being made in providing oxygen to patients. Machines called oxygen concentrators are now available and can be more cost-effective than the traditional oxygen tanks. The advantage is an ability to use ambient air in the patient's room to produce the required oxygen. The potential disadvantage is that, unlike the bulky and unsightly tanks, the oxygen concentrator must have a continuous supply of electricity.

Medications can include digoxin (Lanoxin®), which acts directly on the heart muscle to increase the force of contraction. This is an extremely powerful medication that may cause severe side effects in the elderly when the level of the medication becomes too high in the blood. Confusion or severe behavioral changes may indicate this is occurring (Gambert, p. 21).

To avoid fluid buildup, *diuretics* are also often prescribed to aid the body in eliminating toxic wastes and fluids that have accumulated (Crow, p. 45). Some of the more powerful diuretics deplete the body's supply of important electrolytes, such as sodium and potassium. Low levels of potassium can be particularly dangerous for the elderly patient, who is especially vulnerable to such imbalances. Potassium supplements are frequently prescribed, in addition to dietary supplements, to increase the blood level of this naturally occurring mineral.

5.3.2 Respiratory System

The chief function of the respiratory process is providing the body with oxygen, while removing excess carbon dioxide. These processes occur during breathing, when air enters and exits the body through the nose and mouth. The air that enters the body is rich in oxygen, the gas necessary for many of the cells' basic chemical functions. The respiratory and circulatory systems are very closely related, since both are involved with the oxygenation process.

THE OXYGENATION PROCESS

The circulatory system can be envisioned as a train carrying the oxygen in each car or blood cell. The lungs, then, are the depot terminals where the blood cells pick up oxygen and deposit carbon dioxide. The structures in the body that help the respiratory system do its work include the mouth, nose, pharynx, trachea, bronchi, bronchioles, lungs, alveoli, diaphragm, and various respiratory muscles. The respiratory process involves all of these structures to promote the inhalation and exhalation of air that transports gases to the blood cells and diffuses oxygen into the body (Rosendorff, p. 223).

After the air is inhaled through either the nose or mouth, it travels through the trachea which leads to the bronchi of the lungs. There, the two bronchi, the main airways into the lungs, divide and subdivide numerous times before ultimately forming the bronchioles (see Figure 5-3). The bronchioles are the smallest airways in the lungs and eventually terminate in the numerous alveoli that are the basic respiratory units (see Figure 5-4).

Alveoli are many air-filled sacs that are the site of the actual oxygen–carbon dioxide exchange. In this transaction oxygen is absorbed by the blood, and carbon dioxide is released into the air as the breath is exhaled. Much of the volume within the lungs is taken up by blood undergoing this stage of the oxygenation process.

Because the respiratory and cardiovascular systems are closely related, any damage to one of these systems is likely to directly affect the other (Kart et al., p. 128). A number of other structures are essential for breathing, including the diaphragm and associated respiratory muscles of the chest. These structures aid the lungs in expanding and contracting with each inhalation and exhalation.

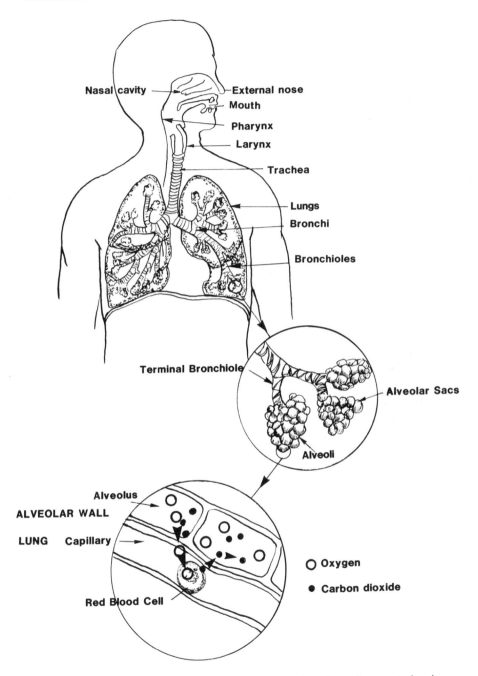

FIGURE 5-3. The respiratory tract. Oxygen–carbon dioxide exchange at alveolar wall where permeation of oxygen and carbon dioxide cells occurs.

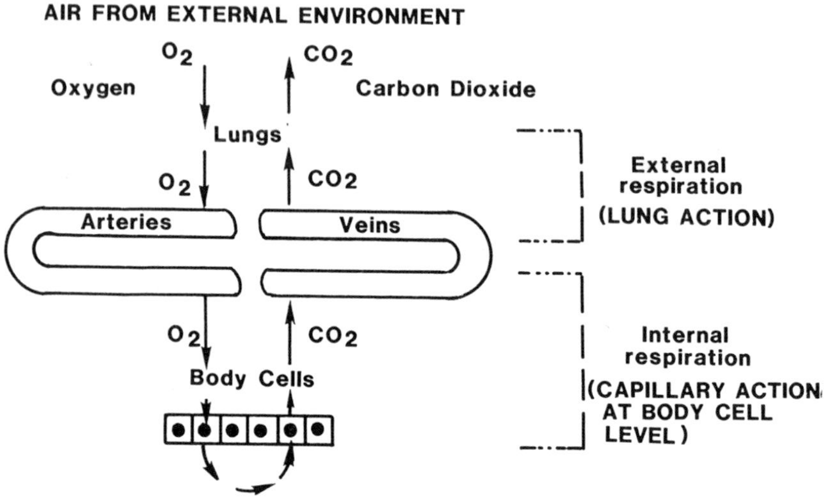

AIR FROM EXTERNAL ENVIRONMENT

FIGURE 5-4. Diagram of events occurring simultaneously during respiration.

AGE-ASSOCIATED CHANGES

Changes associated with the aging process do occur. However, in the elderly person without any significant disease, the overall result of these changes should not be incapacitating or prevent him/her from carrying on the daily routine or activities (Kart et al., p. 129).

One of the reasons for this is that the lung, unlike the heart, has a remarkable ability to repair itself after infection or damage. These repairs normally leave only minor traces that could later be mistaken for degenerative changes (Woodruff & Birren, p. 432). A list of changes due to aging that do affect the respiratory system includes the following (Kenney, p. 42):

- decreasing size (and therefore capacity) of the alveoli
- loss of elasticity of lung tissue
- stiffening of the ribs (requiring muscles to work harder to pump air in and out of the lungs)
- changes in the shape of the chest
- decreased resistance to infection

The decreased capacity of the alveoli is not in itself enough to cause any dramatic changes in the breathing process. However, this does reduce the efficiency of the breathing mechanism and may lead to disability and respiratory problems over time (Weg, p. 270).

The elderly are more prone to infections than the rest of the population (explained further below). When these additional factors are coupled with the fact that the lungs receive foreign materials continuously from the outside air, it is not surprising that many elderly persons suffer from some form of lung disease.

INFLUENCE OF THE ENVIRONMENT ON THE LUNGS

Since the lungs are in almost direct contact with the air outside, the environment may play a more important role in the development of lung disease than in any other body system. Environmental exposure to a lung irritant over a prolonged period of time often produces the type of changes that result in respiratory disease. Some examples are miners' exposure to coal dust, welders' to asbestos, and chronic cigarette smokers' to tar and nicotine.

CHRONIC RESPIRATORY DISEASE

Approximately 6% of nursing home residents suffer from some type of chronic respiratory disease. The most common classification of lung disease is chronic obstructive lung disease (COLD) or chronic obstructive pulmonary disease (COPD). There is no cure for these diseases, but there are a variety of treatments available.

The main complication brought on by COPD is that the body is unable to rid itself of the air containing carbon dioxide. This may be because of a disruption of the alveoli or because the bronchial tubes are not expanding and permitting the gases to escape during respiration.

Chronic bronchitis and emphysema are two diseases of this type that are most commonly seen in the nursing home patient. The signs, symptoms, and treatment of the respiratory diseases mentioned are very similar, since they all affect the lungs. The symptoms listed following the discussion of the next two diseases will apply to all the diseases in the remainder of this section.

Chronic Bronchitis

As the name suggests, chronic bronchitis is caused by a continuing irritation of the bronchii (the two airways into the lungs). The inside of these airways swell and become clogged with mucus secretions, making it more difficult to breathe. This may be due to something irritating from the environment or a recurrent infection. Chronic smokers are the ones most likely to develop bronchitis. This disease is the most common respiratory condition found in the elderly.

Emphysema

Emphysema results in a loss of elasticity in all of the lung tissue. As a consequence, the lung is less able to hold as much air, but the alveoli tend to have air trapped inside causing carbon dioxide to build up. The increasing amount of carbon dioxide only worsens the respiratory condition because the body is triggered to obtain more and more oxygen to compensate for this imbalance.

The causes of emphysema are similar to those for bronchitis, the most common one being a recurrent infection or chronic irritant to the lung. Emphysema is much more serious than bronchitis, and usually patients with this disease die from heart failure as a result of prolonged stress on the cardiovascular system.

Symptoms common for most lung diseases are chronic cough, increased production of thick white mucus, and some shortness of breath. These symptoms are a result of the body attempting to rid itself of whatever is irritating the respiratory tract. Irritation of the inner lining of the respiratory tract results in the increased production of mucus, which is intended to coat the cause of the irritation and assist its excretion from the body.

A cough is another way the body has of rejecting whatever is causing the irritation. When this irritation is chronic, these mechanisms are continually being triggered.

These lung disease symptoms can be found in more severe forms:

- stress on the entire cardiovascular system with related symptoms
- enlarged heart
- heart failure (with emphysema)
- thick mucus plugs blocking the smaller airways within the lung
- alveoli that have become overinflated and eventually burst, decreasing the amount of space available for oxygen exchange
- barrel-shaped chest
- poor appetite
- weight loss
- dizziness

Treatments include medications for the purpose of minimizing airway irritation and obstruction, such as *bronchodilators*—to relax the breathing tubes, widening them and thus improving air flow—and *expectorants*, to thin the mucus so that coughing is more successful.

Pneumonia

Pneumonia is an infection in the lungs caused by either a virus or by bacteria. Patients with chronic obstructive lung disease (COLD) are much more susceptible to this infection because bacteria grow in stagnant areas like those where the mucus is collecting. This infection further complicates the elderly person's ability to breathe, and causes disruptions in other systems.

The **signs and symptoms** are very similar to those already described and may include a fever or very weak condition resulting from the infection. **Treatment** generally includes some type of antibiotic therapy when bacteria are the cause of this infection.

Chronic Tuberculosis

Tuberculosis is an infectious disease more commonly found in nursing home residents because of their higher risk of infection, resulting from multiple chronic diseases.

Tuberculosis may infect a person while he/she is young, but many times a healthy immune system wards off the disease, which goes into a dormant state. As a person ages, this immunity may break down with an infection, and the dormant disease may become active.

Signs and symptoms are similar to those listed for COLD, except that the secretions contain the tuberculosis bacteria. The disease is termed infectious because it may easily be transmitted through the secretions or when a patient coughs.

One of the most important **treatments** then is to isolate the patient as long as he/she is coughing and producing sputum. To prevent the spread of infection, staff and the patient's visitors generally are required to wear masks and gloves when in contact with the patient or in his/her room (see infection control diagram).

Lung Cancer

Lung cancer is a chronic lung disease and is among the leading causes of death for American men. It is also the most prevalent form of cancer found among nursing home patients. Since the disease affects the lung, **symptoms** are similar to those of COLD.

Generally, the nursing home resident is receiving palliative treatment (just enough therapy to make him/her comfortable). Other types of **treatment** include radiation, chemotherapy, or surgery, depending on the size and location of the tumor.

5.3.3 Nervous System

One of the body's most important mechanisms is the nervous system, which acts as its control center by coordinating functions and maintaining order. The brain can be thought of as a computer system with the nerves and spinal cord transferring input and output messages to and from each part of the body.

Some of its specific functions of the nervous system for control of the body include responding to events outside the body through the five senses, performing voluntary activities such as walking, and storing memories, ideas, and emotions so they may be used at a later time for various thought processes. The nervous system also performs automatic responses such as breathing, maintaining heart rate, and controlling temperature.

COMPONENTS OF THE CENTRAL NERVOUS SYSTEM

The central nervous system is composed of the *brain, spinal cord,* and *nerves.* The brain is considered by some to be the most important organ in the body because it is accorded a high level of priority among body functions. When the body is undergoing a great deal of stress, other organs will reduce nutrient intake so that more nutrients can be directed to the brain.

The brain is protected by the skull and surrounded inside by a protective layer of cerebrospinal fluid. This organ is very specialized, with different areas responsible for different body functions.

The *cranial nerves* connect the brain with the areas of the body responsible for sensory perception (identifying what is outside the body through the senses, including taste, smell, and hearing). The base of the brain is called the *medulla.* It is primarily responsible for controlling motor activity or movement. It is this area that connects the brain to the spinal cord.

The spinal cord looks like a tree trunk, with the nerves representing the branches of the tree and eventually leading to the blood vessels, muscles, and/or organs throughout the body.

The brain itself is made up of many specialized cells that are unique to the individual areas of the brain in which they are found. Because the brain cells perform complex processes, they need large amounts of oxygen to function continually. A lack of oxygen to the brain causes the cells and their tissues to die within minutes.

The nerves are composed of many individual fibers that are encased in a fatty substance called *myelin* for the same reason that electrical wires are covered with a plastic coating: to prevent them from "shorting out." These individual fibers are composed of neurons, which are the nerve cells. Unlike the heart cells, nerve cells can be replaced or regenerate themselves, although at a very slow rate.

The nerve fibers form an intricate network that is responsible for carrying a variety of messages to the brain. These messages are carried in the form of electrical impulses that stimulate the appropriate area of the brain, triggering either an involuntary response reaction (reflex) or a thought (cognitive) process.

The nerve fibers form a complex series of pathways that impulses travel along to reach the brain. It is important to remember that the left side of the brain controls the functions on the right side of the body, and the right side of the brain controls functions on the left side of the body.

POSSIBLE EFFECTS OF AGING

The effects of aging on the nervous system are most commonly believed to be the result of a change in the cerebrovascular system that reduces the oxygen supply to the brain cells. This can lead to permanent alterations to those cells which are so sensitive to the level of the oxygen supply (Woodruff & Birren, p. 263).

Apparently the weight of the brain decreases with age, possibly because of some loss of brain cells and nerve fibers (Kenney, p. 65). Researchers, using refined instruments, have been able to detect changes in the neurological system of the elderly when observing the speed with which impulses are transmitted to the brain. But this change is not directly associated with a slowing down of functioning in the thought process. It is probably a myth that older people's thought or cognitive process is much slower than other age groups.

PERCEPTUAL CHANGES

One of the perceptual changes commonly attributed to the aging process is a decreased sensitivity to touch (Kenney, p. 72).

Some of the visual changes associated with age include loss of range of vision for near objects, decreased flexibility of the lens of the eye, and reduced clarity of vision, or the "dusty windshield" effect of the lens of the eye, accompanied by a loss in ability to distinguish pastels.

There may be a change in the central processing of sound in the inner ear. This has not been proved as yet, so patients who are hard of hearing are not necessarily that way just because of age. There does appear to be loss of ability to hear high-pitched sounds; speaking to patients in deep tones can help compensate for this loss.

In many elderly individuals the taste buds appear to have degenerated, and the amount of saliva produced also appears to be diminished, producing a change in the capacity to taste different flavors. Abuse of salt may result from patient efforts to "improve" or increase taste sensations. Ability to taste sweets is apparently unaffected, which may explain the preference of many elderly patients for eating dessert first.

There may also be an age-related decrease in neurons responsible for smell, resulting in the loss of smell for different odors.

Some of the elderly also appear to dream less and have increased periods of wakefulness thoughout the night (Libow, p. 7).

Diseases associated with the nervous system include those that affect sensory components, impair mobility and communication processes, and affect the ability to distinguish reality from fantasy (Steffl, p. 303).

THE EYE

The eye is a complicated structure, with muscles holding it in place. The retina is the innermost layer of the eye and contains receptor cells that actually generate electrical nerve impulses when hit by light. These impulses are carried to the brain on the nerve fibers that leave the retina and form the optic nerve. This nerve leads to the area of the brain responsible for vision. The retina is protected by the lens covering the eye.

The lens can be thought of as a layer of skin except that all of the old cells on the lens cannot be discarded like old layers of skin, and they are continually compacted within the eye (Corso, p. 39). The aqueous humor is a substance that bathes the eye and protects it as well.

Presence of Eye Problems

Approximately 33% of all nursing home residents experience some form of visual impairment, and 5.5% of these patients are blind. About 61% were found to wear some type of eyeglasses to correct their vision (Hing, p. 17).

The aging process may result in an overproduction of aqueous humor, resulting in a large amount within the eye. When this happens, glaucoma may result.

Glaucoma. Glaucoma is a chronic condition that is actually a complex of many different symptoms. This condition is not a direct result of the aging process, but the incidence of the disease is definitely greater among older individuals (Corso, p. 5).

There are four different types of glaucoma: (a) chronic, (b) acute, (c) secondary, and (d) congenital. In each of these, the primary problem is that *fluids within the eye undergo increasing pressure changes*. These fluids are continually being formed but not draining from the eye chamber because of some disruption in the drainage system. As a result, the eyeball itself becomes very hard. This also causes an extremely painful pressure in the eye, which can lead to a range of other conditions.

Symptoms of glaucoma can include acute pain in the eye, elevated blood pressure, blurred vision, and halos seen around lights. Untreated glaucoma can lead to blindness.

Treatment usually varies with the form or stage of disease, but initially medical therapy is used to promote the drainage of excess fluids from the eye. As a rule, medications are the critical variable in preventing blindness from glaucoma (Steffl, p. 54).

Mydriatics are a kind of medication that usually comes in the form of eyedrops that act to dilate the pupil of the eye, helping to drain off some of the excess fluid.

Cataracts. A cataract is a cloudiness that affects the transparency of the lens to the extent that light cannot get through to the retina of the eye. The retina is the area of the eye that transforms light into the objects seen. Usually cataracts form in both eyes.

The major **symptom** of cataracts is increasingly blurred vision, with perceptions of "shadows." **Treatment** usually consists of eyeglasses or contact lenses. The lens can be surgically removed and replaced with a new one (lens implant).

Importance of Vision Among Patients

When older persons with visual impairments are assisted to see better through intervention, they adapt much better to the area around them. Interventions do not need to be complex. They can include provision of large-type books, magazines, and newspapers; painting color-coded boundaries and walkways throughout the facility for easy identification; using large letters and numbers in all visual displays such as doors, elevators, and clocks.

HEARING

The structures of the *outer ear* include those portions of the ear external to the eardrum (tympanic membrane). The *middle ear* contains three small bones that conduct the sound waves; they are called the incus, the malleus, and the stapes.

The *inner ear* contains the cochlea, which transmits sound waves to nerve impulses that travel down the auditory nerve (the eighth cranial nerve) to the auditory center of the brain.

Hearing Impairments

Presbycusis is the term used to describe any hearing impairment in old age. Approximately 26% of nursing home residents suffer some hearing impairment, and it has been estimated that 5% of the residents are deaf (Hing, pp. 17, 63). However, only 6% of residents use hearing aids (which, in any case, are not invariably helpful).

Hearing impairments can also be due to a buildup of wax in the ear or to what is known as a conductive or sensorineural hearing loss. Conductive disorders and ear wax are the only ones that may be treated effectively. Usually surgery or hearing aids are prescribed for those with a conductive loss. The sensorineural disturbances result from a disruption in the structure of the inner ear or the nerve pathway to the brain stem.

Symptoms of hearing impairment can include tinnitus (an intermittent, sometimes constant ringing in the ears), progressive hearing loss, and increased inability to hear high-frequency sounds, including shouting, warning bells, or buzzers.

Treatment can include a hearing aid when appropriate; sign language; lipreading; speech reading; slow, well-enunciated communication; always facing the patient when speaking to him/her; and providing appropriate warning signals to communicate the presence of fires or other dangerous occurrences within the facility.

MOBILITY AND COMMUNICATION

A *cerebrovascular accident* (CVA), also known as a stroke, can be one of the most debilitating conditions that an elderly person faces. It is believed that 16% of nursing home residents have suffered from some form of stroke. The cause of stroke is lack of oxygen to the brain, usually resulting from the blockage of a major blood vessel or the leakage of blood from a vessel that has ruptured.

Warning signs can include weakness of some muscles, depression, and a tingling in the arm or leg.

Degrees of Disability

The degree of disability resulting from a stroke may range from only a slight impairment to complete immobility and loss of voluntary muscle control. *Signs following a stroke are usually specifically related to the area of the brain affected.* These symptoms may include the following:

muscle weakness on one side of the body (hemiplegia)
difficulty standing or walking
poor balance
pain in arms and legs
fatigue
poor vision
confusion
difficulty in spatial judgment, distortion
complete loss of muscle control (quadraplegia)
paralysis of the body below the upper extremities (paraplegia)
difficulty speaking (aphasia)

Aphasia.   Aphasia is the term used to describe an inability to interpret and formulate language. Specifically, such problems may be seen as a slowdown in ability to retrieve vocabulary and inappropriate use of grammar or words, as well as problems in understanding what is being said.

Usually this occurs because the area of the brain responsible for speech is damaged during the stroke. There are many different types of aphasia, with the most severe resulting in an individual being unable to understand what others are saying to him/her (receptive aphasia).

Other types of aphasia result in an inability to express in words what the individual really wants to communicate (expressive aphasia). Other times, inappropriate words or vulgar language is uttered as if the individual had no control of what he/she says.

Dysarthria.   Dysarthria (literally, imperfect articulation of speech) is a speech rather than a language abnormality that may accompany paralysis, weakness, or uncoordination. This deficit can be a frustrating experience for the patient who has all other mental capacities intact. This frustration often leads to emotional upset. The most important need that patients have at this time is the ability to communicate. The incidence of these disorders may exceed 50% in a skilled nursing facility (Corso, p. 211).

Individually designed rehabilitative therapy is the most usual form of **treatment**. The ability of a nursing home patient to recover from a stroke is best correlated with the cause. Lower brain stem damage from a stroke has a more favorable prognosis than any assault on the upper part of the brain (Adams, p. 145).

Rehabilitation therapy usually focuses on standing, ambulation, taking initial steps, and walking with a cane or another appliance. Physical and occupational therapists are integral members of the rehabilitation team for these patients.

Parkinson's Disease.   Parkinson's disease is actually a group of symptoms that can progressively lead to complete disability in those severely affected. Scientists believe that selected groups of neurons (nerve cells) in the brain are lost as a result of this disease, but the cause of this loss remains a mystery.

Symptoms of Parkinson's disease can include tremor, or trembling, of any of the limbs while at rest, rigidity or muscle stiffness, and bradykinesia (a slowness in body movements). Additional symptoms may include the following:

- stooped posture while standing
- walking with short, shuffling steps
- garbled speech
- illegible handwriting
- sad, lifeless facial expression
- facial droop
- mood swings
- dementia (an impairment in intellectual ability)

There is no cure for Parkinson's disease, so the treatment is determined by the specific symptoms and degree of physical impairment in functioning.

Often patients with Parkinson's disease suffer from mental disturbances similar to those seen in patients with Alzheimer's disease, and physicians are finding it difficult to distinguish one from the other. Alzheimer's patients have the additional diagnosis of dementia.

Dementia.   More than one-half of nursing home residents may have some form of dementing illness (Gwyther, p. 435). Dementia is usually thought of as senility in an elderly person and may include behaviors such as forgetfulness, a deterioration in personality, and a decrease in intellectual functioning.

A common misperception is that these behaviors are all a normal result of the aging process. But none of these senile behaviors are considered to be normal aging effects and are instead due to some type of disease or disruption.

Hardening of the arteries due to arteriosclerosis is a disease that may lead to dementia in the elderly patient. In this situation, the arteries do not allow enough oxygen to pass through to the brain, with the result that areas of the brain die. This condition is also referred to as multi-infarct dementia and may affect 20% of elderly patients.

Alzheimer's Disease.   Alzheimer's disease is the most common form of dementia seen in persons over 60 years old; its incidence increases dramatically after that age. The Alzheimer's patient displays an intellectual impairment that is irreversible. The disease progression varies from patient to patient and can extend from 1 year to over a decade (Schneck et al., p. 171). The cause of Alzheimer's is not yet known.

Three distinct phases of Alzheimer's disease have been identified as: I— forgetfulness or early stage, II—confusion or mild stage, and III— dementia or terminal stage (Schneck et al., p. 166; Gwyther & Matteson, p. 93).

The **signs and symptoms** of the disease vary with each stage, but some, including memory loss and behavioral changes, progress in severity until they become profound in the final stage. The following list of signs and symptoms reveals the progressive nature of the disease:

Stage I
  memory loss
  time disorientation
  anxiety
  irritability
  lack of spontaneity
  behavior and personality change
  agitation
  inability to concentrate for long periods of time
Stage II
  excessive hunger
  aphasia
  temper tantrums
  restlessness
  muscle twitching
  aimless wandering, sometimes getting lost
  inability to read, write or do arithmetic calculations
  obsessional behavior (e.g., constantly washing and rewashing hands)
  repetitive movements (e.g., tapping, chewing, lip licking)
Stage III (usually the shortest phase)
  bedridden
  unable to form purposeful movement, i.e., walk
  poor appetite
  poor articulation
  incontinent
  emaciation
  frequent seizures

There is no cure for Alzheimer's disease. The goal of treatment for these patients is to achieve the highest quality of life while maintaining physical function.

Unlike Parkinson's disease, there is no one medication that can significantly alter the signs and symptoms associated with the disease. Those that are prescribed serve only to relieve them. Usually tranquilizers are used to relax the patient and relieve any agitation or violence. Antidepressants are also prescribed to improve the overall mood.

5.3.4 Digestive System

Digestion is the process through which the body breaks down food into needed nutrients. These nutrients are further broken down into particles small enough to pass through tissues and enter the bloodstream for delivery to the appropriate tissues and organs. After absorbing necessary nutrients, the leftover materials or waste products are discarded from the body.

The digestive system is commonly referred to as the gastrointestinal or alimentary tract in reference to the various organs that participate in the digestive process (see Figures 5-5 and 5-6).

MOUTH

Digestion begins when food enters the mouth. Chewing the food is an important step in preparing it for digestion. Saliva, produced by salivary glands in the mouth, contains *enzymes* that begin breaking down food substances while they are still in the mouth.

ESOPHAGUS

After food is swallowed, it enters the esophagus. The esophagus is the tube (made of smooth muscle) connecting the mouth to the stomach. When food is swallowed, the gastric (stomach) sphincter relaxes to allow food into the stomach. Swallowing initiates a wavelike movement of the esophagus (called peristalsis) that propels food toward the stomach.

STOMACH

The next phase of digestion begins in the stomach. The stomach has sphincters (muscles) at both ends that close when the stomach is full, enabling the stomach acids to have sufficient time to break down the food. The digestive process in the stomach is controlled by the brain through the nerves, which constantly carry impulses directing the digestion process.

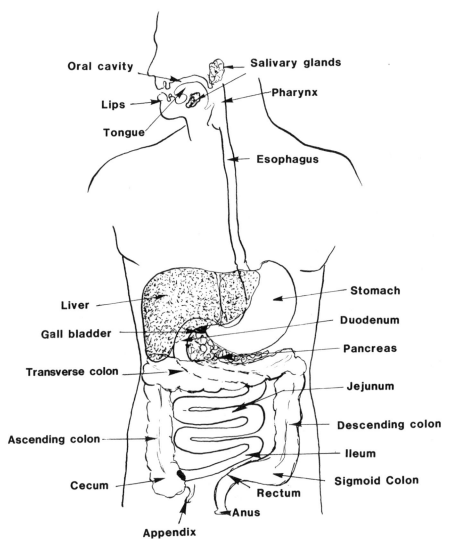

FIGURE 5-5. Organs involved in the digestive processes.

INTESTINES

The intestines may be thought of as a long tube. The intestines are also referred to as the bowels or lower gastrointestinal tract (lower GI). Despite its name, the small intestine is actually much longer than the large intestine.

When the digestive contents enter the small intestine (duodenum), further chemical digestive actions occur. The food is in liquid form at this

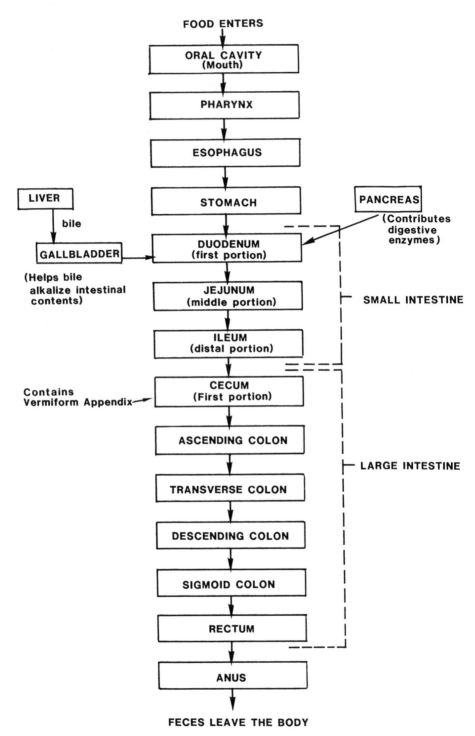

FIGURE 5-6. Diagrammatic representation of the path of food through the digestive system.

stage and contains powerful enzymes that break down certain substances. The intestines are also filled with a supply of bacteria that help to digest some of the food substances. These same bacteria are very harmful to any other part of the body if allowed to escape.

Like the stomach, the intestines also have nerves carrying impulses to and from the brain. These nerves are especially important in stimulating the bowel to move the waste materials along the intestinal tract. As in the esophagus, the intestines contract in snakelike movements (peristalsis), propelling the food along the digestive tract.

If for some reason the brain does not send the appropriate impulses to the intestines, the waste moves much more slowly through these organs. Unlike the esophagus, the intestines do not have the added force of gravity to assist in this process.

LARGE INTESTINE

The large intestine is a continuation of the small intestine and plays its own role in the digestive process. One function of the large intestine is to store the waste so that the body can absorb excess fluids and nutrients before elimination.

By the time waste materials are excreted from the body, they are in a solid form, often referred to as feces or stool. It is important to note that normally patients have voluntary control over when they choose to eliminate these waste materials because the sphincters at the very end of the digestive tract are within the realm of voluntary control.

POSSIBLE EFFECTS OF AGING

Mouth

The amount of saliva secreted by the salivary glands may decrease. The saliva also may become thicker, until it is almost like mucus (MacHudis, p. 400). The loss of teeth may also cause digestive complications (Libow, p. 314).

Esophagus

In some elderly persons food may not travel as quickly through the esophagus. Causes for this appear to be (a) a reduction in the effectiveness of the swallowing mechanism helping foods move toward the stomach, and (b) the gastric sphincter failing to relax as quickly as before (Kenney, p. 61).

Stomach

The lining of the stomach can decrease in thickness with age. This decreased thickness of the lining may allow the size of the stomach to increase. The amount of acid produced by the stomach may decrease (Sklar, p. 206, Kenney, p. 62).

DIGESTIVE DISEASES

The digestive tract is an area of the body about which elderly nursing home patients often complain. Physicians use the general diagnosis of "gastro-intestinal distress" to describe a range of diseases affecting this system.

Esophagus

The esophagus may be a common site of discomfort for the elderly patient. *Esophagitis* (inflammation or irritation of the esophagus) is another name for heartburn, a frequent problem for elderly individuals. Often this sharp, burning pain may be confused with chest pain and may become worse when the patient lies flat, allowing stomach contents to reenter the esophagus.

Dysphagia is difficulty in swallowing or transferring food from the mouth to the esophagus. Persons with neurological damage may be subject to this problem. Persons who have recently suffered a stroke can be at increased risk because without this function they may aspirate (inhale particles of) food into their lungs.

Stomach

Peptic ulcers may occur anywhere in the gastrointestinal tract. Two of the most common types are *gastric ulcers* that affect the mid-stomach and *duodenal ulcers* that involve the lower stomach.

An ulcer is a wearing away of the inner lining of the stomach wall and is due to a chronic buildup of excessive levels of acid. Excessive stress, inactivity, prolonged bed rest, severe trauma, and irritating drugs may all serve to cause or irritate this condition.

Ulcer **symptoms** can include sharp burning abdominal pain 1 to 4 hr after eating, nausea, weight loss, blood in vomitus, and blood in stools.

The goal of **treatment** is to prevent any complications arising from the initial ulceration, thus allowing it to heal. Medications, including antacids, are prescribed to relieve the condition.

Intestines

Constipation is an irregularity in or lack of elimination of waste materials from the body. Twenty-four percent of all nursing home residents have reported this to be a problem, and in one study more than 34% of elderly patients used laxatives at least once a week (Hing, p. 23; Meza, Peggs, & O'Brien, p. 695).

Constipation may initially be a decrease in the number of stools passed, progressing to a complete lack of stool or bowel movements. When the patient has not been able to pass stool for a long period of time, an *impaction* (blockage) has probably occurred. The waste in the large intestine has accumulated in one area and become hard because much of the fluid content has been reabsorbed by the body.

Treatment of constipation can include laxative medications, which are commonly prescribed for nursing home patients. Bulk laxatives, osmotic laxatives, suppositories, and enemas are the different forms of medications that may be prescribed. Increased activity is one of the best treatments.

Hemorrhoids are another painful disturbance that can affect the elimination of waste materials from the body. A hemorrhoid is a vein in either the rectum (internal) or around the anus (external) that becomes enlarged. The external type are usually more painful for the patient. Hemorrhoids may either be the cause or result of chronic constipation.

Incontinence is the inability to control the timing of elimination. Some of the causes of this dysfunction may be a neurological disturbance due to disease or trauma to the brain and spinal cord, anal surgery, chronic diarrhea, or mental disturbance. Urinary incontinence is often caused by impaction.

5.3.5 Nutrition

Food provides the body with the nutrients necessary to cell functioning. Adequate nutrition can be of value in the maintenance of fitness and independence as well as prevention of disease (Franz, p. 40).

In the above section on digestion, the digestive process was described as the time when foods are initially broken down into nutrients so they can be absorbed by the body. The next phase of nutrition is the *metabolic process* whereby the remainder of the nutrients are absorbed, helping to produce energy and/or control the various body functions.

Metabolism is the transformation process in which nutrients undergo various chemical reactions throughout the body, producing energy while also helping cells perform necessary functions. *Calories* are the units of measurement for determining the amount of energy that is contained in foods or used by the body. Below is a list of some of the nutrients considered essential to the body. All of these occur naturally in foods and can be obtained from a well balanced diet.

Protein is a nutrient that can be broken down into components called *amino acids.* Protein is necessary for growth, repair of damaged tissues, transporting nutrients and chemicals throughout the body, and producing various hormones and enzymes.

Carbohydrates can be broken down quickly into readily available fuel for the body. Two common sources are starches and sugars. The brain is especially sensitive to any decreased levels of carbohydrates in the body and may be permanently damaged whenever the level is reduced for a period of time.

Fats are considered to be the body's source of energy reserve. Fat forms a protective padding around the major organs, prevents heat loss from the body, and carries vitamins A, D, E, and K, helping with their absorption.

Minerals needed by the body include

> *Calcium*—used to build bones and teeth, giving them their hard structure; also helps to clot blood.
> *Iron*—important in building healthy red blood cells that are able to carry oxygen.
> *Sodium*—acts as a buffering mechanism, helps dissolve substances in the bloodstream, monitors the amount of fluid in the body.
> *Potassium*—contained in fluids and tissues; important in muscle contraction, maintains the body fluid balance, and also acts as a buffering mechanism in the bloodstream.

Vitamins act to control certain body functions and regulate the body's utilization of other foods.

FLUIDS

Internally, the body is bathed in fluids that help to eliminate wastes and assist the cells with chemical reactions. Fluids help maintain the integrity of the body by protecting the skin and distributing nutrients to promote healing. Some major body fluids include

> *Plasma*—carries red blood cells and essential nutrients throughout the body.
> *Cerebrospinal fluid*—protects the brain and spinal cord.
> *Lymphatic fluid*—carries white blood cells and fluids from the tissues.

In all phases of life, adequate nutrition sustains the building-up processes of the body and impedes the wearing-out processes (Albanese, p. 20). However, elderly patients suffering from multiple chronic diseases may need even more nutrients than the healthy adult.

POSSIBLE EFFECTS OF AGING

The elderly are believed by some researchers to require fewer calories in the diet because of reduction in body weight, a decrease in the metabolic rate, and often a decline in physical activity (Albanese, p. 23; Franz, pp. 41–42). However, at the same time that it may be desirable to reduce the amount of carbohydrates and fats, the elderly person has an increased demand for nutrients to enable him/her to resist the effects of disease. Thus, the appropriate diet for an older person is complex.

Osteoporosis, a softening of the bones, is a concern among numerous elderly persons. It has been observed frequently in women over 40. A lack of sufficient amounts of calcium may contribute to a softening of the bones, making some nursing facility residents especially susceptible to bone breakage in falls or other accidents.

Dehydration may occur more easily among older persons if they reduce their fluid intake. Smaller proportions of fat under the skin may permit body fluids to evaporate more readily than previously. Dehydration can occur quickly when an elderly person has a fever.

Aging may affect other structures that aid in digestion. Loss of teeth can result in changes in the types of foods eaten. Loss of weight generally causes problems with fitting of dentures; refitting is often necessary.

A loss in the overall number of cells and muscle mass may decrease body weight. In this situation the body may no longer need as many calories to provide sufficient energy.

As with any person, consumption of more calories than needed while remaining relatively inactive can lead to obesity—more and more fat being stored in the tissues as reserve energy. Obesity has been referred to as a frequent form of malnutrition in the elderly (Foley, p. 295).

PRESCRIBED DIETS

Although the majority of nursing facility residents will eat normal diets, some residents will have special nutritional needs. Chronic disease and the effects of institutionalization on appetite pose a challenge.

Physicians often prescribe special therapeutic diets for this group. The following are among the most common:

Soft diet—for patients who need a diet that is low in fiber, soft in texture, and mild in flavor.

Mechanical soft diet—same as above, except texture is either chopped, pureed, or ground to make foods easier to chew.

Strict full-liquid diet—consists of foods and liquids that are liquid at body temperature but can include cold ice cream and hot soup.

High-fiber diet—to provide bulk; similar to regular diet but with foods that are difficult to digest, e.g., fruits, vegetables, whole-grain breads and cereals, nuts, and bran.

High-calorie–high-protein diet—may include milk shakes, meats, and similar foods, to provide additional sources of protein.

When patients cannot eat normally, nasogastric, esophagostomy, or gastrostomy tube feeding may be prescribed by the physician.

Nasogastric tubes are inserted through the nose and enter the stomach. Esophagostic tubes pass through the neck into the esophagus. Gastrostomy tubes are surgically inserted directly into the stomach.

Gastrostomy tubes may be preferred for patients needing long-term tube feeding, e.g., a cancer patient, because they can be more comfortable and there is no chance for fluids to flow into the patient's lungs (aspiration) when the tube is mistakenly inserted into the trachea (lung cavity) instead of the stomach cavity. These tubes also will not irritate the lining of the upper gastrointestinal tract as may nasogastric tubes.

Enteral feeding is a recent innovation using such products as Osmolite or Ensure. In this case the feeding tube is inserted nasogastrically but continues into the duodenum (past the stomach into the opening of the small intestine). A pump feeding tube similar to an IV arrangement delivers the nutrients to enter the duodenum.

The obvious advantage is to reduce the possibility of aspiration occurring, since the nutrients are introduced into the small intestine itself. The disadvantage is that a permanently inserted tube between the stomach and duodenum must be inserted with the use of an X-ray machine, usually in a hospital setting. If it gets stopped up or is pulled out by the patient, an immediate trip to the hospital is required for reinsertion.

ANEMIA AND DIABETES: TWO METABOLIC DISEASE PROCESSES

Two of the most common diseases that disrupt the metabolism of important nutrients are anemia and diabetes.

Anemia is a condition in which hemoglobin is deficient, resulting in the body not getting enough oxygen. The red blood cells contain a substance called hemoglobin, which carries the oxygen. *Diabetes* occurs when the body is unable to metabolize glucose (sugar) because of a problem with a hormone, called insulin, that is produced by a ductless gland called the pancreas.

Anemia

Various types of anemia are found in the nursing facility. It is thought to be due to disease, not old age (Freedman, p. 136), and the therapy for each type of anemia is varied. About 5% of nursing home residents probably suffer from some form of chronic anemia (Hing, p. 56).

Anemia is the result of a significant decrease in the number of red blood cells produced. Having multiple chronic diseases can lead to anemia. Symptoms of anemia are similar to those for heart disease because they also result in a problem with oxygenation. When anemia is combined with other diseases, such as peripheral vascular disease or coronary artery disease, it may be very serious as well as painful for the patient.

Diabetes

Diabetes affects about 15% of all nursing home residents (Hing, p. 56). It results from an inability to convert carbohydrates in the body to forms the body can utilize.

Normally, the pancreas produces the hormone insulin, which helps the cells convert sugars (or glucose) into a form for energy use or storage. Diabetics either produce insufficient amounts of this hormone or have some difficulty in utilizing insulin. The result is large amounts of sugar continually circulating in the bloodstream, causing the condition known as *hyperglycemia* (high blood sugar).

Chronic hyperglycemia can damage many of the tissues in the body. Hyperglycemia can cause complications and disabilities in other systems in the body. In its more extreme form diabetes is a factor in the cause of blindness and amputation for elderly patients.

There are two different classifications of persons with diabetes: *insulin dependent* and *non-insulin dependent*. Insulin-dependent diabetics have generally had the disease since childhood and require daily doses (or the equivalent) for control of the disease. About 10% of the nursing home diabetic population fall into this category (Bazzare, p. 257). Non-insulin–dependent diabetics, usually diagnosed while adults, are generally able to control the disease by dietary restrictions and the use of oral hypo-glycemics (Bazzare, p. 258).

Much of the **treatment** provided to nursing home residents involves monitoring the blood sugar levels. Fasting blood sugar tests determine the blood sugar content. Another method is to measure the amount of glucose in the resident's urine at specific times of the day.

5.3.6 External and Internal Defense Mechanisms

The body is equipped with special defense mechanisms to protect it from harmful disruptions in the environment. Two different types of defense mechanisms serve the body.

THE BARRIER SYSTEM OF DEFENSE

The first type acts as barriers preventing harmful substances from entering the body. The largest organ acting as a barrier is the *skin*. While protecting the body from harmful organisms, the skin also seals in essential body fluids and regulates the body temperature. The respiratory, intestinal, and urinary tracts also have barrier-like components to protect the body from foreign materials that may enter through their systems.

In the respiratory tract, thousands of cilia (small hairlike elements) line the passageways and help propel outward any foreign materials that may be inhaled from the air. Coughing expells these particles from the body and back into the air.

Two additional barrier-like protections are the acid composition of gastric juices and urine, which also act to protect each of those systems from the entrance of harmful organisms.

THE CHEMICAL DEFENSE SYSTEM

The immune system is often referred to as the second line of defense; it protects the internal structures of the body. Whenever foreign material or an antigen enters the body, the components of the immune system recognize this and mobilize for an attack response. Most often, the foreign material is a small bacterial or viral microorganism.

Different types of antibodies have various means of fighting an infection and use a much more complex interaction than that seen in the cell-mediated response.

INFECTIONS

When bacteria or viruses are successful in penetrating the defense mechanisms in large numbers or are allowed to enter areas of the body where they are not normally found, the resulting disruption is known as an *infection*. Nursing home residents are more prone to infections than other population groups because of:

- age-related changes in their bodies
- the presence of multiple chronic diseases (weakening the defenses)
- associated use of multiple medications with side effects that may compromise the body
- increased incidence of immobility and incontinence
- frequent use of invasive devices such as indwelling urinary catheters

These factors all increase nursing home residents' susceptibility to infections and also serve to weaken their body's own natural defense mechanisms.

Nosocomial Infections

Infections that are associated with institutionalization or acquired while in a health care facility are called nosocomial infections. Nursing home residents are considered to be at a particular risk of developing these infections because of the high levels of group interaction and activities among residents (Garibaldi, Brodine, & Matsumiya, p. 734).

Farber, Brennen, Punteri, and Brody found that half of all infections in the chronic-care facility they studied may be due to nosocomially acquired pneumonia or urinary tract infections and that these two infections are commonly responsible for morbidity (illness) in the elderly population (p. 502). Some of the other types of nosocomial infections often seen in the nursing home include infections of the skin, soft tissues, and gastrointestinal tract (Farber et al., p. 514; Nicolle, McIntyre, Zacharias, & MacDonald, p. 646).

The Inflammation Response

Inflammation occurs in the physical responses by the other body systems when fighting off infection or some external threat. The blood vessels dilate (expand) bringing more cells to combat the unwanted component. This is often the cause of redness surrounding areas of skin that may become infected. The debris from the antigen often become pus, which may drain from the infection as well (Groenwald, p. 647).

Special Difficulties in Identifying Infections

Infections in the elderly may be more difficult to diagnose because it is possible to confuse the symptoms with those of other chronic diseases. Also, even when symptoms are present, the elderly resident may be reluctant to complain about these disruptions, so they are less likely to be reported (Beck & Smith, p. 273).

Most infections are not considered to be chronic diseases because they respond to treatment, and their damage to the body can often be reversed. Some of the possible effects of aging on the immune system are discussed below.

Possible Effects of Aging

The skin contains collagen fibers that change as a person ages. These changes may make the skin and other connective tissue drier and less resilient (Kenney, p. 34).

Skin, nail, and hair cells, which are among the fastest to grow during younger years, often do not replace themselves as quickly when persons age (Carter & Belin, p. 532). Together, these changes help explain why many elderly people have some degree of tough, dry, wrinkled skin (Kenney, p. 37). Kligman also suggests that these types of changes work to diminish the barrier function of the skin as a person ages (p. 40).

A study by Tindall and Smith of 163 persons 64 years of age and older showed that 94% of those elderly individuals studies had "lax" skin, secondary to changes in connective tissue, which contributed to wrinkling and other related manifestations (p. 1039).

The greatest change of the internal immune system is the involution (decrease in size) of the thymus gland; (Weksler, p. 53; Smith, p. 69; Felser & Raff, p. 803). This change is suspected to influence the function of the immune system, but it is still too early to determine the full range of implications this may have on the health of elderly individuals. However, Weksler notes that some impairment of the immune response makes elderly individuals more susceptible to infection (pp. 56–57).

DISEASE PROCESSES

Some of the more prevalent diseases or disruptions that affect either of the body's defense mechanisms are discussed below. Tuberculosis and pneumonia have already been dealt with in greater detail.

Facility Responses to the Presence of Infections: the Infection Control Committee

The federal Conditions of Participation in the Medicare program require skilled nursing facilities to establish infection control committees to monitor facility performance in this area.

Depending on the nature of the infection, various isolation precautions need to be taken to protect other patients, staff, and visitors from acquiring the infection as well. The administrator must also make sure that residents with certain communicable diseases are reported to the state health department. Each state, in cooperation with the U.S. Public Health Service, specifies diseases that must be reported to the state health department.

Infections complicate the elderly residents' disease status and may even increase their chance of death (mortality). Besides this risk, infections may increase the likelihood that a resident will need to be transferred to a hospital for more intensive care (Irvine, VanBuren, & Crossley, p. 107).

These are all reasons why the nursing home administrator needs to understand the dynamics of the elderly resident's defense mechanisms and the subsequent need for adequate infection control practices. Below are some of the more common diseases affecting residents' defense mechanisms.

Skin Disease

Herpes Zoster (shingles). One of the diseases that primarily affects elderly individuals is herpes zoster, more commonly called shingles. This infection is caused by the herpes varicella virus (not to be confused with herpes simplex), which travels along nerve pathways to infect skin cells (Becker, p. 41). Skin covering the chest region and areas surrounding the eye are among the areas more commonly affected by this disease. Residents who suffer from a debilitating disease, such as cancer, are also at greater risk of developing this infection.

Signs and symptoms include itching, usually preceding a rash, reddened areas of the skin (usually along a nerve pathway), vesicles (fluid-filled pimples) often erupting over reddened areas, and burning accompanied by stabbing pain.

At present there is no cure for this form of herpes infection, so **treatment** consists of attempts to alleviate the associated symptoms rather than effect a cure. Steroids are often used to reduce inflammation, which may shorten the length of the infection and provide comfort. Antibiotics are sometimes prescribed to prevent secondary infections, and analgesics to relieve pain.

Decubitus Ulcers

Bed sores, pressure sores, and stasis ulcers (ulcers resulting from tissue death due to reduced blood flow) are all different names describing the same process—tissue breakdown. Stasis ulcers are the sores that result from extremely poor peripheral circulation or peripheral vascular disease.

Tissue breakdown often occurs over a bony prominence (buttocks, elbow, heel, hip, shoulder). These ulcers do not develop from an infection but rather from some form of constant unrelieved pressure on one area of the body.

With all of these ulcers the end result is the same: tissues do not receive an adequate amount of oxygen, so they break down and begin to die. This process is similar to what happens to the heart muscle in coronary artery disease.

Residents at most risk for developing these ulcers are those chronically immobile (paralyzed) because of a stroke or some other incapacitating illness and those experiencing poor nutritional status, constant pain, incontinence or dementia (Husain, p. 347). These ulcers often enlarge to form cavities of dead tissue prone to the development of infection and once enlarged, they are difficult to heal (Kart et al., p. 41).

Decubitus Ulcer Formation. The formation of an ulcer usually occurs when the weight of the body exerts pressure on internal soft tissues by compressing them between skeletal bone and another hard surface. Patients who are immobilized or unable to move by themselves are particularly at risk for developing bedsores. Because these patients cannot, on their own, change position frequently, there is the danger of continuous pressure on one area of their body.

Many of these patients spend much of their time lying on their back, also known as the decubitus position ("decubitus" means lying down). When this occurs, the areas most likely to develop sores are the buttocks, hips, heels, shoulders, ears, and elbows. Similarly, residents who spend long periods sitting up in a chair without moving are also at risk of developing these sores.

Signs and symptoms of decubitus ulcers include

tingling, pale skin color, or other signs that there is a loss of circulation to an area
reddened area of skin over a bony prominence
a sore that will not heal
edema (swelling) of the lower legs and shiny skin

However, these signs are often difficult to recognize before tissue has already died and the ulcer itself has already developed (Rowe & Besdine, p. 51).

Following are some of the main **treatments** the facility may use:

providing special equipment, such as a water mattress
keeping the resident clean and dry

eliminating the source of pressure

working to improve patient's circulation

assuring frequent position changes (at least every 2 hr) for those who are unable to do so themselves

padding feet, elbows, and other areas at high risk of tissue breakdown

frequently assessing the integrity of a patient's skin

changing diet to include foods higher in protein, Vitamin C, and calorie content to promote healing

preventing infection by applying dressings and dispensing antibiotic medications as prescribed

using elastic stockings or Ace wrap bandages, which are often prescribed for the patient with peripheral vascular insufficiency (poor blood circulation in their arms and legs).

Both pressure sores and stasis ulcers are significant disruptions of the skin's protective barrier defense. A study by Garibaldi et al. concluded that 32% of infections originated from this source (p. 733). One of the most severe types of infections that may result is called *sepsis*, a condition in which the circulating bloodstream carries infectious organisms throughout the body.

Attention of the Administrator.   Good nursing care is the best form of overall treatment. Lehman identifies the administrator's role as assuring that evaluation and screening for residents at high risk for developing these ulcers is routinely done.

Approximately two-thirds of these ulcers develop within the first weeks that a patient is institutionalized (Lehman, p. 22). Decubitus ulcer rates are often one of the three or four yardsticks by which the quality of the care given in the facility is judged.

Hypothermia

Hypothermia (low body temperature) is an issue of special concern to nursing home staff. Normally, the body temperature is maintained between 97 and 99 degrees Fahrenheit. Patients in a nursing home facility may be endangered by subtle changes in temperature (Collins et al., p. 353). The elderly resident often may have less insulation from body fat, increasing the risk of hypothermia.

Hypothermia is the sudden appearance of a low body temperature (less than 95 degrees). Often it is difficult to diagnose hypothermia because symptoms may be similar to those of a minor stroke.

When the body temperature drops below 95 degrees, residents are no longer able to feel cold and may be suffering from confusion, so they are often unable to complain of other symptoms, such as skin that is pale, dry, and cool, with low pulse or blood pressure.

Many complications may result from hypothermia, including dehydration, renal failure, pneumonia, and/or cardiac arrhythmias. Treatment is aimed at slowly rewarming the patient back to a normal body temperature, usually with blankets. Residents with multiple chronic diseases may not survive an episode of hypothermia.

Because of the threat of hypothermia, loss of heat in the nursing facility can be a life-threatening situation for the patients.

Cancer

Cancer is actually a group of chronic diseases that affect different areas of the body (Birchenall & Streight, p. 230). Approximately 5% of nursing home residents suffer from some form of cancer (Hing, p. 56). Cancer is discussed here as a disorder of the immune system because cancer cells act as antigens and are known to attack many organs or cells throughout the body.

The growth of cancer cells is markedly different from that of normal cells. They grow much more rapidly and are often released or break out from their initial area of growth (tumor) and travel into the bloodstream or lymphatic channels and then throughout the body. Damage may result either from this rapid cell growth, depleting normal cell food supply, or from actual expansion and crushing of the organ affected.

Another mode for cancer growth occurs when cancerous cells travel from the initial growth to new sites, forming *metastases* or other cancer sites throughout the body. Metastasis is the transfer of disease from one organ or part of the body to another not directly connected with it, due either to transfer of pathogenic microorganisms or transfer of cells.

The cause of cancer is still unknown, but among the different factors believed to play possible roles in this disease are environmental exposure to harmful substances, chronic chemical or biological irritation (drugs, alcohol, smoking, viral infections, radiation), inherited genetic predisposition to the disease, dietary factors, and even behavioral factors.

It has been suggested that some combination of these factors probably best explains the cause of cancer (Fraumeni, p. 61). Often these factors may expose the body to a substance known as a carcinogen, which alters the body's immune response capabilities and allows these substances to enter the body and promote the growth of cancerous cells.

According to Birchenall and Streight (p. 225), the leading types of cancer seen in nursing facility residents, listed in order of prevalence by sex, are

Males—lung, colon, rectum, and prostate
Females—breast, colon, rectum, and lung

Variations in Cancer Treatments.   Different physicians may choose to manage cancer patients with different forms of treatments, depending on the specifics of the disease. Surgery, radiation, and use of chemical therapy are the three most common forms of cancer treatment. There are more than 250 different kinds of cancer; forms of treatment will vary for individual patients according to the severity of their illness.

Problems Associated with Cancer Treatments.   There are many problems associated with cancer treatment. The patient with colon cancer may have undergone surgery to remove the diseased portion of the bowel. If a large enough area has been removed, then the patient will usually also have a *colostomy*, which is an opening on the abdomen where the end of the bowel is brought to the surface and digestive waste materials are collected in a bag attached to an appliance surrounding the site. Depending on the level of independence, residents with colostomies may require additional assistance with this special type of elimination process.

The two other types of cancer treatment (radiation and chemotherapy) may be quite painful for residents because of their associated side effects. One of these is anorexia (continual lack of appetite). When this persists, physicians may prescribe special high-calorie food supplements to maintain the patient's strength and energy, as well as treatments for pain and nausea.

5.3.7 Musculoskeletal System

The muscles and skeleton working together provide two important functions: (a) a supporting framework for all of the other body structures, and (b) mobility, which is closely related to the nursing facility resident's degree of independence and autonomy.

THE SKELETON AND MUSCLES

One of the basic elements of the supporting framework of the body is the skeleton, which is composed of the many bones that meet to form joints. The muscles are attached to the skeleton. The skeleton also protects soft tissues and organs inside the body. This framework dictates an individual's posture, directly affecting personal appearance.

JOINTS

In the body there are 68 joints, which are the points where the ends of two bones meet. These joint bones are covered by cartilage and surrounded by a capsule containing fluid that lubricates the area to enhance movement. The joint is held in place by ligaments.

MOVEMENT

In order for movement to occur, the muscles must first receive a nerve impulse from the brain directing them to contract, then relax. Since the muscles are attached to the bones, when they move, the bone moves also. The joints respond like mechanical levers to assist in completing this movement. Thus, mobility requires coordination between both the nervous and musculoskeletal systems.

POSSIBLE EFFECTS OF AGING

The individual bones contain an inner component—bone marrow—that produces the red blood cells. The remainder of bone consists of a network of fibrous tissue containing salts, which are primarily minerals, such as calcium, that serve to harden and strengthen the bone.

There is some consensus that during the aging process the total amount of bone in the body is decreased. However, to determine the loss, one needs to have measured the amount of bone the individual had at age 35 (Heaney, p. 76).

Higher Risk for Women

Women are at a high risk of experiencing some degree of bone loss following menopause. It has been established that this loss results from a withdrawal of estrogen, which apparently helps promote the body's use of dietary calcium for the purpose of bone growth (Heaney, p. 78).

When bone loss occurs, some of the observable changes are shortened stature and a slumped posture due to a compression of the vertebrae (bones in the spine) and the cartilage discs between them (Grob, p. 236). Often, because of these changes, elderly individuals become stooped and appear to have a hump back. These individuals are also more likely to fracture one of their bones.

While a certain amount of bone loss is associated with aging, much of it in the elderly is a result of *osteoporosis*. There is considerable controversy over the extent to which these changes in the bone can be attributed to normal aging rather than osteoporosis, which will be described below.

Both muscles and bones are made up of connective tissue and collagen. Similar to the collagen-related changes associated with age, muscles also become less elastic as a result of this same process. The most significant age-related muscle change for the elderly is a decrease in the amount throughout the body. In addition, degenerative changes in the nervous system may disturb impulses, decreasing muscle skills. However, it is unclear to what extent, if any, these changes in bone and muscle size and strength are related to age, rather than to the possible effects of decreased activity (Weg, p. 236).

DISEASE PROCESSES

The discussion of age-related changes in the musculoskeletal system reflects the considerable uncertainty as to whether the changes in bones are a manifestation of the aging process or a distinct disease process (Barzel, p. 179).

The term *rheumatism* has often been used by the elderly to describe any painful disorder of the muscles, joints, and their surrounding areas (Agate, p. 75). Following is a discussion of some of the common disruptions of musculoskeletal functioning as experienced in the nursing home population.

Osteoporosis

Osteoporosis has already been described as a condition of decreased skeletal mass without alteration of any chemical components of bone (Rossman, p. 285). Thus, while there may be less total amount of bone, the components of bone are still present in necessary proportions.

The cause of osteoporosis remains unclear, but the mechanism of bone loss apparently is through increased resorption of bone tissue by the body. Osteoporosis may result from prolonged use of medications, immobility, or some other underlying disease (Spencer, p. 296).

Symptoms of osteoporosis include bone pain, often in the lower back, recurrent bone fractures, and frequent falls and related injuries.

Treatment can include managing the symptoms of pain, treating complications such as fractures, rehabilitation to correct physical inactivity, and increasing protein and vitamin intake. Medications often used are calcium supplements and hormones, usually estrogen, to improve the body's ability to absorb calcium.

Arthritis

Arthritis is an inflammation of a joint. Nearly 25% of nursing home residents suffer from some form of this disease. However, there are many different types of arthritis; two that commonly afflict nursing home residents are listed below.

Osteoarthritis. This is the most prevalent form, also called degenerative joint disease. As the disease progresses, the cartilage and other components of the joint begin to wear away or degenerate. The joints that bear most of the weight on a continual basis are most commonly affected, including the knees, hips, and ankles.

Symptoms include aching pain in the affected joint, most often a backache, and decreased mobility because the pain becomes worse following exercise.

Treatment consists of relieving symptoms. Continual degeneration of the hip joint may require a surgical replacement if the patient still has good walking skills.

Rheumatoid Arthritis. This is a much more serious form of arthritis. It can affect any age group. This is considered an *autoimmune disease* because it is thought the body begins to attack it's own cells in the joint, causing an inflammatory reaction.

Signs and symptoms include

symmetric inflammation of joints on both sides of the body
frequent flare-ups and remissions of pain
stiffness and joint swelling, usually in the hands
pain, often occurring in the morning hours and decreasing with exercise

Treatments include

a balance of rest and exercise
physical therapy
heat and cold applications
whirlpool baths

Medications include

aspirin, to decrease the inflammation
analgesics, to relieve the pain

FALLS

More than 70% of deaths that result from all falls occur among persons over 65 years of age. *Falling is a major cause of disability and death in the elderly* and may be due to factors such as chronic illness or orthostatic hypotension (decreased blood pressure upon standing).

Patients in the facility dining room who have just finished a large meal are especially vulnerable. It appears that the blood supply is being routed to the digestive system, causing even lower blood pressure when the resident stands up from the meal.

Osteoporosis, gait disorders, and decreased blood supply to the brain (Rodstein, p. 115) may also be found in the typical nursing home resident, leaving them more prone to falls than the noninstitutionalized elderly population.

FRACTURES

Frequently, when facility residents fall, they fracture one of the bones in their body. Often this is in either the spine or the hip. When a nursing home resident fractures the hip, two treatment approaches are used.

One is to place the resident on bed rest. Lyon and Nevins suggest that this conservative form of treatment is safer and less likely to lead to further mental decline or other complications (p. 391). The other approach is for the resident to have surgery to repair the hip. Often the patient is provided with an artificial prosthesis. The physical therapist has a key role to play in the recovery of fracture patients.

AMPUTEES

Amputees are another group of nursing facility residents who need special assistance when walking.

Three-fourths of all amputations are performed on patients 65 years of age and older (Vallarino & Sherman, p. 148). The most common type of amputation is the removal of the leg either above or below the knee (abbreviated as AKA or BKA). An amputation is the treatment of last resort for residents with a severe infection, peripheral vascular disease, or injury that is often related to diabetes.

CONTRACTURES

Often patients with chronic rheumatoid arthritis develop contractures in their hands. Contractures are a deformity that result when the muscle has shortened and pulls the adjacent joint into a flexed position. After a period of time the joint becomes fixed in this position and results in a permanent deformity in which the joint cannot be straightened. Contractures are another disruption likely to occur in the immobilized resident.

Other joints that are likely to develop contractures, besides those in the hand and wrist, include the foot, hips, and legs.

The best form of treatment for contractures is to help prevent them by exercising the joints of those who are unable to do so for themselves. These are called passive range-of-motion exercises and can be taught to the resident's family. Proper positioning in bed helps prevent the development of these contractures. Special devices and splints are available for that purpose.

5.3.8 Genitourinary (Renal) System

The renal system consists of the two kidneys, which filter wastes from the blood, and two ureters, which transmit the filtered materials (urine) from the kidneys to the bladder, where the urine is stored until discharged through the urethra.

In addition to removing waste materials from the bloodstream, the kidneys also help regulate the amount of fluids in the body. At the same time, the kidneys also monitor the level of important electrolytes including sodium (Na), potassium (K+), and calcium (Ca++).

Channels within the kidney filter the blood and collect a concentration of waste products and excess fluids. The newly filtered blood supply is returned to the general circulation by the renal vein and the concentration of waste materials or urine travels from within the kidney to the bladder by connecting tubes (ureters).

The bladder is a balloon-like muscular structure that serves as a holding tank for the continuous stream of urine produced by the kidneys. When a sufficient amount of urine has collected in the bladder, signals are sent to the brain identifying the need to urinate.

Individuals have voluntary control over the bladder in responding to this need to urinate. A nerve impulse sent back to the bladder signals it to contract and expel urine through the urethra, at which point it leaves the body. See Figure 5-7 for an illustration of the location of the renal system for both men and women.

EFFECTS OF AGING ON THE RENAL SYSTEM

The average 80-year-old adult, according to some studies, has approximately one-half of the renal function of a normal 30-year-old (Lindeman, p. 286).

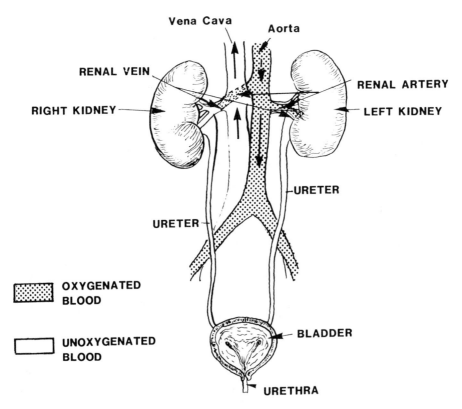

FIGURE 5-7. Diagram of the urinary system.

Because the kidneys are so closely associated with the circulatory system, age-associated atherosclerotic (hardening) changes in blood vessels can also affect the kidney. Because of the location of the renal organs, age-related changes in the reproductive organs also influence their ability to function.

Studies have shown that the ability of the kidneys to concentrate urine probably decreases with age (McLachlan, p. 143). A progressive loss of renal mass (size) is also believed to occur (Rowe, p. 223). However, these changes have not been associated with an overall decline of kidney function. Since the bladder is a muscle, its capacity to hold large amounts of urine also seems to decrease with age.

Alterations in Renal Function

Disruptions in renal function may be caused by problems in an associated system or systems, such as arteriosclerotic changes in blood vessels, and changes in body nutrients, as in diabetes, leading to renal failure.

A disruption may also be due to a malfunction of the kidney itself or to some type of internal blockage within the kidney and ureters, as with kidney stones or tumors. Approximately 10% of nursing home residents are estimated to have kidney problems (Hing, p. 56).

Chronic Renal Failure

Renal failure is the inability of the kidney to filter out body waste products. This can be either an acute (short-term) or more likely, a chronic (long-term) process.

Chronic renal failure may be caused by cardiovascular changes leading to a decreasing amount of blood being filtered through the kidneys. This decrease in blood flow can result in permanent damage to some of the kidney's internal filtering mechanisms (nephrons) that require continual use for optimal functioning. The most obvious physical sign of renal failure is *uremia*, or a decrease in urine output, which may progressively lead to *oliguria*, or no urine output.

The **symptoms** of chronic renal failure, much like the disease itself, develop gradually. Some of the initial symptoms include dehydration, electrolyte imbalance, osteoporosis, nocturia (producing much urine at night), and anemia.

When little or no urine is produced by the body, toxic waste materials may build up, which could damage other organs and cause painful symptoms, including itching and dry skin, mental confusion, weakness, muscle cramps, nausea, vomiting, and diarrhea.

End Stage Renal Disease

Chronic renal failure that has progressed to the stage where little or no urine is being produced is called end stage renal disease (ESRD). The two most common forms of **treatment** are kidney transplantation and dialysis.

Kidney dialysis (hemodialysis, i.e., filtering the blood) requires special equipment that performs much like the kidney in filtering unwanted waste materials and fluids from the blood. The process is normally performed in special clinics and takes several hours. The patient's blood is circulated externally through a small machine that filters the blood in much the same fashion as the kidney itself. Feinstein and Friedman (p. 234) report that from the inception of hemodialysis it has been successful when used for older patients.

Peritoneal dialysis may be performed for the bedridden patient; it involves filtering out excess fluids from the peritoneum, which lines the abdominal organs (i.e., the serous membrane lining the walls of the abdominal and pelvic cavities, containing the viscera). This procedure is similar to kidney dialysis. The waste products are filtered out through dialyzing the peritoneal cavity instead of the kidneys themselves.

Renal Calculi

Kidney stones, or renal calculi are formed in the kidney as a result of an imbalance in body chemistry. These stones are hard crystalline stonelike substances that become a problem when they block urine flow out of the kidney or block any other area of the renal system.

The group of residents most at risk for developing kidney stones are those unable to move or those on chronic bed rest. In the previous section we discussed how these residents are likely to suffer from increased osteoporosis. The extra calcium that the body absorbs may also form kidney stones when enough of this mineral is filtered.

Symptoms are blood in urine, decrease in urine outflow, and pain in the back or side. **Treatment** consists of relief of pain symptoms and medications to relax ureters, allowing the stones to pass. If retrieved, the stones are analyzed to determine their composition and the necessity for any further treatment.

Urinary Incontinence

Urinary incontinence is the inability to control the timing of urination. There are many reasons why a resident may become incontinent, including neurological damage, chronic constipation, and impactions. A defect in the nervous system (stroke patients who lose nervous control of the bladder), urinary tract infections, constant pressure on the bladder from other disorders such as constipation all may cause incontinence.

Problems in mobility that prevent the resident from reaching the toilet in time may also lead to incontinence (Keegan & McNichols, p. 262; Williams & Fitzhugh, p. 903). The nursing staff must be prompt in assisting the resident to the bathroom on a regular schedule. The resident is more able to empty the bladder if placed on the commode.

Bladder retraining is used to assist the resident in using the bathroom at appropriate times. There are several types of bladder retraining programs. Once assurance has been obtained that there is no impaction, the nurses monitor the amount of fluid consumed by the resident and assist the patient to use the toilet about 2 hr afterward.

Residents who are unable to use a bathroom are *catheterized* (release of urine) intermittently about every 2 hr following fluid intake. Special devices are also used to assist the resident in voiding (urinating). These include bedpans, urinals for men, and bedside commodes for the resident who can get up out of bed.

If none of the above treatments is successful, some type of drainage system can be ordered for the resident. Men may use either a condom-like or an indwelling type of catheter. Women may use only the indwelling catheter, which is inserted into the urethra and threaded up into the bladder. Urine flows out of the bladder and through the catheter. It is then collected in a clear plastic drainage bag. This is a closed system to attempt to control the introduction of bacteria or other harmful microorganisms into the urinary tract, but it is a last choice because urinary tract infections are associated with this approach.

Urinary Tract Infections

According to Kurtz, of all age groups, the elderly most frequently have urinary tract infections (UTI) and associated illnesses (p. 54). Together, urinary tract infections and pneumonia were found to be responsible for more than half of all infections in a chronic-care facility studied (Farber et al., p. 518).

The most commonly associated causes of UTI, as identified by Bjork and Tight, include lack of handwashing between patient contacts (an example of poor infection practices by staff), close proximity of residents with catheters, and the prevalence of residents who have indwelling urinary catheters (p. 1675). Other causes, such as poor insertion techniques and poor positioning of drainage bags, have been identified as causes of infection.

Since all indwelling catheters are assumed to eventually cause UTI, residents with catheters are especially at risk of infection (Kurtz, p. 56). A study by Garibaldi et al. found 12% of skilled-nursing-facility residents surveyed had indwelling catheters (p. 732). Residents with urinary catheters often show no symptoms associated with the initial stages of this infection. Residents who do not have indwelling catheters may complain of **symptoms,** including burning and painful urination, cloudy and foul-smelling urine, fever, and chills.

An initial form of **treatment** is to obtain a sample of urine which may be studied to determine the organisms present. Antibiotic therapy is usually held off for as long as possible. There is only a limited number of antibiotics available to treat UTI, and residents with chronic indwelling catheters are likely to become resistant to these antibiotics quickly, at which point there is little alternative treatment available. As many as 50% of urinary tract infections are recurrent.

In an effort to avoid overuse of antibiotics, a new trend among geriatric physicians is to treat UTI only if it is symptomatic, i.e., burning discomfort or pain; not treating when the culture is positive but the patient is asymptomatic.

UTI is an ongoing treatment challenge in the nursing facility. New approaches are constantly being sought. Practical experience suggests that no matter how careful or sterile the procedures, infection often spreads, not on the inside but up the outside of the inserted tube. Despite every staff effort an incontinent female patient may be at risk of infection within minutes after incontinence occurs.

5.3.9 Reproductive System

The reproductive system in the younger adult has the capacity to promote the creation of new life and facilitate the expression of intimacy through human contact. Some of the most notable changes in the elderly include the woman's loss of reproductive capabilities following menopause (change of life), whereas a man retains reproductive capabilities. However, both sexes have continued needs to express their sexuality throughout the life span.

The first part of this section is a description of the reproductive organs and age-associated changes for each sex; the second is a discussion of sexuality and the nursing home resident.

WOMEN

The reproductive organs in women include the ovaries, which produce eggs that travel down the fallopian tubes to the uterus about once every month. Hormones act to control these reproductive cycles. Estrogen is the female sex hormone that directs most of these processes.

The organs of the lower reproductive tract are the cervix, the uterus, and the vagina. The *cervix* is the opening of the *uterus* leading into the **vagina.** The vagina is a barrel-shaped organ that leads to the external genitals in the female reproductive tract, such as the labia and the clitoris. During midlife most women go through menopause (cessation of egg production and therefore of menstruation) and are no longer fertile.

Diseases of the uterus tend to decrease with age (Rossman, p. 334). Changes in the reproductive system are closely related to decreases in secretions of the hormone estrogen.

Some of the physical changes that may be experienced by elderly women include a loss of tone and elasticity in the breast, uterus, cervix, and vagina; a thinning and drying of the vaginal walls, which may cause uncomfortable irritations; infections and bleeding; decrease in size of the uterus, fallopian tubes, and vagina; loss of pubic hair; and decrease in the number of ducts or milk glands of the breasts (Butler & Lewis, p. 115; Kart et al., p. 172; Kay & Neeley, p. 39; Kenny & Kenny, p. 85; Goldfarb, p. 336; Stillwell & O'Conner, p. 596).

Elderly women do not tend to suffer from diseases of the uterus or reproductive tract per se (Rossman, p. 334). However, the incidence of *breast cancer* does continue to rise with age, and it remains the most common type of cancer affecting elderly women. The **signs and symptoms** of breast cancer are a hardened lump or thickening in the breast, change in size of the breast and the nipples. **Treatment** depends on the extent of the disease and may include surgery, radiation, or chemotherapy, as well as the relief of associated symptoms.

Another age-related change is *genital prolapse*. This occurs when the tone of the genital organs becomes so weakened that they begin to drop and may seem to fall out of the vagina. Women with weak muscles are at risk. Some of the *signs and symptoms* associated with genital prolapse include constant pressure on the bladder, incontinence of urine, and a sense of weight in the pelvis. Usually this disorder can be repaired surgically.

Decrease in the production of the female sex hormone estrogen may also lead to osteoporosis (discussed under the musculoskeletal system).

MEN

The primary organs of the male reproductive tract are the testes, scrotum, prostate, and penis.

The *testes* are encased within the *scrotum* and produce the male hormone testosterone and sperm cells. These cells mature as they travel through the surrounding *epididymis* until released into the *vas deferens*. The sperm travel through the vas deferens until they are released from the ejaculatory ducts into the *urethra*. Nearby ducts secrete seminal fluid from the *prostate gland*, which provides food for the sperm as well as enhancing their motility. When the male ejaculates, the sperm travel down the urethra through the *penis*, and are emittted from the body.

Some of the age-related changes in the male reproductive tract are an enlargement of the prostate gland, decreased production of testosterone, which may result in slight decrease in sexual desire, and a reduction in muscle bulk and strength. Sperm production continues into advanced old age, so males continue with the ability to impregnate into old age (Kay & Neeley, p. 40).

Problems with the prostate gland are a major concern for many elderly men (Kart et al., p. 152). Enlargement of the prostate is a common age-related change in men (Kart et al., p. 152; Reichel, pp. 304, 596; Rossman, p. 328). For some men, this enlargement may interfere with the ability to urinate or may cause incontinence. *Prostatitis* is an inflammation of this gland that often develops following the initial enlargement of the prostate gland and can be very painful. Other **symptoms** include painful urination and blood in the urine.

This enlargement may develop into *cancer of the prostate,* which is the second most common form of cancer in elderly men. Cancer of the prostate is considered a "geriatric disease," with 95% of all cases seen in elderly men (Rowe, p. 156). The initial **symptoms** for this disease are the same as those experienced with prostatitis, including a decrease in urination and discomfort. Surgery is usually performed to remove the cancerous or extremely large prostate. Chemotherapy or hormone treatments may also be used.

COPING WITH SEXUALITY

Sexual needs persist into old age, with continued activity considered healthy and health-preserving (Snowden, p. 55; Griggs, p. 1352). The elderly nursing home resident, like those in the community, continues to have needs for a positive self-image and self-esteem, which are closely associated with the needs for intimacy and sexuality (Butler, p. 116; Griggs, p. 1352). Too often, society and individuals discourage sexual activity in the nursing home because of existing stereotypes and misunderstandings about sex and old age (Wasow & Loeb, p. 73).

Sexuality is not achieved exclusively by sexual intercourse but may also incorporate a variety of activities related to touch and displays of affection. Older people may be more likely to express their sexuality in these more diffuse and varied terms (Boyer & Boyer, p. 422).

Impotence, or the inability to perform sexually, is more often attributed to the male. The extent of this disorder in old age is not known, but a 1972 American Medical Association report revealed that, rather than organic problems, anxiety and internalization of society pressures account for most of the problems related to impotence, (Kay & Neeley, p. 40). Nursing homes are often perceived as disapproving and as actively discouraging displays of love or affection among residents. A frequent suggestion in the literature is that nursing home staff be educated concerning sexuality in old age and that more efforts be made to deal with problems of morality that may arise.

Stillwell and O'Conner (p. 596) attempt to dispel some of the myths concerning sexuality with the observations that

older people do remain interested in sex
older people finds each other physically attractive
sexuality contributes to overall well-being

Contrary to public perceptions, the incidence of a heart attack or stroke during sexual intercourse is actually very low, and sexual activity is sometimes recommended for patients with diseases such as arthritis because of the therapeutic effects of exercise and intimacy.

One research study suggests allowing for privacy of some residents to develop closer relationships (Kay & Neeley, p. 45). Another encourages the development of programs to deal with quality-of-life issues such as loneliness and isolation that are important to residents. Sexual expression would be only one component of this type of effort.

5.3.10 Emotional and Mental Well-Being

A number of the physical system disruptions discussed above can have profound effects on the mental well-being of the nursing home resident.

EFFECTS OF AGING

Differences of opinion exist as to whether *intelligence* declines with age. One difficulty is the use of tests that may not be appropriate measures for the elderly (Botwinick, p. 249).

Aging is associated with special problems that may not be as disruptive for younger individuals. Burnside identifies two of these as *behavioral problems* and *mental illness* (p. 63). The range of behaviors residents employ to cope with these problems will vary, but studies often show that many of the recurrent problems in a nursing home are related to behavioral problems (Stotsky, p. 172).

When residents are admitted to the facility, they may display initial symptoms of anxiety and apprehension regarding their new surroundings (discussed below). Chronic illness and the process of dying are anxiety-provoking and necessarily are an aspect of life with which nursing home residents must constantly cope.

Anxiety may be experienced by most individuals, and each copes with it in a particular way. Some manifestations of anxiety include fantasizing, hostile or dependent behavior, avoidance of eye contact, fidgeting, insomnia, and isolation from others.

INSOMNIA

Insomnia, or sleep disorders, is common among the elderly. Studies of human sleep patterns have shown that the elderly spend more time in bed, have more difficulty getting to sleep, or tend to awaken during sleep periods (Dement, Miles, Bliwise, p. 180; Busse & Pfeiffer, p. 138).

Sleep problems may result from the use of multiple medications as well as from anxiety. To assist the residents to cope, sleeping medications may be prescribed, along with increases in daily activities and attempts to alleviate the source of anxiety.

LONELINESS

Behaviors associated with loneliness are similar to those of a mild depressive mood and include isolation, constipation, weight loss, insomnia, fatigue, and loss of appetite.

Treatment for these residents is to discern the cause of depression and try to help them cope effectively with those feelings. If these behaviors persist and worsen, the resident may be progressing toward mental illness. Antidepressive medications may also be prescribed in these cases.

MENTAL ILLNESS

Some studies have revealed that about 10% of elderly citizens have severe mental illness (Palmore, p. 43), and the incidence of mental illness tends to increase as people age (Butler, p. 56). It is estimated that the rate of mental illness in nursing homes is somewhere between one-fourth and one-half of all residents. This high prevalence of mental illness may be a result of preexisting problems (Birren, p. 254).

Often the term *senile* is used to describe a variety of behaviors in mental illness, ranging from slight forgetfulness to a generalized decline in mental functioning of the elderly. Butler and Lewis describe two different groups of older persons suffering from mental illness as (a) those with a history of mental illness and (b) those who develop mental illness for the first time in late life (p. 53).

Those with a history of mental illness often have been transferred to the nursing home following deinstitutionalization from a psychiatric facility, a phenomenon brought about by the development of psychotropic drugs in the 1950s and 1960s. This population may also be suffering from mental retardation.

Psychotropic drugs are those that exert an effect on the mind. They are normally used to calm and control patient behavior. Equipped with these new medications and a belief that mentally ill persons are better cared for in the community setting, most states dramatically reduced the number of persons held in the state mental hospitals. *It is believed that a significant portion of persons who were deinstitutionalized during this movement have entered the nursing home as a substitute for the mental hospital.*

The second group of mentally ill patients often become emotionally disturbed because they are no longer able to cope with the physical and social changes associated with the aging process.

Who is mentally ill? What is mental illness? These are difficult questions in the setting of the nursing facility. The changes brought about by chronic physical illnesses and by the "normal" social changes faced by older persons are powerful enough to overwhelm even the best adjusted person. The line between disabling mental illnesses and the day-to-day effects of attempting to cope with aging is often blurred.

ORGANIC BRAIN SYNDROME

Organic brain syndrome, dementia, brain failure, and senility are all different words describing the same disorder (Burnside, p. 107). Dementia and Alzheimer's disease have already been discussed as a problem of the nervous system.

The two most common causes of organic brain syndrome are (a) Alzheimer's disease, and (b) cerebrovascular insufficiency or reduced blood flow to the brain. The brain tissue responds to any impairments resulting from these disorders with a variety of symptoms that initially can involve memory loss, leading to levels of disorientation and confusion and to difficulty following even simple directions. These symptoms of confusion progress until the resident is no longer aware of reality.

Affected residents may engage in such problematic behaviors as suicidal threats or attempts, destructiveness, hostility, noisiness, and wandering off (Busse & Pfeiffer, p. 173). These behaviors can become especially troublesome in the group setting of a nursing home. Psychiatric consultation is usually desirable in these instances.

Treatment can include

- reality orientation (continually reminding residents of the date, time, and place to keep them oriented to their environment)
- choosing compatible roommates and company for these residents
- avoiding sudden changes or surprises
- increasing the amount of assistance available to these residents to perform the activities of daily living
- providing a supportive environment

DEPRESSION

Depression is probably the most common mental illness in the elderly (Blumenthal, 1980, p. 34). Residents must be assessed to determine whether they are merely in a depressed mood or if the disease has progressed to a mental illness (Lazar & Karasu, p. 49). Often depression may be associated with another underlying chronic disease (e.g., arthritis or Parkinson's disease) or may be a result of a reaction to medications (Blumenthal, 1980, pp. 35–36; Lazar & Karasu, p. 49). Busse and Pfeiffer also implicate depression as a cause or precursor of other chronic diseases (p. 148).

Additional **signs** of depression include loss of appetite resulting in weight loss, feelings of sadness, loss of interest in people, and a sense of great effort needed to perform daily activities (Blumenthal, 1980, p. 34). Elderly persons may also complain of symptoms that are actually attributable to depression.

Treatment of depression can include the use of antidepressant medications, usually tricyclic antidepressant drugs. These drugs themselves, however, also have strong side effects.

Electrocortical shock treatment (ECT) is a powerful form of treatment used to stimulate a specified area of the brain. Blumenthal suggests that ECT may be safer than drug therapy (1980, p. 43). However, use of electro shock treatments for depression and other mental disorders has been a subject of intense controversy for decades.

Counseling, group activities and social functions appear to be productive therapeutic techniques available to the nursing home staff (Busse & Pfeiffer, p. 120; Shore, p. 353).

In essence, efforts by the staff to restore a sense of worth and importance to the resident may be among the most powerful tools available. Some of these include daily exercise, such as aerobics geared to the resident's level of physical capacity, dance therapy, recreation therapy, work therapy, and bibliotherapy (reading books).

5.3.11 Medications

EXTENT OF DRUG PRESCRIPTIONS IN THE NURSING FACILITY

Medications are among the most common types of treatment prescribed by physicians for the nursing home resident. According to the 1977 National Nursing Home Survey, 95.9% of nursing home residents receive at least one or more medications (Hing, p. 23). This is not surprising, since admission normally depends on being ill and in need or continuing treatment. However, another study revealed that more than half of nursing home residents receive three to seven different medications a day (USDHEW, p. 13).

ROUTES USED IN DRUG ADMINISTRATION

Some of the most commonly prescribed medications have already been discussed in previous sections. Basically, these drugs function in the body after being absorbed, usually through the digestive tract, into the bloodstream, following a pathway similar to that traveled by nutrients from food.

Drugs may be administered several ways, intramuscularly (IM) by an injection; or directly on skin (topically); on membranes or other tissue, such as being held under the tongue (sublingually); or as suppositories. Usually medications eventually become inactive in the liver and are removed from the body by the kidney.

THE FIVE BASIC DRUG ACTIONS

The following are the five basic types of actions that drugs will produce (Poe & Holloway, pp. 14–15):

- blocking nerve impulses
- stimulating nerve impulses
- working directly on living cells
- working to replace body deficiencies
- any combination of the above

Every person is affected by drugs differently because of individual body chemistries, so every patient must be monitored to determine the appropriateness of different dosages.

As a result of age-related changes in the liver, kidney, and other organs throughout the body that alter the normal utilization of drugs, *the elderly are at a much greater risk of suffering from drug reactions,* which are often the result of a buildup or excess amount of drugs in the body. In addition, there may also be an increase in the occurrence of side effects that are commonly associated with most medications.

Policy Implications

Because nursing home residents are more likely to suffer from multiple diseases and, as suggested above, use multiple medications, these drug combinations can produce dangerous drug interactions. These same residents are also at a much greater risk of suffering from an adverse drug reaction, many of which are the result of chemical imcompatibilities between the different medications.

For these reasons, the nursing home administrator must assure that drug regimens in the facility are appropriately monitored. Special precautions can be mounted to prevent the consequences of illness or disability from drug reactions.

Use of prn

Often, physicians rely on what is commonly referred to as prn (*pro re nata*, literally meaning "as the thing is necessary") approach. These "prescribe as needed" orders allow licensed nurses to determine when to administer a particular medication. A study of nursing home medication practices by Segal, Thompson, and Floyd revealed that approximately 46% of medications were prescribed on a prn basis (p. 117). These practices, while functional and probably desirable, nevertheless need to be monitored closely.

A policy of involving the facility pharmacy consultant and medical director, along with the nursing staff in a constant monitoring of drug regimens is required by the Conditions of Participation. However, closer and more active monitoring seems appropriate, inasmuch as undesirable drug interactions are a major ongoing concern in facility administration.

The five rights of medication administration include identifying

- the right medication
- the right dose
- the right time for administration
- the right route (oral, shot, etc.)
- the right patient

GENERIC AND BRAND NAMES

Familiarity with some of the more commonly prescribed medications by both the generic (chemical) names and brand (manufacturing) names can be useful. In the following discussion the generic names are mentioned first, with the brand names following in parentheses. Brand names are often used among health professionals unless a particular medication, e.g., aspirin, is produced by a number of companies. Some of the more frequently prescribed medications are discussed below.

ANTIANXIETY AND ANTIPSYCHOTIC MEDICATIONS

Antianxiety and antipsychotic medications act on the central nervous system to enable patients to deal with changes in their own behavior or stressful and anxiety-provoking changes in their environment. The two major classes of this type of drug are tranquilizers and sedatives/hypnotics.

These medications act directly on the major control center—the brain—and should be administered very cautiously. Many of the drug-related fatalities among the elderly are associated with these medications (Basen, p. 44).

Some of the most commonly prescribed tranquilizers and sedatives/hypnotics used in the nursing home are thioridazine and chlordiazepoxide. Thioridazine (Mellaril®) is a major tranquilizer and/or antipsychotic drug prescribed for mild to moderate anxiety relief. This medication has been used for long-term alcoholics to control their illness. Chlordiazepoxide hydrochloride (Librium®) is a minor tranquilizer prescribed for relief of anxiety.

The **side effects** associated with these medications include drowsiness, dizziness, disorientation, and allergic reactions.

VITAMINS AND MINERALS

Vitamins and minerals are the most common classes of medications prescribed for the elderly nursing home resident, according to the National Nursing Home Survey (Hing, p. 23). Ferrous sulfate, which is an iron supplement, and multivitamins are among the most popular in these categories.

A common **side effect** of iron supplements is irritation of the gastrointestinal tract, which may cause patients some stomach upset. Other frequently prescribed minerals include calcium and potassium supplement.

ANALGESICS

Analgesics are often administered for pain relief. Acetylsalicylic acid, or aspirin, may be relatively safe, except for nursing home residents with kidney problems and ulcers. Aspirin may also act as an anti-inflammatory agent for arthritic patients. Such medications serve to reduce the amount of damage to the joints, and to lessen the painful side effects associated with the inflammatory process.

Some of the **side effects** associated with aspirin include stomach upset, ringing in the ears, deafness, dizziness, confusion, and irritability (Gotz & Gotz, p. 1349).

Acetaminophen (Tylenol®) is an analgesic similar to aspirin but without anti-inflammatory properties, and hence it may serve only as a pain reliever. Some **side effects** associated with it are redness and itching of the skin and possible liver damage.

Another group of much stronger analgesics are the narcotics. Federal regulations require that they be kept under lock and key in a safe place because of their potential for abuse. A dangerous **side effect** with these drugs is the potential to depress breathing and respiratory functions that are controlled by the central nervous system. Alterations in consciousness or blood pressure may also occur. Some of the more commonly prescribed narcotic analgesics include codeine (Methylmorphine®), meperidine (Demerol®), morphine sulfate, and oxycodone terephthalate (Percodan®).

LAXATIVES AND GASTROINTESTINAL AGENTS

Gastrointestinal agents are among some of the more commonly prescribed medications for nursing home patients. Laxatives are also referred to as cathartics. This category includes suppositories, such as bisacodyl (Dulcolax®), bulk laxatives like plantago seed (Metamucil®), and stool softeners such as milk of magnesia (Cooper, p. 25).

Often these agents are prescribed with other medications to neutralize their irritating effects on the gastrointestinal tract. Antacids, one of the most commonly indicated for this purpose, unfortunately may also cause **side effects** such as diarrhea. Milk of magnesia is frequently prescribed for gastrointestinal problems.

CARDIOVASCULAR AGENTS

Various groups of cardiovascular agents have already been mentioned. Two of them, antihypertensives and diuretics, work to reduce blood pressure by different actions.

Methyldopa (Aldomet®) is an antihypertensive that works directly on the central nervous system to lower blood pressure. Orthostatic hypotension, or decreased blood pressure upon standing, may be associated with this medication and increases the likelihood of patients falling (Gotz & Gotz, p. 1350).

Diuretics work by forcing the body to excrete excess fluids. Furosemide (Lasix®) and hydrochlorothiazide (Esidrix®) are commonly prescribed. But they cause the body to excrete potassium, and this may result in muscle weakness, lethargy, and muscle cramping.

Other medications act directly on the heart muscle. Digoxin (Lanoxin®) acts to slow down the heart rate by decreasing the speed of impulses traveling along muscle fibers. Propranolol hydrochloride (Inderal®) is another medication that works to block chemicals from increasing the heart rate. Some **side effects** from these medications include a loss of appetite, nausea, vomiting, confusion, blurred vision, and arrhythmias.

Antianginal medications work to alleviate the pain associated with a decreased oxygen supply to the heart muscle. Nitroglycerin (NTG), works as a vasodilator to increase the size of blood vessels so they will carry more oxygen. This medication is administered sublingually (under the tongue).

ANTIDEPRESSANTS

Amitriptyline hydrochloride (Elavil®) is one of the most commonly prescribed drugs for elderly residents in a skilled nursing facility (Cooper, p. 25). This medication also acts as a tranquilizer. The extent of its use is not surprising, considering that depression is one of the most common forms of illness. Depression is also common among patients suffering from other chronic ailments, especially Alzheimer's and Parkinson's diseases.

Some of the **side effects** associated with antidepressant medications such as Elavil® include confusion, drowsiness, decreased blood pressure, constipation, dry mouth, heart flutter, rashes, and retention of urine.

ANTI-INFECTIVES

Anti-infectives kill or decrease the growth of infectious organisms, complementing the natural body defense mechanisms.

Antibiotics are one of the more notable groups of medications within this class. Among the different types are the penicillins, cephalosporins, and tetracyclines. One of the most important **side effects** associated with these medications are allergic reactions, which are often identified by skin rashes.

Some antibiotics may be used to combat fungal and viral infections. Intravenous (IV) therapy is introduced when dealing with the more resistant organisms.

MISCELLANEOUS MEDICATIONS

Respiratory agents: Expectorants, including ammonium chloride (Robitussin®), terpin hydrate, and acetylcysteine (Mucomyst®) are used to break up and expel mucus from the respiratory tract. The first two medications are taken orally; the third is usually administered by inhaling it in the form of a vapor. Tetracycline and ampicillin can be effective antibiotics for patients with respiratory tract infections due to chronic bronchitis (Rodman & Smith, p. 251).

Optical medications: Mydriatics are often used for patients with glaucoma. Pilocarpine and physostigmine are two commonly prescribed medications. They act to decrease the fluid buildup in the eye resulting from glaucoma. These medications are administered as eyedrops. Some of the more common **side effects** are headaches, diarrhea, and sweating.

CONTROLLED DRUGS SCHEDULES

Condition of Participation 405.1124 Nursing Services, Standard I, addresses the storage of drugs. All drugs and biologicals are to be stored in locked compartments. Separately locked, permanently affixed compartments are required for Schedule II drugs listed in the Comprehensive Drug Abuse Prevention and Control Act of 1970.

Formerly, drugs were regulated under the 1914 Harrison Narcotic Act, which placed them into classes A, B, X, and M narcotics. Subsequently, each state passed drug acts. Today pharmacists and nursing facilities must meet the individual state drug laws and the federal drug law. Most states have passed a State Uniform Controlled Substances Act, some with six instead of five drug group classifications.

The federal government has classified drugs into the following five schedules.

Schedule I Drugs: drugs with a high abuse potential and no accepted medical use in the United States, e.g., heroin, marijuana, LSD, peyote, mescaline, and certain other opiates and hallucinogenic substances.

Schedule II Drugs: drugs with accepted medical use in the United States, having high abuse and dependency potential, e.g., opium, morphine, codeine, methodone, cocaine, amphetamine, secobarbital, methaqualone (Quaalude), and phencyclidine ("angel dust"). These were formerly Class A narcotics.

Schedule III Drugs: drugs with less abuse potential than schedules I and II drugs. Several compounds are included, e.g., Empirin compound with codeine, Tylenol® with codeine, and Phenaphen® with codeine. These were formerly Class B drugs.

Schedule IV Drugs: drugs with less abuse potential than Schedule III drugs, e.g., barbital, meprobamate (Equanil® and Miltown®), Librium®, Valium®, Dalmane®, Darvon®, and Talwin®.

Schedule V Drugs: drugs with less abuse potential than Schedule IV drugs. These typically are compounds containing limited quantities of narcotic drugs for antitussive (anti-cough) and antidiarrheal purposes. Examples are Lomotil®, Actifed-C® expectorant, Phenergan® expectorant with codeine, and Robitussin®A-C syrup. These were formerly Class X (exempt narcotics) under the Harrison Narcotic Act.

5.4 Patient Needs: Personal and Social Aspects of Institutional Living

5.4.1 Admission

Admission to a skilled nursing facility for a long term of care, usually interpreted as "for life," is a time of radical change at a juncture when the typical prospective patient is least able to tolerate change.

Studies of stress reveal that an individual is generally capable of absorbing and adjusting at any moment to one major change such as divorce, death of a spouse, loss of a job. These same studies have also shown that when more than one major stress factor of this magnitude occur together, the stress level becomes almost intolerable.

Admission to a skilled nursing facility with the expectation that the change is permanent can be a similarly traumatizing period of time.

LOSSES, ADJUSTMENTS AND GAINS

Figure 5-8 shows what we consider to be the potential losses, adjustments, and gains associated with the move to a long-term-care facility.

Variations among Patients

Every patient's personal circumstances before entering a long-term-care facility are unique to that individual. One person may be leaving 80 years

LOSSES ⟶	ADJUSTMENTS ⟶	GAINS
FAMILIAR SURROUND-INGS—"home" whatever it was.	ADAPT TO NEW ROOM, ROOMMATE(S)	AN ENVIRONMENT ADAPTED TO THEIR NEEDS
LOSS OF FAMILY CONTACTS or caregiver contact pattern	ACCEPT NEW CAREGIVERS AS NEW "FAMILY"	PERSONNEL AVAILABLE 24 HOURS, WHO TRY TO CARE
LOSS OF CONTACT PATTERN WITH FRIENDS	REDUCED CONTACT, ESPECIALLY IF FRAIL	NEW FRIENDS ONE'S OWN AGE AND CONDITION
LOSS OF CONTROL OVER ONE'S LIFE, INCLUDING medications	NOT ALLOWED TO GIVE ONESELF ONE'S MEDICINES	EXPERT CAREGIVERS WHO TAKE OVER THIS FUNCTION
meal timing choice of snacks	ACCEPT THE SNF'S FOOD CHOICES	PREDICTABLE MEALS, SNACKS, 24 HRS.
RANGE OF DECISION MAKING LOSSES independence, e.g., eat or not, take medicines or not	ACCEPT PHYSICIAN'S NEARLY TOTAL CONTROL OVER DIET, ACTIVITIES	AN ARRAY OF CONCERNED STAFF, ASSISTING DECISION MAKING
PERSONALIZATION LOSSES in clothing, life style, timing, daily living activities	CONFORMITY TO SNF'S TIME SCHEDULE, FOOD CHOICES, DAILY SCHEDULE	NOT MUCH—**AN INTENSE STRUGGLE TO REPERSONALIZE ONESELF IN A POTENTIALLY DEPERSONALIZING INSTITUTIONAL ENVIRONMENT**

FIGURE 5-8. Losses, adjustments and gains of patient admitted for long-term care.

of life on a rural farm far from the closest neighbor, in which case admission to a long-term care facility can be a radically new (literally uprooting) experience.

The next patient admitted may have lived in the neighborhood of the facility and even been a volunteer or visited relatives residing there. This person may face a less radical transition. On the other hand, being admitted could have equally devastating psychological impacts on both of these individuals.

Similarities among Patients

Recognizing that every person entering the facility brings a unique personal background, there are, nevertheless, certain aspects of institutionalization to which all patients must adjust, no matter what their background. Some of these are presented in Figure 5-8.

LOSS OF FAMILIAR SURROUNDINGS

The surroundings that have been called "home" are lost. That environment may have a lifetime of emotional associations, or it may be more recent, perhaps living with one's children for the 5 months prior to entering the facility. For all persons entering the facility, "home," whatever it represents to the person over his/her lifetime to that point, is left behind.

To leave home behind is a major life adjustment. It means adapting oneself and one's life-style to living in one room. The room may be private; or if two or more persons have beds in this room, one must adjust to living with one or more unfamiliar persons.

What the person entering the long-term care facility gains is an environment that is adapted to his/her needs and physical disabilities. Each aspect of the physical environment in the nursing facility accommodates to the goal of providing a safer physical environment for the residents.

LOSS OF FAMILY CONTACTS

For most persons entering a facility, a reduced amount of contact with family or caregivers may follow admission. Visits by family members and former caregivers may be frequent, at least at first, but the reality for most persons is that the staff of the facility become, to some extent, a substitute family.

In place of more frequent family or caregiver contacts, the person gains the nursing facility personnel who try to care and who are available on a 24-hr-a-day basis.

LOSS OF CONTACT PATTERN WITH FRIENDS

Inevitably, a reduction in contact with friends is likely, especially if the person's friends are themselves frail elderly who ordinarily do not drive or get out. Many frail elderly persons have already experienced loss of friends; reduced contact with those few remaining may be an especially difficult adjustment.

To partially replace the potential reduction in contacts with friends, the facility offers the opportunity to form new friendships with persons of one's own age and physical condition.

The potential value of this adjustment is not to be underestimated. The same set of values has led more than 50,000 persons to move to Sun City, Arizona, a suburb of Phoenix, where the rules exclude anyone under age 50. Everywhere one goes in Sun City the average age is well advanced, whether in the beauty parlor or in the grocery stores. Here the residents have made the positive choice to live among persons of similar age and condition.

LOSS OF CONTROL OVER ONE'S LIFE

To move into a long-term-care facility is to experience a loss of control over one's life: to become institutionalized. This loss of control may take many forms, two of the more obvious relating to medications and eating habits.

A person is seldom allowed to control his/her personal medications in the nursing facility. One reason patients are usually not allowed to keep medicines in their rooms is to prevent others from finding and taking them. One is powerless in even the simpler aspects of one's life when, on entering a nursing facility, one must obtain permission for an aspirin or an antacid.

In place of the freedom to use, and sometimes misuse, medications, the facility provides expert caregivers who are trained in administering and monitoring the total medication regimen for possible adverse side effects or adverse interactions among them. Experts take over this function.

Loss of control over one's personal eating habits and food preferences, after a lifetime of choosing one's food and eating it when one wishes, is to lose a valued power of choice. The new resident has to accept the food choices made by the facility personnel, whose taste, food preferences, and food preparation may be markedly different from his/her own.

However, in place of what for some older chronically ill persons had become a pattern of random eating and missed meals, the facility offers a predictable meal schedule with snack food available 24 hr a day. There is no need to shop for groceries, plan a balanced meal, prepare it, and wash the dishes. Life is a hotel—if not a cabaret.

LOSSES IN RANGE OF DECISION MAKING

Independence, the capacity to decide to eat or not, to take prescribed medicines or ignore them, or to take them only half as often or twice as often as prescribed, is replaced by near total control by the attending physician over the range of choices allowed the new resident.

Thus, the new resident must adjust to the physician's having nearly complete control over matters of diet, medications, and even the amount of activity allowed. The potential gain for the new resident is an array of concerned staff who, along with the physician, assist in making decisions within the permitted, but greatly narrowed, range.

LOSS OF A MORE PERSONALIZED EXISTENCE

Entering a long-term care facility as a resident/patient can be a depersonalizing experience. Choices in clothing, in the timing of the activities of daily living, and in one's own personal life-style may be more restrictive. These are *potential* effects of institutionalization.

5.4.2 Reactions at Admission

At about 2 o'clock on Tuesday afternoon, a long, unrelenting wail began coming from the lobby. The emotions carried in the wail seemed to blend simultaneously anger, anxiety, fear, mourning, hopelessness. The uncontrollable high-pitched wailing lasted over half an hour. An elderly woman, being admitted to the facility, sitting in a wheelchair near the admissions office door, was the source.

The degree of change introduced is potentially overwhelming to most persons at admission to what is expected to be life care. Understandably, the person has feelings of anger and fear. Mourning for one's former capacities and powers may, for most, be inevitable.

ANGER, ANXIETY, DEPRESSION

Anger and anxiety associated with being admitted can, and typically do, lead to admission-associated depression. Dealing with the depression, that is usually a result of the anger and feelings of helplessness and hopelessness persons may feel at admission is one of the major tasks of the nursing facility staff.

Not all admissions, of course, bring an intense level of anger and depression. For some, admission may be a fundamentally positive experience. We have pointed out that the facility offers meaningful substitutes for nearly all of the losses the person may experience in being admitted to a nursing facility.

However, it must be remembered that persons are admitted to skilled nursing facilities because they do need that type of care. This means that the typical person who is admitted has one, usually several, chronic diseases or other circumstances that limit his/her ability to perform for him/herself the activities of daily living satisfactorily.

To a very real extent, then, the new patient gains access to a needed environment that has been carefully designed to meet his/her special needs. For many, the facility provides a level of security and capacity to meet their needs that make admission a welcome experience. Even for them, however, adjusting to facility life is potentially disturbing.

5.4.3 Living in an Institution: Some Aspects of Institutional Living

To institutionalize is to require some degree of conformity in those who are institutionalized. It is to reduce the degree of choice that the individual retains in even the simpler aspects of daily living.

The institution has the power to require conformity to its decisions for the patient about

- what and when to eat
- when to bathe
- when to take medication
- when to get up and go to bed
- when to dress and in what clothes
- what possessions to keep
- when to have recreation choices offered
- when visitors are welcome
- when to have snacks
- what the noise level in the environment will be
- and often, when to go to the bathroom

The skilled nursing facility *can* assume nearly total control over what are called the activities of daily living. Being a patient *can* mean submitting to others' control over even the most intimate aspects of one's personal life.

5.4.4 Dealing with the Effects of Institutionalization: Person-Centered Administration

The task of the nursing facility staff is to accept the validity of the patients' feelings about institutionalization, and provide needed emotional support to assist him/her in establishing a new personalized existence in the facility.

This is an immensely complex task. The key to the process is for the staff to minimize the depersonalizing effects of living in the skilled nursing facility. This can be accomplished by staff efforts to retain for the patients as much control over their lives as is feasible, given the constraints of being in an institution required to conform to all of the federal, state, and local nursing home regulations. Person-centered administration means focusing on the quality of patient life in the facility.

QUALITY OF PATIENT LIFE

Nursing home inspectors may focus their review on quality of nursing care and similar measures of facility performance. In our view, this is not what the nursing facility is fundamentally about. The nursing facility is a living community. The more appropriate question for the administrator to ask is, What is the quality of patient life in this facility?

Asking the Right Question

Granted, the administrator must continually focus on the degree to which his/her facility is meeting federal, state, and local standards for good patient care. This is institution-centered administration. The focus is on running an acceptably conforming institution, but this is only the minimum condition for operating a nursing facility. It is only the floor or base on which the administrator can build a person-centered facility.

Staff attention must be focused on two principles that contribute importantly to the quality of patient life in each facility: reserving to the patients as many choices as possible and maintaining as positive and optimistic an atittude toward everyday life as is possible under the circumstances.

FOCUSING ON THE RESIDENT

Person-centered administration means that the needs of the resident prevail rather than, as is too often the case, those of the institution itself.

What the facility can offer the new resident is a caring, structured environment. Every resident's immediate previous environment is unique, but for many who enter a skilled nursing facility there have not previously been enough caregivers to interact throughout each day with him/her. Many will be changing a life-style from one in which they were increasingly left to their own devices but which was progressively less meaningful and, especially, detrimental to their health.

The facility offers a structured environment in which the patient has multiple human contacts throughout the day and a dependable schedule. The nursing home can offer a comfortable, human, unconfusing life-style. For many persons who have been struggling with depression and loneliness, the structure of the nursing home day offers a sense of security and desired predictability. For persons in advanced old age with multiple chronic illnesses, this is highly beneficial.

A nursing facility exists to serve persons in need of this care. Excellence in care is not necessarily equated with a facility run smoothly and in conformity with all rules and regulations, but rather is achieved when the quality of life experienced by its residents is optimized.

The most intractable of the negative effects of institutionalization is its depersonalization: a person is deprived of control over his/her life and experiences powerlessness, which diminishes feelings of self-worth. We believe that consciously reserving to the patients as much power and personal choice over their lives as they can absorb will help minimize the more negative aspects of institutional living.

This can be achieved by giving each patient discretion to decide in as many areas of daily living as possible, within organizational constraints. Practically speaking, this means treating each patient with respect as an adult whose wishes are to be honored to the degree feasible.

Administrative Mind Set

The mind set is the basic behavioral stance taken by the administrator toward the patient population. The staff of the facility take cues from the facility administrator.

If the administrator treats the residents as consenting adults whose ideas and wishes are to be taken seriously, the staff will tend to regard the residents similarly. If the staff senses that the administrator treats residents as persons who are not expected nor, for the most part, permitted to make decisions over their lives, the staff will treat the residents with similar paternalism.

Paternalism

Paternalism can be an all too frequent characteristic of the behaviors of institutional officials. The most obvious illustration is the military. From the general down to the master sergeant, there is the expectation that all the persons lower in rank will do as told, when told. The private is not expected to think on his/her own, nor to exercise any power.

Officials tend to make decisions for the good of their constituencies, typically without consulting them. For example, various state governments have complained in recent decades that the federal government is treating them too paternalistically. They have detected an implicit assumption in federal regulations that if the federal government does not force the states to do such things as to give adequate welfare payments or medical assistance to the poor, it will not be done acceptably, i.e., to the federal government's satisfaction.

The 50 states regard themselves as sovereigns who have delegated particular powers to the federal government in order to accomplish certain things that are better done on a collective basis. National defense or maintaining the national borders are examples. All powers and authority not delegated by the states to the federal government are presumed to be reserved by the states to themselves.

This is a useful model for nursing facility administrators to follow. The residents/patients have delegated certain rights and authority to the nursing facility for the purpose of obtaining needed health care. The residents/patients retain to themselves, however, authority over their own lives to the extent they are able to exercise it, given the condition of their health.

WHOSE NEEDS ARE TO DOMINATE?

At the heart of the issue is this: Whose needs predominate? The administrator and staff are in positions of true power over the patient population. Most staff have a need to feel in power and in control of things that occur in the facility.

Nursing home staff members all too often permit their own needs to influence their behavior toward the patients, who become trapped in the staff struggle to gain control and exercise power. Patients, for example, are expected to conform to the staff's time schedule for bathing. When there is a contest between the staff and the patients, the staff will tend to win because they are obviously more powerful than the patients.

What we are suggesting is a conscious effort on the administrator's part to increase the range of choices available to residents/patients. The level of cooperation and satisfaction among patients can rise markedly when they feel they have some influence over their own lives.

Residents versus Residents

Sometimes the administrator may be pitted against a group of residents. For example, in one facility the administrator's policy was to permit any resident, who so desired and could be physically present, to eat in the facility dining room. Residents who were more ambulatory and who did not "make unsightly messes" when eating resented the administrator permitting these less capable patients to eat in the dining room.

The administrator understood and sympathized with the more ambulatory patients, who were disturbed at the sight of "messy" residents, primarily, it is suspected, because the sight reminded them too poignantly of the condition in which they might find themselves in a few months or years.

The administrator persisted, however, with the original plan, with the result that, although more competent residents continued to find the sight unpleasant, they understood that should they themselves reach a similar state, their dining wishes would be similarly honored by the administrator.

In decisions such as these, the administrator can demonstrate to the staff and residents a commitment to respecting the preferences of all residents to the extent possible.

5.5 Patient Care Planning

Patient care planning is one of the standards under Condition of Participation 405.1124, Nursing Services (see page 389). This federal requirement mandates a written care plan for each patient. The plan must be developed and maintained by the nursing service in coordination with the other patient care services. It must include the care to be given, the goals to be sought, and a designation of the staff members responsible for achieving each part of the plan.

This Standard also calls for review and update of the plan by all of the professional personnel involved in the care of the patient, as necessary. States frequently specify care planning in more detail, generally announcing the duration of intervals between revisions.

The federal standard does not require that the patient or the patient's family be involved in formulating his/her care plan. Federal Condition of Participation 405.1121, Governing Body and Management, Subpart K, states patients' rights but does not mention a right to be involved in one's own care plan.

In the federal view the entire patient care planning process could be done *for* the patient by the professionals who know what the patient needs. This federal model tends toward a professional–medical approach of doing for and deciding for the patient. We prefer a more social model in which the patient, to the degree feasible, is involved in his/her care plan.

The federal standard mandates that all of the patient care services and the professional personnel involved with any patient participate in the care plan. In most facilities this takes place in patient-care conferences attended by all staff persons involved with each case. In these planning conferences the group leader receives reports and makes a record of the extent to which the goals previously set have been accomplished. New goals are then proposed for the upcoming period. The role of each person to be involved is specified in writing.

ACCOMPLISHMENTS OF PATIENT CARE PLANNING

Patient care planning accomplishes several things. It focuses staff attention on identifying and deciding how to meet the specific care needs of each resident. In one sense the patient care plan becomes a contract among the caregivers, a commitment to care for each specific patient. By requiring that all concerned staff participate in the planning, these sessions can initiate exchanges of information that otherwise might not occur.

The process helps focus the staff's attention on *patient needs* as opposed to staff or facility needs. The patient care plan assists the staff to personalize the response of the organization to each resident.

"On Demand" Patient Care Planning

The formally scheduled patient-care conference plays an important role. But patient and family or sponsor needs and feelings do not always fit a planning conference schedule. The administrator, director of nurses, and other staff members must be ready to have impromptu patient-care planning conferences with the patient and/or family at their request.

When they want to talk with the care providers, the true feelings and concerns of the patient or family are more likely to be communicated to the staff. It is important to be available and to listen attentively. Human needs know no routine patient-care conference timetable. When the patient is ready to communicate, the facility must be ready to listen and learn.

An Optimistic, Cheerful Community

A major requirement for establishing a caring atmosphere for persons admitted to skilled nursing facilities is *cheerfulness*. Administrators should assure that their nursing home facility is a community for living, not for dying.

Nursing homes have unusually high levels of morbidity (prevalence of illnesses) and mortality (death rate among the population). This is natural and normal. Persons are admitted to the facility because they have illness(es) that require 24-hr nursing care.

Being cheerful is a matter of attitude and values. To be cheerful is to have an upbeat outlook on life. There are skilled nursing facilities in which one does feel the glass is half empty instead of half full. In successful nursing facilities the staff focuses on assisting the patients to remain involved, at whatever level they may be capable, in living.

When the residents and patients have the feeling that their needs come first, even when on occasion it may inconvenience the staff or the institution, there is reason to be positive about living.

REFERENCES TO PART FIVE

Adams, G. (1981). *Essentials of geriatric medicine* (2nd ed.). Oxford: Oxford University Press.

Agate, J.N. (1979). *Geriatrics for nurses and social workers* (2nd ed.). London: Heinemann Medical Books.

Albanese, A.A. (1980). *Nutrition for the elderly*. New York: A.R. Liss.

American Medical Association. (1967). *The extended care facility: A handbook for the medical society*. Chicago: AMA.

Anderson, W.F. (1976). *Practical management of the elderly* (3rd ed.). Oxford: Blackwell Scientific Publications.

Barzel. U. (1983). Common metabolic disorders of the skeleton in aging. In W. Reichel (Ed.), *Clinical aspects of aging* (2nd ed.) (pp. 360–371). Baltimore: Williams and Wilkins.

Basen, M. (1977). The elderly and drugs—problem overview and program strategy. *Public Health Reports, 92*(1), 43–48.

Bazzare, T. (1983). Nutritional requirements of the elderly. In J. McCue (Ed.), *Medical care of the elderly: A practical approach*. Lexington, MA: The Collamore Press.

Beck, S., & Smith, J. Infectious diseases in the elderly. *Medical Clinics of North America, 67*(2), 273–289.

Becker, L. (1979). Herpes zoster: A geriatric disease. *Geriatrics 34*(9), 41–47.

Birchenall, J.M., & Streight, M.E. (1982). *Care of the older adult* (2nd Ed.). Philadelphia: J.B. Lippincott.

Birkmayer, W., & Riederer, P. (1983). *Parkinson's disease: Biochemical, clinical, pathology and treatment*. New York: Springer Verlag.

Birren, J. (1964) *The psychology of aging*. Englewood Cliffs, N.J.: Prentice-Hall.

Bjork, D., & Tight, R. (1983). Nursing home hazard of chronic indwelling urinary catheters. *Archives of Internal Medicine, 143*(9), 1675–1676.

Bleckner, M. The place of the nursing home among community resources. *Journal of Geriatric Psychiatry, 1*(67), 135–144.

Blumenthal, H.T. (1968). Some biomedical aspects of aging. *Gerontologist 8.*

Blumenthal, M. (1980). Depressive illness in old age: Getting behind the mask. *Geriatrics, 35*(4), 34–43.

Botwinick, C. (1978). *Aging and behavior: A comprehensive integration of research findings*. New York: Springer Publishing Co.

Boyer, G., & Boyer, J. (1982). Sexuality and Aging. *Nursing Clinics of North America, 17*(3), 421–427.

Bozzetti, L. (1977). Contemporary concepts of aging: An overview. *Psychiatric Annals, 7,* 16–43.

Breschi, L. (1983). Common lower urinary tract problems in the elderly. In W. Reichel (Ed.), *Clinical aspects of aging* (2nd ed.) (pp. 302–318). Baltimore: Williams and Wilkins.

Brocklehurst, J. (1971). Dysuria in old age. *Journal of the American Geriatrics Society, 19,* 582.

Brocklehurst, J. (1979). The urinary tract. In I. Rossman (Ed.), *Chinical geriatrics* (2nd ed.) (chap. 16). Philadelphia: J.B. Lippincott.

Brocklehurst, J.C. & Hanley, T. (1981). *Geriatric medicine for students.* London: Churchill Livingstone.

Burch, G.E. (1983). Interesting aspects of the aging process. *Journal of the American Geriatrics Society, 31*(12), 766–779.

Burnside, I. (Ed.). (1981). *Nursing and the aged.* New York: McGraw-Hill.

Busse, E., & Pfeiffer, E. (1973). *Mental illness in later life.* Washington, DC: American Psychological Association.

Butler, W. (1975) Psychology and the elderly: An overview. *American Journal of Psychiatry, 132,* 893–900.

Butler, R., & Lewis, M. (1977). *Aging and mental health* (2nd. ed.). St Louis: C.V. Mosby.

Caird, F.I. (1979). *Assessment of the elderly patient* (2nd ed.). Philadelphia: J.B. Lippincott.

Cape, R.D. (Ed.). (1983). *Fundamentals of geriatric medicine.* New York: Raven Press.

Carter, D., & Balin, A. (1983). Dermatological aspects of aging. *Medical Clinics of North America, 67*(2), 531–534.

Collins, K., Dore, C. et al. (1977). Accidental hypothermia and impaired temperature homeostasis in the elderly. *British Medical Journal, 1,* 353–356.

Cooper, J. (1978). Drug therapy in the elderly: Is it all it could be? *American Pharmacy, 18*(7), 25–33.

Corso, J. (1981). *Aging: Sensory systems and perception.* New York: Praeger.

Crow, M. (1984). *Pharmacology for the elderly.* New York: Teachers College Press.

Dement, W., Miles, L., & Bliwise, D. (1982). Physiological markers of aging: Human sleep patterns. In M. Reff & E. Schneider (Eds.), *Biological markers of Aging.* (pp. 177–187) Washington, DC: NIH Pub. No. 82–222/. Public Health Service. pp. 177–187.

DeVita, V. (1982). *Cancer treatment.* Washington, DC: Public Health Service. (Medicine for the Layman Series, No. 82–1807).

Dimond, M., & Jones, S.L. (1983). *Chronic illness across the life span.* Norwalk, CT: Appleton-Century-Crofts.

Duvoisin, R. (1984). *Parkinson's disease: A guide for patient and family.* New York: Raven Press.

Ernst, N.S., & Glazer-Waldman, H.R. (1983). *The aged patient: A sourcebook for allied health professionals.* Chicago: Year Book Medical Publishers.

Farber, B., Brennen, C., Punteri, A., & Brody, J. (1982). Nosocomial infections in a chronic care facility. *Journal of the American Geriatrics Society, 32*(7), 513–519.

Feinstein, E., & Friedman, E. (1979). Renal disease in the elderly. In I. Rossman (Ed.), *Clinical geriatrics* (2nd ed.) (chap.12). Philadelphia: J.B. Lippincott.

Felser, J., & Raff, M. (1983). Infectious diseases and aging. *Journal of the American Geriatrics Society, 31*(12) 802–806.

Finch, C., & Hayflick, L. (1977). *Handbook of the biology of aging.* New York: Van Nostrand Reinhold.

Finley, M. (1971). *Good eating: Meeting nutritional needs for aged persons in residential care home.* Sacramento, CA: State of California, Human Relations Agency, Department of Social Services.

Foley, C. (1981). Nutrition and the elderly. In L. Libow (Ed.), *The core of geriatric medicine: A guide for students and practitioners* (chap. 13). St. Louis: C.V. Mosby.

Franz, M. (1981). Nutritional requirements of the elderly. *Journal of Nutrition for the Elderly, 1.*

Fraumeni, J. (1979). Epidemiological studies of cancer. In A. Griffin & C. Shaw (Eds.) *Carcinogens: Identification and mechanism of action.* Symposium on Fundamental Cancer Research, 31st M.D. Anderson Hospital + Tumor Institute, 1978. (pp. 53–66). New York: Raven Press.

Freedman, M. (1982). Anemias in the elderly: Physiologic or pathologic? *Hospital Practice, 17*(5), 121–136.

Freeman, J. (1979). Aging: its *history and literature.* New York: Human Sciences Press.

Gallis, H. (1984) Infectious diseases in the elderly. Covington & Walker (Eds.), *Current geriatric therapy* (chap. 7). Philadelphia: W.B. Saunders Company.

Gambert, S.R. (1983). A clinician's guide to the physiology of aging. *Wisconsin Medical Journal, 82*(8), 13–15.

Garibaldi, R., Brodine, S., & Matsumiya, S. (1981). Infections among patients in nursing homes. *New England Journal of Medicine, 305*(13), 731–735.

Goldfarb, A. (1979) Geriatric gynecology. In I. Rossman (Ed.), *Clinical geriatrics* (2nd ed.) (chap. 17). Philadelphia: J.B. Lippincott.

Gotz, B., & Gotz, V. (1978, August). Drugs and the elderly. *American Journal of Nursing, 78*(8), 1347–1350.

Griggs, W. (1978, August). Sex and the elderly. *American Journal of Nursing, 78*(8), 1352–1354.

Grob, D. (1983). Prevalent joint diseases in older persons. In W. Reichel (Ed.), *Clinical aspects of aging* (2nd ed.) (chap. 25). Baltimore: Williams and Wilkins.

Grocer, M., & Shekleton, M. (1979). *Basic pathophysiology—a conceptual approach.* St. Louis: C.V. Mosby.

Groenwald, S. (1980). Physiology of the immune system. *Journal of the Heart and Lung, 9*(4), 645–650.

Gwyther, L. (1983). Alzheimer's disease. *North Carolina Medical Journal, 44*(7), 435–436.

Gwyther, L., & Matteson, M.A. (1983). Care for the caregivers. *Journal of Gerontological Nursing, 9*(2).

Hayflick, L. (1965). The limited in vitro lifetime of human diploid cell strains. *Experimental Cell Research, 37*(3), 614–636.

Heaney, R. (1982). Age related bone loss. In M. Reff & E. Schneider (Eds.), *Biological Markers of Aging* (pp. 161–167), Washington, DC: USDHHS, NIH, Public Health Service.

Hickey, T. (1982). *Health and aging.* Monterey, CA: Brooks-Cole.

Hing, E. (1977). Characteristics of nursing home residents' health status and care received. USDHHS, PHS, Office of Health Research Survey and Testing, National Center for Health Statistics. (National Nursing Home Survey, Series 13, No. 51) Washington, DC: U.S. Government Printing Office.

Hogstel, M. (1981). *Nursing care of the older adult.* New York: John Wiley & Sons.

Horstman, B. Importance of physical therapy in fostering independence. *American Health Care Association Journal, 9*(3), 51–57.

Husain, T. (1953). An experimental study of some pressure effects on tissues with reference to the bed sore problem. *Journal of Pathology and Bacteriology*, 66, 347.

Irvine, P., VanBuren, N., & Crossley, K. (1984). Causes for hospitalization of nursing home residents: The role of infection. *Journal of the American Geriatrics Society, 32*(2), 103–107.

Jarvik, L., & Greenblatt, D. (1981). *Clinical pharmacology and the aged patient.* New York: Raven Press.

Kames & Sherman F. (1981). In L. Libow (Ed.), *The core of geriatric medicine: A guide for students and practitioners* (pp. 305–329). St. Louis: C.V. Mosby.

Karasu, T., & Lazar, I. (1980). Evaluation and management of depression in the elderly. *Geriatrics, 35*(12), 47–56.

Kart, C. Metress, E., & Metress, J. (1978). *Aging and health: Biological and social perspectives.* Menlo Park, CA: Addison-Wesley.

Kay, B., & Neeley, J. (1982). Sexuality and aging: A review of current literature. *Sexuality and Disability, 5*(1), 38–46.

Keegan, G., & McNichols, D. (1982). The evaluation and treatment of urinary incontinence in the elderly. *Surgical Clinics of North America, 62*(2), 261–269.

Kenney, R. (1982). *Physiology of aging: A synopsis.* Chicago: Year Book Medical Publishers.

Kleiger, R. (1976). Cardiovascular disorders. In F. Steinberg (Ed.), *Cowdry's: The care of the geriatric patient* (5th ed.) (pp. 66–78). St. Louis: C.V. Mosby.

Kligman, A. (1979). Perspectives and problems in cutaneous gerontology. *Journal of Investigative Dermatology, 73*(1), 39–46.

Kurtz, S. (1982). Urinary tract infection in older persons. *Comprehensive Therapy, 8*(2), 54–58.

Lazar, I., & Karasu, T. (1980). Evaluation and management of depression in the elderly. *Geriatrics, 35*(12), 47–53.

Leaf, A. (1973). Getting old. *Scientific American, 229*(3), 44–53.

Lehman, K. Administrator's role in prevention and care of decubitus ulcers. *Journal of Long Term Care Administration, 11*(2).

Levine, A. (1984). The elderly amputee. *American Family Physician, 29*(5), 177–182.

Libow, L. (1981). *The core of geriatric medicine: A guide for students and practitioners.* St. Louis: C.V. Mosby.

Lindeman, R. (1983). Application of fluid and electrolyte balance principles to the older patient. In W. Reichel (Ed.), *Clinical aspects of aging: A comprehensive text* (2nd ed.) (pp. 286–301) Baltimore: Williams and Wilkins.

Lotzkar, S. (1977). Dental care for the aged. *Journal of Public Health Dentistry, 37*(3), 201–207.

Louis, M. (1978). Falls and their causes. *Journal of Geriatric Nursing, 4* (6), 143–144.

Lyon, L., & Nevins, M. (1984). Management of hip fracture in nursing home patients: To treat or not to treat? *Journal of the American Geriatrics Society, 32*(5), 391–395.

MacHudis, M. (1983). In W. Reichel (Ed.), *Clinical aspects of aging: A comprehensive text.* (2nd ed.) (chap. 38). Baltimore: Williams and Wilkins.

McLachlan, M. (1978). The aging kidney. *Lancet, 2*, 43.

Meza, J.P., Peggs, J.F. & O'Brien, J.M. (1984). Constipation in the elderly patient. *Journal of Family Practice, 18* (5), 695–703.

Nicolle, L., McIntyre, M., Zacharias, H., & MacDonald, J. (1961) Twelve months of surveillance of infections in institutionalized elderly men. *Journal of the*

American Geriatrics Society, 9(4), 654–680.

Ostfeld, A., & Gibson, D. (Eds.) (1972). *Epidemiology of aging: Summary report and selected papers from a research conference.* Washington, DC: USDHEW, NIH, PHS. (Publication No. 75–7111).

Palmore, E. (1973). Social factors in mental illness of the aged. In E. Busse and E. Pfeiffer (Eds.), *Mental illness in later life* (pp. 41–52). Washington, DC: American Psychological Association.

Phair, J.P. (1979) Aging and infection: A review. *Journal of Chronic Disease, 32,* 535–540.

Poe, W. & Holloway, D. (1980). *Drugs and the aged.* New York: McGraw-Hill.

Reichel, W. (Ed.). *Clinical aspects of aging: A comprehensive text* (2nd. ed.). New York: Williams and Wilkins.

Rodman, M., & Smith, D. (1977). *Clinical pharmacology in nursing.* Philadelphia: J.B. Lippincott.

Rodstein, E. (1983). Falls by the aged. In I Rossman (Ed.), *Fundamentals of geriatric medicine* (pp. 109–116). New York: Raven Press.

Rosendorff, C. (1983). *Clinical cardiovascular and pulmonary physiology.* New York: Raven Press.

Rossman, I. (Ed.). *Clinical Geriatrics* (2nd ed.). Philadelphia: J.B. Lippincott.

Rowe, J. (1982). Renal function and aging. In M. Reff & E. Schneider (Eds.), *Biological markers of aging* (chap. 25). Washington, DC: USDHHS, NIH, Public Health Service.

Rowe, J., & Besdine, R. (1982). *Health and disease in old age.* Boston: Little, Brown.

Rubin, P. (1981). Management of hypertension in the elderly. In F. Ebaugh (Ed.), *Management of common problems in geriatric medicine* (chap. 16). Menlo Park, CA: Addison-Wesley.

Rux, J. (1981). Thoughts on culture, nutrition, and the aged. *Journal of Nutrition for the Elderly, 1.*

Sartor, R., & Nuzum, C. (1983). Constipation. In McCue (Ed.), *Medical care of the elderly: A practical approach* (pp. 65–73). Lexington, MA: The Collamore Press.

Segal, J., Thompson, J., & Floyd, R. (1979). Drug utilization and prescribing patterns in a skilled nursing facility: The need for a rational approach to therapeutics. *Journal of the American Geriatrics Society, 27*(3), 117–122.

Shinnar, S. Use of adaptive feeding equipment in feeding the elderly. (1983). *Journal of the American Dietetic Association, 83*(3), 321–322.

Shore, H. (1978). Group programs in long term care facilities. In I. Burnside (Ed.), *Working with the elderly: Group process and techniques.* North Scituate, MA: Duxbury Press.

Sinex, F.M. (1977). The molecular genetics of aging. In C. Finch & L. Hayflick (Eds.), *Handbook of the biology of aging* (pp. 37–62). New York: Van Nostrand Reinhold.

Sklar (1983). Gastrointestinal diseases in the aged. In W. Reichel (Ed.), *Clinical aspects of aging: A comprehensive text* (2nd ed.) (chap. 17). Baltimore: Williams and Wilkins.

Smith, W. (1982). Infections in the elderly. *Hospital Practice, 17,* 69–85.

Snowden, J. (1983). Sex in nursing homes. *The Australian Nurse's Journal, 12*(8), 55–56.

Spencer, H., & Lender. M. (1977). The skeletal system. In I. Rossman (Ed.), *Clinical geriatrics* (2nd ed.) (pp. 460–473). Philadelphia: J.B. Lippincott.

Starr, I. (1964). An essay on the strength of the heart. *American Journal of*

Cardiology, 14(b), 771–783.

Steffl, B. (Ed.) (1984). *Handbook of gerontological nursing.* New York: Van Nostrand Reinhold.

Stillwell, E., & O'Conner, C. (1983). Sexuality, intimacy, and touch. In W. Reichel (Ed.), *Clinical aspects of aging* (2nd ed.) (pp. 596–599). Baltimore: Williams and Wilkins.

Stotsky, B. (1973). In E. Busse & E. Pfeiffer (Eds.), *Mental illness in later life* (chap. 10). Washington, DC: American Psychological Association.

Strehler, B. (1962). *Time, cells, and aging.* New York: Academic Press.

Tindall, J., & Smith, J. (1963). Skin lesions of the aged. *Journal of the American Medical Association, 186,* 1037–1040.

U.S. Department of Health, Education and Welfare, Public Health Service, Office of Long Term Care. (1976). Physician drug prescribing patterns in skilled nursing facilities. Washington, DC: DHEW. (Long Term Care Facility Improvement Campaign Monograph No. 2).

Vallarino R., & Sherman, F. (1981). Stroke, hip fractures, amputations, pressure sores, and incontinence. In L. Libow (Ed.), *The core of geriatric medicine: A guide for students and practitioners* (pp. 127–168). St. Louis: C.V. Mosby.

Wainwright, H. (1978). Feeding problems in the elderly disabled patient. *Nursing Times, 74,* 543–545.

Wasow, M., & Loeb, M. (1979). Sexuality in nursing homes. *Journal of the American Geriatrics Society, 27,* 73–79.

Weg, P. (1983). Changing physiology of aging. In D. Woodruff & J. Birren (Eds.), *Aging: Scientific perspectives and social issues* (2nd ed.) (chap. 2). Monterey, CA: Brooks/Cole Publishing.

Weksler, E. (1981). The senescence of the immune system. *Hospital Practice, 16,* 53–58.

Williams, M., & Fitzhugh, C. (1982). Urinary incontinence in the elderly. *Annals of Internal Medicine, 97,* 895–907.

Woodruff, D., & Birren, J. (1975). *Aging—scientific perspectives and social issues.* New York: D. Van Nostrand.

PART SIX

Marketing the Long-Term Care Facility

6.1 The Turn to Marketing

Why, one might ask, should the nursing facility administrator be concerned with marketing? High occupancy rates seem guaranteed for the foreseeable future. Most nursing facilities have patient waiting lists (Midgett, p. 77). The proportion of Americans who will need nursing facility care is expected to increase yearly at least through the middle of the 21st century. Patient waiting lists are becoming even longer in response to Medicare's prospective payment method (the DRGs) placing more and more pressure on hospitals to rapidly discharge acute care patients to nursing facilities or into home health care where expenses are lower. However, a number of factors are coming together which may threaten the seeming guarantee of high occupancy rates.

FORCES LEADING TO COMPETITION

Narrowed Profit Margins.   Government Medicaid and Medicare regulations, services offered by the facility, and sources of patient payment all affect the ability of a facility to survive. Over the past decade government regulators who pay for the care offered under the Conditions of Participation for Medicare and Medicaid patients have narrowed the margins of profit to achieve mandated government cost savings. One result is that the economic well-being of the typical nursing facility will become more and more tied to an ability to attract private paying patients.

End of Federal Planning.   The federal Conditions of Participation, along with state regulations, have tended to control the shape of the long-term care industry. The payment policies of the state Medicaid offices, along with Medicare claims authorities, have tended to set prices charged in the industry (Ting, p. 62). Product design in nursing facilities, i.e., the mix of services, has mostly been shaped by product and price decisions made by these government agencies. Now, the affluent elderly are beginning to shape the product mix.

6.2 A New Market Base: The Affluent Older American

Two major forces are coming into play simultaneously: (1) the end of federal health planning and (2) the emergence of more affluent older Americans as a major market base.

Federal health planning agencies, and the certificates-of-need they required before new beds could be built (in all states but Texas), ended October 1, 1986. These agencies tended to keep demand for nursing home beds high by using the certificate-of-need program to restrict the number of beds which could be built. As described in Part Four, a number of states, too, are ending state certificate-of-need programs. This will allow freer competition among some nursing home providers. The future in most states may become like those in Texas, where free competition has been allowed over the years and competition has resulted in an oversupply of beds leading to an average 70% occupancy rate in nursing facilities.

The emergence of more affluent older Americans is a second force that will encourage future nursing home administrators to develop marketing plans for their facility. Future elderly will be more able to purchase nursing facility care privately. A number of factors are contributing to this. Postretirement income is expected to come closer to matching preretirement income through social security benefits and an increasing number of private pensions. Forty percent of families with persons aged to 65 to 69 received pension benefits in 1979. This proportion is expected to increase to 80% by the year 2004 (Scanlon & Feder, p. 34).

Increases in Discretionary Income

To be over 65 will mean less and less often to be with reduced discretionary income. The 1986 federal law forbidding mandatory retirement at any age may also allow increasing proportions of elderly persons to continue to have a steady income stream into their seventies and, for some, into their eighties.

Americans 65 and older control vast amounts of wealth. Close to 30% of all discretionary income in the United States belongs to households headed by persons 65 and older (Berkowitz, Kerin & Rudelius, p. 69; Scanlon and Feder, p. 19). Seventy percent of persons 65 and older own their own homes. Eighty percent of these homes are mortgage-free (Rice and Taylor, p. 33). The federal program of encouraging Individual Retirement Accounts (IRAs) is also expected to place more buying power into the hands of the elderly.

Absence of Catastrophic Care Programs

Currently, the United States has neither a public, nor private financing mechanism to pay for extended long-term care needs of anyone except the impoverished. To be eligible, a person must be financially destitute: having remaining assets of $1200 or less is required for Medicaid and/or Supplemental Security Income (SSI) assistance. Once on Medicaid and/or SSI, the older ill individual has little hope of ever regaining economic solvency. Medicare, the reader will recall, pays only for short-term acute illnesses. The private insurance industry is only now beginning to offer long-term care insurance.

Coverage for Catastrophic Care Costs

Mechanisms are becoming available that will protect older persons from economic impoverishment due to extended long-term care costs. The federal government is exploring ways to provide catastrophic health care coverage under Medicare. New private insurance industry plans will allow more and more persons to protect themselves against the costs of extended stays in long-term care facilities.

The result of all these forces is the emergence of an older population better equipped to pay for extended long-term facility costs. The proportion of patients who will be private paying patients can be expected to rise. The long-term care patient of the future will be increasingly better educated, better equipped to pay for care, and more discriminating about the services received in addition to basic quality care in the nursing facility. As the proportion of these private paying patients rises, ability to compete successfully for their health care dollars will become a skill required of most long term care administrators.

6.3 "Marketing" Health Care

In 1977 the U.S. Supreme Court ruled illegal any self-imposed restrictions by health and other professionals against advertising services or prices which have the result of keeping the public ignorant or of inhibiting the free flow of commercial information (Kinnear & Bernhardt, p. 669). As a result, over the past decade the marketing of professional health services has become an increasingly accepted practice.

Health care professionals, led by hospitals, spent 3.7 million dollars on television spots in 1977. They were spending 41 million by 1983, 11 times as much. During the first half of 1986, health care television ads showed a 40% increase over the rate of television advertising in 1985 (Hospitals, p. 16).

In the year 1978, one year after the U.S. Supreme Court ruling, hospitals employed a total of three marketing executives. In 1985 hospitals employed over 2,000 marketing executives (Califano, p. 121).

HOSPITALS BEGIN TO "MARKET"

Hospitals have turned to marketing because the occupancy rates across the United States have fallen in each of the past several years, standing at about 66% nationwide in 1986. This is too low for cost-effective operation of a hospital. To get their occupancy rates up, hospitals have begun to compete with each other for patients. Hospitals are attempting to distinguish themselves from their competitors (Inguanzo & Harju, p. 62).

Competition for patients among public, not-for-profit and for-profit hospitals, is a new experience. Administrators in nursing facilities, which may be two to four years behind hospitals in being subjected to these same competitive market forces, are also beginning to feel the need to "market" their services.

Definition of Marketing

In 1985 the American Marketing Association defined marketing as the process of planning and executing the conception, pricing, promotion, and distribution of ideas, goods, and services to create exchanges that satisfy both individual and organizational objectives (Kinnear & Bernhardt, p. 10). The nursing facility is in the business of marketing services. In the mid-1980s, 47 cents out of every dollar spent by U.S. consumers went to services (Berkowitz, Kerin, & Rudelius, p. 608).

Levey and Loomba, in *Health Care Administration: A Managerial Perspective,* included a chapter on marketing in their second edition published in 1984. Healthcare marketing began, they argue, with a spate of articles first appearing in 1973. They comment that the spread of marketing to hospitals and nursing facilities was inevitable due to forces such as lowered occupancy rates and increasingly marginal income margins due to lowered Medicaid reimbursement rates (Levey & Loomba, p. 347). Marketing is now regarded as a central consideration in health care management.

Marketing is the effort to improve the interaction between the organization's goals and the persons whose needs the organization seeks to serve. The steps in marketing are often described as

- the audit
- market segmentation
- choosing a market mix
- implementing the plan
- evaluation of results
- control (Levey & Loomba, p. 350)

This should sound familiar. It is a restatement of the steps in planning described in Part One. The primary difference is the degree to which the administrator's attentions, when setting the organization's goals, is focused outward on analyzing and meeting the needs of potential patients.

Marketing as Managerial Thinking

Marketing is a variation on managerial thinking, focusing sharply on the idea that success of the facility will depend on bringing about a voluntary exchange of values (services) with the target persons, i.e., the market to be served. Traditionally, the focus of health care providers has been on designing a quality hospital or nursing facility, assuming that if it is built it will become filled to capacity with patients (Fine, p. 66). This is "seller's" market thinking. Marketing of health care today is the recognition that health care services are increasingly a "buyer's" market.

Auditing is the process of identifying, collecting and analyzing information about the external environment. *Market segmentation* is the step of using the audit information to divide the potential persons served into identifiable subgroups, such as longer-termed patients and shorter-termed patients who come for rehabilitation then return home, or into groupings such as private-pay patients and public-pay patients. Deciding which patients to seek and in what proportions is determining the *market mix*. *Implementation* is the process of managing organizational behaviors and outreach activities to attract patients in the proportions desired, e.g. the balance desired between the proportion of private-pay and public-pay patients. Evaluation and control of the marketing program is no different from the evaluation and control process described in detail in Part One. If, for example, the desired proportion of private-pay patients remains below target (evaluation of results achieved), new control steps are taken to reach the desired balance.

6.4 Marketing the Long-Term Care Facility

Deciding who the facility will serve is critical. A variety of differing organizational goals are available from which to choose. As mentioned above, the administrator may consciously seek to serve longer term care patients. Or the administrator may concentrate on providing rehabilitation services, thus seeking a large proportion of short-term rehabilitative patients. The facility may seek to serve an entirely private-paying patient population, an entirely public-paid patient population or any ratio of the two. The facility may seek to admit only light care patients, only heavy care patients, or any mix of the two. The facility might seek to serve as a subacute care facility for one or more hospitals. The administration of each facility, then, must set organizational marketing goals as to the type(s) of patient population(s) it seeks to serve. This is called market segmentation.

Numerous market segments exist in the long-term care field. For example, an emerging new market in the long term care continuum is the life care community which provides care from entrance into the community as an ambulatory well person through final care, if necessary, in the same institution's nursing facility.

Creating awareness among potential consumers that the services exist, assisting them in deciding, and assuring that they are satisfied with the quality of services provided by the facility is the process of marketing implementation (King, p. 39).

The Marketing of Services

According to Berkowitz, Kerin, and Rudelius, services have four characteristics which differentiate them from durable goods, e.g. a car: intangibility, inconsistency, inseparability and inventory.

Intangibility. Services cannot be touched, sat in, or driven like a car: they are intangible. Health care that the consumer expects will be given in a nursing facility cannot be directly experienced before entering the facility. Nursing facilities can, however, make services appear more tangible, e.g., a television advertisement portraying atttentive care being given to a resident at the facility (Berkowitz, Kerin, & Rudelius, p. 609).

Inconsistency. Marketing services differs from marketing tangible goods like an automobile because the quality of service can be inconsistent from day to day. Quality that endures over time can be built into an auto through consistent assembly line procedures, but the service received at the hands of the nurses or orderlies on any given day can vary widely depending on the mood of the employee.

Inseparability. A third characteristic of marketing services is that the consumer does not separate the service from the deliverer of the service or the setting in which service is given. The nursing home may be giving excellent nursing care, but if the bathrooms are smelly and dirty the patients' and visitors' perceptions of the facility, including the quality of nursing care, are affected. The services given and the service provider are inseparably linked in the consumer's mind.

Inventory. Idle production capacity, i.e. the presence of an unoccupied bed in a health care facility, is a fourth characteristic of service marketing. Inventory carrying costs of empty nursing home or hospital beds is high, the empty bed costing as much as 70% of the costs of occupied beds due to the fixed and semivariable costs (discussed in Part Three).

The Case Mix

In the text (edited by Winston) *Marketing Long-Term and Senior Care Services*, Matthew Midgett asserts that "by carefully proportioning the number of subsidized and private-pay patients, nursing homes can provide better accommodations and services for both" (p. 78). This is true because in many states the public reimbursement rates for care are set so close to break-even that it becomes necessary to achieve a case-mix consisting of both private paying and subsidized patients (Sinioris & Butler, p. 42).

Consumers: Deciding on the Basis of Services Offered

Marketing texts typically characterize consumer decision making as: problem recognition, information search, alternative evaluation, purchase decision, and postpurchase evaluation (Berkowitz, Kerin, & Rudelius, p.

98). This process is not unlike that employed by the facility administrator as described above.

Definition of Service.   The nursing facility's business is providing health services to the patient. A *service* can be defined as an identifiable and essentially intangible activity that provides the recipient with performance satisfaction, but does not involve ownership (Kinnear & Bernhardt, p. 654). Consumer decisions are based on their image of whether the service provided by the nursing facility will meet their needs (Kotler, p. 117; Goldsmith & Leebov, p. 83). Research suggests that physicians typically have a major influence on patient decisions (Smith, p. 105). Recommendations of the facility from local physicians can provide the facility with a sustainable advantage (Ghemawat, p. 55).

Personal tours through the facility, and meeting the staff and patients is one of the most effective marketing tools available to the facility administrator (Skelley, p. 58; Butler, p. 48). During the visit or visits the potential client(s), usually the children or close friends of the prospective patient, are gathering impressions on which they will judge the facility. Often, subliminal perceptions become key factors. *Subliminal perceptions* are factors of which the decision maker is not consciously aware, such as general appearances of the facility, the friendliness of the staff, the appearances of the patients, the cleanliness of the bathrooms (Robertson, Zielinski & Ward, p. 186).

As one writer has put it, image is credibility (Peterson, p. 36). Numerous ways of creating a positive image for the facility in the community are available. Developing a community advisory board, hosting neighborhood openhouses, publicizing enthusiastic families and volunteers, and cosponsoring community events such as local arts festivals are but a few of the avenues available to facilities (Anderson, p. 50; U.S. DHHS, p. 30; Ruff, p. 46; Jerstad & Meier, p. 60; Sweeney & Lewis, p. 70).

As the proportion of patients, and/or those who pay for the patients' care come from the private paying segment of the market, the wants and needs of patients will become ever more important in deciding what services are to be offered along with basic nursing care. The days are passing when hospitals and nursing facility staffs feel themselves better qualified than the public itself to determine what the patient needs (Hauser, p. 76; Rosenberg & Van West).

6.5 Emerging Marketing Strategies

Nursing facilities are beginning to offer special services and amenities to patients. A transition is being made from what has been called "hospital" type nursing facility care toward "hospitality" type care (Ting, p. 70). Stiff competition for attracting new patients is coming from service oriented groups like experienced hotel chains which are entering the field of long-term care services. These chains practice what is called "aggressive hospitality," assuring that all members of their staff play active roles in positive patient relations (Riffer, p. 51).

Some examples of additional services being made available in nursing facilities are cable television; separate recreational activities, e.g., trips; varying levels of accommodations, e.g., quality of furniture; special meal services, i.e., menus carrying selections for which the resident pays extra.

Some providers are renovating facilities in order to attract larger portions of private-paying patients. Others offer clearly differing levels of accommodations within the same facility, according to the ability and willingness of the patient to pay. It is not yet known how much dissension may be caused by creating two or more classes of services within a single facility. It may be that larger providers will offer different classes of services by establishing separate facilities for each class of service (Ting, p. 70). This process is already far advanced among life care communities, where entrance fees, hence the level of services, can vary from $15,000 to as much as $250,000 or more.

There is also a trend for large providers to prefer to build new facilities in the newer more affluent areas of towns rather than buying preexisting facilities which may be in "less desirable neighborhoods," i.e., likely to have lower proportions of private-paying patients.

6.6 Ethical Concerns

Inevitably, as facilities cater to the growing private-paying patient population, classes of care are emerging. This problem has already been documented. A major study has shown that in states with larger numbers of beds available per 1000 older persons, more than 90% of persons most in need of nursing facility care were being admitted to nursing facilities. Where beds were in short supply, only half of those most in need, most of whom are Medicaid patients, were being admitted to nursing facilities (Scanlon and Feder, p. 28).

REFERENCES TO PART SIX

Anderson, C.C. (1986, April). Local arts festival raises facility to new heights. *Provider 12*(4) 50–55.

Berkowitz, E.N., Kerin, R.A. & Rudelius, W. (1986). *Marketing.* St. Louis: Times Mirror/Mosby College Publishing.

Butler, R.L. (1986, November). Nursing homes gain consumer confidence. *Provider 12*(11) 48.

Califano, J.A., Jr. (1986) *America's Health Care Revolution.* New York: Random House.

Fine, S.H. (1984). The health product: A social marketing perspective. *Hospitals,* June 16, pp. 66–68.

Ghemawat, P. (1986, Sept./Oct.). Sustainable advantage. *Harvard Business Review, 64*(5), 53–58.

Goldsmith, M. & Leebov, W. (1986). Strengthening the hospital's marketing position through training. *Health Care Management Review, 11*(2) 83–93.

Hauser, L.J. (1984). 10 reasons hospital marketing programs fail. *Hospitals,* September 1, pp.74–77.

Hospitals. (1986). Health care TV advertising up 40% for first half of 1986. October 20, p. 16. Author.

Inguanzo, J.M. & Harju, M. (1985). Creating a market niche. *Hospitals,* January 1, pp. 62–67.

Jerstad, M.A. & Meier, P. Advisory board a valuable 'two-way link' to community. *Provider, 12*(11), 60–63.

King, H. (1983). Effective marketing can maintain census. *Contemporary Administrator,* June, 39–41.

Kinnear, T.C. & Bernhardt, K.L. (1986). *Principles of Marketing,* 2nd Ed., Glenview, IL: Scott, Foresman & Co.

Kotler, P. (1986, March, April). Megamarketing. *Harvard Business Review 64*(2), 117–124.

Levey, S. & Loomba, N.P. (1984). *Health Care Administration: A Managerial Perspective (2nd. ed.).* New York: J.B. Lippincott Co.

Midgett, M. (1984). Skilled nursing facility marketing. In W.J. Winston (Ed.), *Marketing long-term care and senior care services,* (pp. 77–81). New York: The Haworth Press.

Peterson, S.(1986, November). Take note: Image is as image does. *Provider, 12*(11), 36–39.

Rice, J.A., & Taylor, S. (1984). Assessing the market for long-term care services. *Healthcare Financial Management,* February, pp. 32–46.

Riffer, J. (1984). The patient as guest: A competitive strategy. *Hospitals,* June 16, pp. 48–55.

Robertson, T.S., Zielinski, J., & Ward, S. (1984). *Consumer behavior.* Palo Alto: Scott, Foresman and Co.

Rosenberg, L. J., & Van West, J.H. (1984). The collaborative approach to marketing. *Business Horizons,* November–December, pp. 29–35.

Ruff, K.A. (1984, November). Families and friends can help educate. *Provider, 12*(11), 46–47.

Scanlon, W.J. & Feder, J. (1984). The long-term care marketplace: An overview. *Healthcare Financial Management,* January, pp. 18–36.

Sinioris, M.E. & Butler, P. (1983). Basic business strategy: Responding to change requires planning, marketing, and budgeting strategies. *Hospitals, 57,* June 1.

Skelley, G. (1986, November). Is food service a part of your marketing strategy? *Provider, 12*(11), 58–60.

Smith, S.M. (1984). Family selection of long-term care services. In W.J. Winston (Ed.), *Marketing long-term and senior care services* (pp. 101–103). New York: The Haworth Press.

Sweeney, M. & Lewis, C. (1986, November). Neighborhood nursing home program opens the right doors. *Provider, 12*(11) pp. 70–71.

Ting, H.M. (1984). New directions in nursing home and home healthcare marketing. *Healthcare Financial Management,* May, pp. 62–72.

U.S. DHHS Administration On Aging. (1985). On finding, training, and keeping volunteers from dropping out. U.S. DHHS Publication No. 348, p. 30. Washington, DC: U.S. Government Printing Office.

Winston, W.J., (Ed.) (1984). *Marketing long-term and senior care services.* New York: The Haworth Press.

Index